Prescribing Movement as Medicine

The Professional's Guide to Exercise for Health and Longevity

Kevin Carr

HUMAN KINETICS

Library of Congress Cataloging-in-Publication Data

Library of Congress Cataloging-in-Publication information is available. LCCN 2026015311 (print).

ISBN: 978-1-7182-4573-0 (print)

Senior Acquisitions Editor: Michelle Earle; **Developmental Editor:** Amy Stahl; **Senior Managing Editor:** Hannah Werner; **Copyeditor:** Marissa Wold Uhrina; **Permissions Manager:** Laurel Mitchell; **Graphic Designer:** Denise Lowry; **Layout:** MPS Limited; **Cover Designer:** Keri Evans; **Cover Design Specialist:** Susan Rothermel Allen; **Photographs (cover and interior):** Ben Connolly/© Human Kinetics, unless otherwise noted; **Photo Asset Manager:** Laura Fitch; **Photo Production Manager:** Jason Allen; **Senior Art Manager:** Kelly Hendren; **Illustrations:** © Human Kinetics, unless otherwise noted; **Printer:** Versa Press

We thank Mike Boyle Strength and Conditioning in Woburn, Massachusetts, for assistance in providing the location for the photo shoot for this book.

Printed in the United States of America 10 9 8 7 6 5 4 3 2 1

The paper in this book is certified under a sustainable forestry program.

Human Kinetics
1607 N. Market Street
Champaign, IL 61820
USA

United States and International
Website: **US.HumanKinetics.com**
Email: info@hkusa.com
Phone: 1-800-747-4457

Human Kinetics' authorized representative for product safety in the EU is Mare Nostrum Group B.V., Doelen 72, 4831 GR Breda, The Netherlands.
Email: gpsr@mare-nostrum.co.uk

L1346

*To my parents, who first inspired my love for exercise,
and to my wife and children, whose love and support
give me every reason to keep showing up.*

CONTENTS

FOREWORD

It means a lot to me to write the foreword for this book because Kevin is someone I've always looked up to, even though he's two years younger than I am. Kevin and I first met as newbie coaches at MBSC (Mike Boyle Strength and Conditioning) back in 2010. Well, he was a new trainer, and I was a brand-new intern.

Prior to coming to MBSC, I'd trained clients a little bit, and I trained super hard myself, so in my mind I was already an expert. Back then, most of what I learned came through DVDs and magazines, mainly on the topics of bodybuilding and powerlifting. I loved lifting heavy weights, but I hated cardio, stretching, and mobility. So, as any young kid would do, I just stuck to lifting weights and ignored the rest.

Then I got to MBSC and was in for a somewhat rude awakening: They had a much more well-rounded system for training clients, and lifting weights was only part of it. There was stretching, foam rolling, agility ladders, hurdles, and medicine balls all before clients even lifted a single weight. As someone who was used to having clients do just a few arm circles and *maybe* a few warm-up sets before heavy lifting, I didn't love all that other stuff, if I'm honest. But I knew it was important to learn it if I wanted to make it at MBSC, and I also knew that they had a tried-and-true recipe for happy clients, so I went along with it.

And that's where I really gravitated toward Kevin. Relative to most of the staff as MBSC, Kevin was a "meathead" (a huge term of endearment in my book) because he competed in powerlifting. But he was a more evolved meathead than I was because he also knew how to do all the other functional stuff too. He knew more than I did about mobility and movement prep, and he also had a great way of teaching clients things, because he's able to convey complex ideas simply. Plus, he's a just a cool, chill guy.

So I started following Kevin around the gym and trying to learn from him; and now, almost 20 years later, I live on the opposite side of the country, but I'm still always trying to learn from him.

Social media has changed the fitness landscape, because most of the people educating trainers about training don't actually train people. A lot of the biggest fitness influencers (I hate that word, even though some people might consider me to be one) are either failed trainers who then turn all their attention to social media or super-fit people who only train themselves and use their bodies as social proof.

Kevin is a huge breath of fresh air in a polluted fitness world, because everything he teaches people who train clients is based on his real-world experiences, not just theory. He's a master of the practical application, and he has found an amazing system to help clients achieve peak health and performance without having to make fitness their full-time job.

I would've supported any book Kevin wrote just because it's Kevin, but it just so happens that I'm who the trainers who are the target audience for this book will be training. I just turned 40 and just became a new dad, and my training doesn't look like it used to.

I used to be obsessed with how much weight I could lift on whatever exercise was the flavor of the month for me at the time. I have no regrets because I had a blast and learned a lot in the process, but I'm entering a stage of life where my only real fitness goal is to have people think I'm younger than I really am, based on what I'm able to do. When I turn 50, I want people to say, "I didn't realize you were 50!" And then say the same at 60, 70, and beyond. For that to happen, I know I must do all the stuff that Kevin outlines for trainers to teach their clients in this book. Unlike a lot of so-called experts on longevity who make the process overly complicated and time-consuming, Kevin simplifies it down into a system that feels doable and manageable.

I'm proud and lucky to have Kevin as a friend, and he's one of the only trainers in the world who I repeatedly text or call for advice for training clients. And now we're all lucky to have his brain spill out into one amazing book.

—Ben Bruno

ACKNOWLEDGMENTS

This book is the product of many people who have influenced my thinking, shaped my approach, and supported me along the way.

I'd like to thank Mike Boyle and all of the coaches I've worked with at Mike Boyle Strength and Conditioning. The environment at MBSC has played a huge role in my development as a coach and in shaping the ideas presented in this book.

Thank you to my clients, who have trusted me over the years and ultimately shaped my perspective on exercise more than anything else. This book reflects what I've learned from working with you.

Finally, thank you to everyone at Human Kinetics for helping turn this vision into a reality.

PREFACE

From the time I was young, I can remember my parents prioritizing physical activity: my mother following exercise tapes in the basement and my father heading to the gym long before I was out of bed. Even now, in their 60s, they continue to push themselves and reap the rewards of decades spent moving. It was simply part of their life, and because of their influence, it became part of mine, not only personally but professionally.

I chose exercise as my career because I believe it is the most powerful tool we have to change lives. In writing this book, my goal is to pass that gift forward by helping other coaches, trainers, and everyday people harness the benefits of movement as medicine.

The urgency could not be greater. We are living through a health crisis rooted largely in inactivity. Fewer than 25 percent of Americans meet the minimum guidelines for aerobic exercise and strength training. Obesity rates continue to climb, bringing with them increases in diabetes, heart disease, and dementia. The truth is simple: We are not moving nearly enough. And for those who try, the landscape of health and fitness can be confusing, frustrating, and often intimidating.

The media is crowded with extremists selling quick fixes or promoting programs designed for the few, not the many. Even well-meaning professionals sometimes share workouts that overshoot the needs or abilities of the average client. The result is that people do not know where to start, or worse, they give up before they have a chance to succeed.

This book is not a promise of immortality or a six-minute miracle plan. Getting in shape is hard work. Staying in shape as we age is harder still. But the rewards—more energy, more independence, more quality years—are worth every ounce of effort. What I hope to provide in these pages are clear, evidence-based, and practical strategies for building programs that truly change lives.

Every day, our choices are a vote for how we want our future selves to age. That truth applies equally to a 20-year-old athlete, a 40-year-old parent, or an 80-year-old retiree. We are all aging, and thoughtful exercise is the single most effective way to influence that process.

For fitness professionals, this means much more than just writing workouts. It means learning how to prescribe movement intentionally, with an eye toward both immediate results and long-term health. For everyday people, it means building routines that are realistic, sustainable, and adaptable to real life.

In my 18 years as a coach at Mike Boyle Strength and Conditioning, I've trained thousands of clients: athletes chasing peak performance and adults simply trying to feel better, move better, and live better. I think of every session as clients making a deposit into their "health investment account." Every day, we are either adding to or withdrawing from that account. The challenge and the opportunity is to help people tip the balance in their favor.

This book is my attempt to give you the framework to do exactly that. Whether you are a coach guiding clients or an individual taking your first steps, my hope is that these pages make the process less intimidating, more accessible, and ultimately more effective. Movement is medicine, and my aim is to help you prescribe it wisely.

You will find the references for this book online at https://ancillaries.humankinetics.com/PrescribingMovementAsMedicine or by scanning this QR code.

PART I

THE PATH TO LONGEVITY

Chapter 1

Roadblocks to Longevity

Lack of activity destroys the good condition of every human being, while movement and methodical physical exercise save it and preserve it.

—Plato

This book is not meant to sell a magical plan for immortality. The truth is that aging is inevitable. Muscular and skeletal systems weaken, the nervous system slows, the immune system falters, cells fail to regenerate, and the vascular system stiffens and clogs. No matter the efforts, every life ultimately answers to time.

But this reality is not meant to discourage; it should inspire urgency. Since people cannot add endless years to life, our charge as fitness professionals is to add life to the years our clients have. Within the time they are given, they have immense power to shape their health, extend their vitality, and preserve independence—and we, as coaches, are uniquely positioned to guide them there.

While the march of time is unstoppable, the pace and severity of physical decline are not fixed. As personal trainers we hold more leverage over the aging process of our clients than we often give ourselves credit for. Every training session, every program, every cue is a chance to bend the aging curve. The progressive accumulation of daily habits, good or bad, becomes either an investment or a withdrawal from our clients' future health. Some ailments may be unavoidable, but many of the challenges so often dismissed as "just getting older" are not fate at all. They are the predictable results of disuse and inactivity, problems that the right kind of training can prevent, slow, or even reverse.

THE HEALTH SPAN: LIFE SPAN GAP

When longevity is discussed, the focus often is on life span: the total number of years from birth to death. By that measure, the story looks good. Over the past century, people have added decades to the average life through cleaner living conditions, safer food and water, improved sanitation, vaccines, antibiotics, and emergency medicine. Thanks largely to medical advances over the past century, global life expectancy has reached 71.4 years (68.9 for men, 74 for women). In the United States, the averages are even higher: 73.7 years for men and 79.1 for women (World Health Organization, 2024a).

These are remarkable achievements. A child born today is far less likely to die from pneumonia, influenza, or a contaminated water supply than at any other time in human history. If someone is injured in a car accident or suffers a heart attack, emergency medicine can stabilize and save them in ways that were impossible just a few generations ago. By nearly every measure, modern medicine has been extraordinarily successful at extending life.

But life span alone does not tell the whole story. The more important and often overlooked measure is health span: the number of years lived in good health, free from chronic disease and disability. By this metric, people are failing. While people are living longer, they are not necessarily living better.

This contrast is especially stark in the United States, which has the largest health span–life span gap in the world. On average, Americans spend 12.4 years—nearly 30 percent more than the global average—living with chronic disease, pain, and dependence (Garmany and Terzic, 2024). Much of that gap is bridged not by improving underlying health, but by medications that manage symptoms rather than address root causes. The U.S. healthcare system has excelled at extending life span, but it has fallen short in helping people live healthier lives. Figure 1.1 demonstrates the gap between health span and life span.

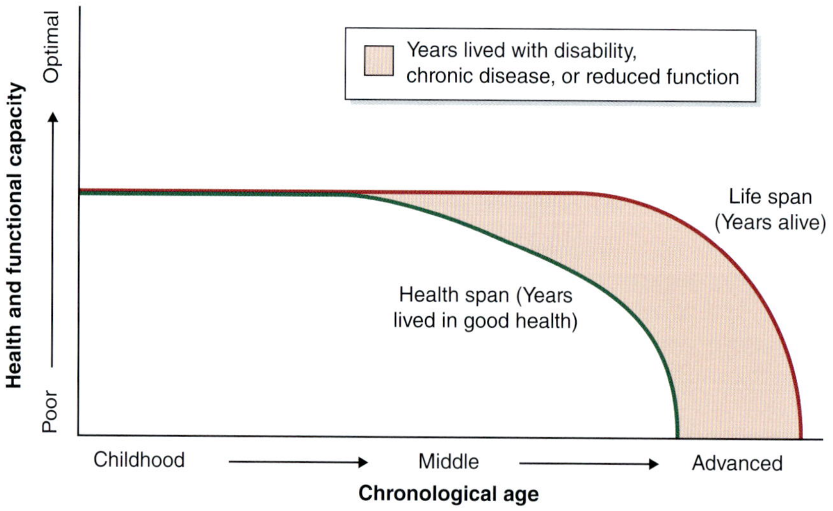

Figure 1.1 Health span versus life span gap.

In the United States, 68 percent of adults take at least one prescription drug daily, and 26 percent take four or more (CivicScience, 2024). Many of these medications are essential and even lifesaving, stabilizing heart conditions, controlling infections, or easing severe pain. But the majority are prescribed for lifestyle-related conditions such as high blood pressure, high cholesterol, type 2 diabetes, chronic pain, and depression (Fuentes et al, 2018; Safer, 2019).

These conditions are largely driven by how people live via their diets, activity levels, sleep, and stress. In many cases, they can be prevented, improved, or even reversed through consistent exercise, better nutrition, and healthier daily habits. Yet instead of addressing the underlying behavioral and lifestyle drivers, the modern healthcare system leans heavily on pharmaceuticals to manage symptoms.

This dependence comes at a cost. The widespread use of multiple medications, known as *polypharmacy*, increases the risk of dangerous interactions, side effects, addiction, and ballooning health care costs (Maher et al., 2014). As chronic diseases accumulate, many individuals are prescribed multiple medications to manage symptoms, creating a cycle in which treatment focuses on controlling disease rather than preventing it or reversing it.

Medication will always be a critical part of health care, but the potential to reduce people's dependence is immense. With the right lifestyle interventions, many of the most commonly prescribed drugs could be delayed, reduced, or avoided altogether.

DISEASES OF DISUSE

Across the globe, and especially in the United States, people are failing to meet even the minimum recommended levels of physical activity. The U.S. Department of Health and Human Services (2018) recommends that adults engage in

- 150 to 300 minutes per week of moderate-intensity aerobic activity, or
- 75 to 150 minutes per week of vigorous-intensity aerobic activity, or
- an equivalent combination of the two,
- *plus* muscle-strengthening activities for all major muscle groups at least two days per week.

Yet fewer than one in four Americans meet these basic standards. Figure 1.2 shows the percentage of Americans meeting the minimum recommended exercise guidelines (Elgaddal et al., 2022).

Falling short of the recommended guidelines represents the single largest missed opportunity to restore people's collective health, and the consequences are deadly. Physical inactivity is a leading lifestyle-related contributor to global mortality and a major risk factor for noncommunicable diseases such as cardiovascular disease, type 2 diabetes, stroke, obesity, and certain cancers (Lee, 2012; Katzmarzyk, 2022). The modern epidemics of cardiovascular disease, diabetes, dementia, and cancer all share a common accelerant: inactivity. Together, noncommunicable diseases account for nearly three-quarters of global

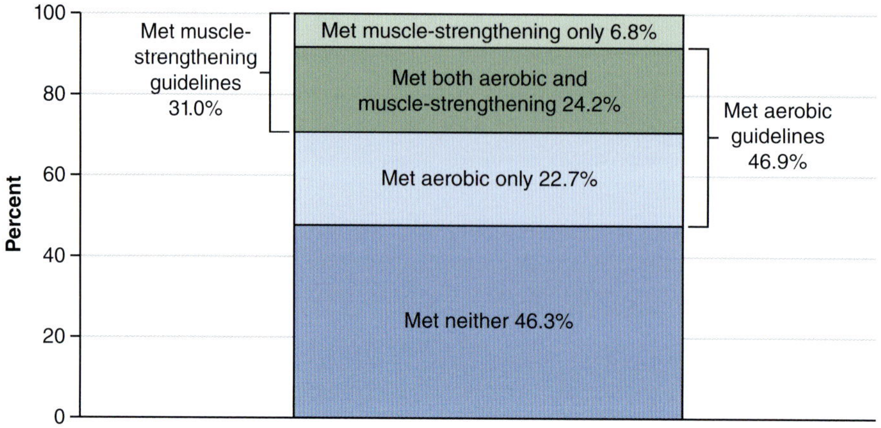

Figure 1.2 Percentage of Americans meeting the minimum recommended exercise guidelines for cardiovascular and resistance training (Elgaddal et al., 2022).

deaths each year, with cardiovascular disease alone responsible for more than 20 million lives annually (World Health Organization, 2024b; Di Cesare et al., 2024). In the United States, 60 percent of adults live with at least one chronic disease, and managing these conditions consumes 90 percent of the nation's $4.5 trillion in annual health care spending (Buttorff et al., 2017; CDC, 2025).

Physical inactivity fuels one of the most visible and widespread consequences of modern living: obesity. In the United States, more than 40 percent of adults and 21 percent of children and adolescents are living with obesity (Bryan et al., 2021). Globally, the World Health Organization estimates that over one billion people now live with obesity, a figure that has tripled in just four decades. This rise parallels sharp increases in type 2 diabetes, cardiovascular disease, and certain cancers, all of which are strongly linked to excess body fat. In fact, obesity alone is estimated to account for five million deaths worldwide each year (Ahmed and Mohammed, 2025).

The tragedy is that much of the global burden of chronic disease is largely preventable. Regular physical activity offers profound protection against heart disease, type 2 diabetes, cancer, and dementia. It is one of the most powerful and cost-effective forms of preventive medicine people have, yet it remains vastly underprescribed and underused. Disuse accelerates the decline of both structure and function in bodies: Muscles atrophy, bones weaken, neural signaling diminishes, joints stiffen, and cardiovascular capacity fades. Beyond lost performance, these changes threaten independence and shorten life span.

Inactivity alters body composition and fuels chronic, low-grade inflammation, damaging blood vessels, disrupting insulin signaling, and accelerating cellular aging. This persistent inflammatory state is now recognized as a unifying mechanism behind many of today's most common killers: It stiffens arteries and drives atherosclerosis in cardiovascular disease (Henein, 2022), impairs glucose regulation in diabetes (Donath and Shoelson, 2011), promotes tumor growth in cancer (Grivennikov, 2010; Hojman et al., 2011), and accelerates neurodegeneration in Alzheimer's disease (Heneka et al., 2015; Hu et al., 2024). Even depression has been linked to inflammation-driven changes in brain chemistry (Osimo et al., 2020; Felger and Lotrich, 2013).

Growing evidence suggests that these conditions do not develop in isolation but instead share common upstream drivers, including chronic inflammation, insulin resistance, and metabolic dysfunction that link muscle loss, glucose dysregulation, and cognitive decline (Xenos et al., 2026). These structural losses and metabolic shifts often create a self-perpetuating cycle: As muscles waste and fitness declines, daily activity becomes harder, movement decreases further, and excess energy accumulates. In turn, inflammation and metabolic dysfunction worsen, accelerating disease progression. From this perspective, sarcopenia, type 2 diabetes, and cognitive decline are not separate age-related conditions but interconnected manifestations of a broader failure in metabolic and inflammatory regulation that progressively erodes both physical and cognitive function when movement is lost. Left unchecked, the cycle compounds over time, transforming disuse into disability and chronic illness. Figure 1.3 provides a visual representation of the inactivity, inflammation, and disease cycle.

Beyond long-term disease risk, inactivity also plays a major role in the development of chronic pain. As physical activity decreases, muscles lose strength, joints stiffen, coordination declines, and the body becomes less tolerant to load and stress. As capacity declines, even normal daily activities can become sources of discomfort.

In many cases, chronic pain is not simply the result of structural damage but a reflection of reduced capacity. When the body is no longer prepared to handle the demands placed upon it, pain emerges as a signal of that mismatch. This creates a self-reinforcing cycle: pain leads to avoidance of movement, further reducing capacity and worsening both pain and dysfunction over time.

The effects of inactivity are not only mechanical but also physiological. A sedentary lifestyle promotes a more pro-inflammatory internal environment, reduces tissue quality, and impairs metabolic health. Physical inactivity has been shown to increase pro-inflammatory cytokines and heighten pain sensitivity, whereas regular activity promotes an anti-inflammatory state and improves pain tolerance (Burini et al., 2020; Jones et al., 2014).

Emerging evidence also suggests that many common musculoskeletal conditions, such as tendinopathy and osteoarthritis, have a metabolic component (Sellam and Berenbaum, 2013; Lai et al., 2024; Zhang et al., 2025). Chronic low-grade inflammation and insulin resistance

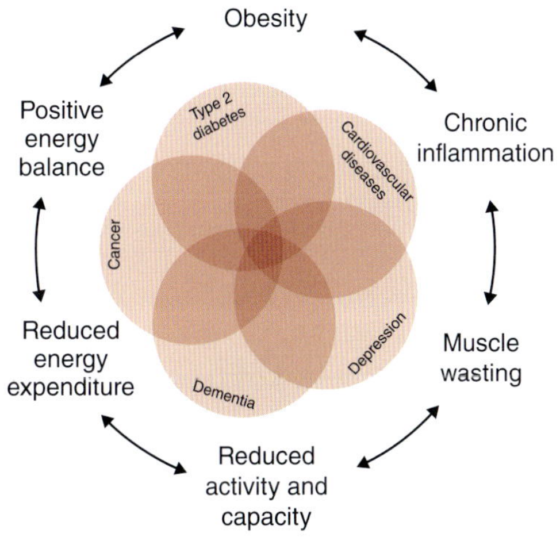

Figure 1.3 The inactivity, inflammation, and disease cycle.

can impair connective tissue health, reduce healing capacity, and increase the likelihood of pain—even in the absence of excessive mechanical load.

In many cases, improving general physical capacity can reduce pain and improve quality of life, even when the exercise itself does not directly target the painful area (Nayab and Bilal Elahi, 2024). By improving the body's internal environment and restoring tolerance to load, movement enhances tissue health and helps break the cycle of pain and inactivity. Exercise and physical activity are among the most effective nonpharmacological interventions for chronic pain. Regular exercise can reduce pain severity, improve physical function, and enhance quality of life when it is prescribed and progressed appropriately based on the client's current capacity and tolerance to load (Geneen et al., 2017; De la Corte-Rodríguez et al., 2024; Núñez-Cortés et al., 2025).

Many chronic diseases often do not fully manifest until people reach later stages of life, but they actually begin to take root much earlier than most people realize. Too frequently, training for longevity is presented as something only relevant to older adults. However, many of the so-called diseases of aging are actually the result of years of inactivity. Muscle and skeletal mass start to decline in people's 30s, vascular stiffness and rising blood pressure can emerge in midlife, and metabolic dysfunction may silently progress for years before any symptoms become apparent. By the time problems show up, the groundwork has already been laid.

This means that the habits people build during early and middle adulthood are just as important, if not more so, than the interventions applied later in life. Longevity training is not just about reactively extending life in later years; it is about proactively protecting quality of life at every stage. Each session of strength training, each mile walked, and each repetition performed is not solely for the 70- or 80-year-old versions of people; it is for the 40- or 50-year-olds who want to remain strong, mobile, and free of chronic disease. When longevity is rethought in this way, it shifts from being an "old person's problem" to becoming everyone's concern. The earlier people start investing in strength, fitness, and health, the greater the compounding benefits they will enjoy throughout their lives.

Regular physical activity preserves both the structure and function of the body, protecting muscles, bones, joints, the cardiovascular system, and even the brain. Exercise does not just slow decline; it actively prevents many of the lifestyle-related diseases that dominate modern health care.

If exercise is the most powerful medicine people have—capable of preventing disease, extending life span, and transforming nearly every aspect of health—the obvious question is this: Why is it not being prescribed, and why are people not taking it?

THE FITNESS PARADOX

The irony of modern health is that at a time when people have more information about fitness and spend more on it than ever before, the population is also sicker and less active than at any point in history. In 2023, the global wellness economy reached a staggering $6.3 trillion, with major spending in areas such as gym memberships, sports and recreation, nutrition, supplements, and apparel (Global Wellness Institute, 2025).

No country invests more than the United States, which leads the world by a wide margin, spending $2.01 trillion (over $6,000 per person each year) on health and wellness. That is more than 7 percent of the nation's gross domestic product (GDP), directed toward activities and products aimed at improving fitness, health, and quality of life (Global Wellness Institute, 2025).

Yet for all this investment, much of it goes unused. About one in four Americans has a gym membership, but many never build the habit of actually going. Dropout happens fast, with up to 63 percent of members stopping participation in the first three months, and fewer than 4 percent maintaining consistent activity for more than a year (Health and Fitness Association, 2024; Sperandei et al., 2016). Research shows nearly half of the people who intend to be physically active never follow through. In a meta-analysis of over 29,000 participants, 47 percent of those who planned to exercise failed to take action (Feil et al., 2023). Expensive gear sits in closets, gym memberships are abandoned, and results never appear, not because people don't intend to exercise but because they can't stick with it.

With the Internet in nearly everyone's pocket, people can also instantly access thousands of free workouts, training plans, and how-to videos from every corner of the fitness world. There is no shortage of expert advice, inspirational content, or step-by-step programs promising to get people in shape. But this flood of information has a downside: Instead of clarity, it often creates confusion. Conflicting messages about the best workout, diet, or program leave many feeling paralyzed before they even start. This overload often leads to decision fatigue, which turns into inaction.

The rise of influencers and wellness companies has turned health into a marketplace of expensive, unrealistic, and often harmful solutions. Common portrayals of fitness are out of touch with the realities of starting and sustaining a program. Many people feel overwhelmed, discouraged, or convinced they cannot succeed without the latest product, gadget, or trend, when in reality, the basics have always worked. People are not short on resources, advice, or opportunities. So what stands in the way?

ROADBLOCKS TO EXERCISE

The most commonly cited reason for avoiding exercise is lack of time. The realities of modern life, such as 40-plus-hour workweeks, commutes, and family responsibilities make it difficult for many people to consistently engage in physical activity. But the challenge runs deeper than busy schedules. Socioeconomic determinants of health such as income, education, occupation, and neighborhood strongly influence a person's ability to exercise. Individuals with higher socioeconomic status often have more access to resources, facilities, and support systems that make being active possible. Those with fewer resources face greater barriers, which helps explain why chronic disease linked to inactivity disproportionately affects lower-income populations.

Layered on top of this is the wellness industry itself. Much of the marketplace is built around products, services, and messaging aimed at higher-income audiences. Fitness is often packaged as a luxury rather than a necessity, leaving those with fewer resources excluded.

Even for those with the means and access, the act of joining a gym or beginning an exercise program can feel intimidating. Many gyms project an environment that seems designed for the already-fit rather than those seeking to become fit. For someone who is untrained, these spaces can feel exclusionary, filled with equipment they do not know how to use, people who seem to know exactly what they are doing, and an atmosphere that suggests that exercise is reserved for those already in shape.

Unfortunately, many coaches and training programs fail to bridge that gap. Instead of creating scalable systems that meet people where they are, programs often cater to the advanced, leaving beginners overwhelmed. The result is that when newcomers do manage to begin, setbacks quickly arise. Extreme portrayals of fitness in media and on social platforms fuel unrealistic expectations, while irresponsible coaching and poorly designed programs push people too hard, too soon. Rather than building confidence and consistency, these approaches often leave people injured, exhausted, or discouraged before they have had the chance to experience progress.

Collectively, these barriers—access, intimidation, poor programming, and unrealistic messaging—create a cycle of confusion and discouragement for the average person trying to improve their health. Breaking that cycle requires a fundamental shift in how we view and deliver fitness. If we want to change the trajectory of society's health, exercise must be positioned as a necessity of life, not a luxury reserved for the wealthy or already athletic.

That shift begins with the modern-day fitness professional. Trainers and coaches are uniquely positioned at the front line of preventive medicine, capable of guiding people safely into exercise, scaling programs to meet individual needs, and helping clients build sustainable habits that extend health span and life span. In many ways, the modern fitness professional is not just a coach but a health care practitioner, an essential partner in preventing disease before it takes root.

The chapters that follow are designed to prepare fitness professionals to meet this challenge. This book provides a clear framework for delivering scalable, sustainable exercise coaching that produces life-changing improvements in health and function. Built on decades of coaching experience and supported by the best available research, this text serves as a comprehensive technical manual for the modern fitness professional. It addresses the full spectrum of skills required for effective coaching, from program design and progression strategies to communication, behavior change, and long-term client engagement. The goal is not simply to improve performance in the gym but to equip coaches with the tools to help clients move better, feel better, and live longer and healthier lives.

Chapter 2

The World's Strongest Medicine

Despite society's struggles to stay active, fitness professionals should feel hopeful about the role they can play in reversing the trend. The personal trainer is uniquely positioned to improve not only performance but also long-term health and quality of life.

Physicians remain indispensable when it comes to saving lives, but when it comes to changing lives, their influence is often limited. According to the CDC's National Center for Health Statistics, the average American visits their physician just over three times per year (CDC, 2024). By contrast, clients who train twice per week will spend more than 100 hours annually with their coaches. This asymmetry of contact time creates a unique opportunity: While doctors are the frontline of reactive medicine, fitness professionals are the frontline of preventive medicine.

And if movement is medicine, no one is more qualified to prescribe it than the fitness professional. Trainers have both the frequency of contact and the strength of relationship to influence behavior in ways that even the best physician cannot. Each repetition, each session, each conversation is a dose that contributes to a client's long-term resilience, independence, and vitality.

As personal trainers, we therefore must move beyond the outdated stereotype of cheerleader or repetition counter and instead see ourselves as true preventive health care providers, guiding people out of inactivity; scaling programs to meet individual needs; and building habits that protect against disease, disability, and decline.

This is not just an inspiring idea; it is one of the most evidence-based truths in health care. Exercise is the most potent, wide-spectrum "drug" ever discovered. No pill, no procedure, and no supplement rivals its impact across so many systems of the body.

EXERCISE AS A POLYPILL

If exercise could be put into a capsule, patented, and sold, it would instantly become the most prescribed, profitable, and sought-after drug on the market. Just consider the recent success of GLP-1 medications such as semaglutide, which have shown impressive results in reducing body weight and improving metabolic health (Wilding et al., 2021; Lincoff et al., 2023). These drugs have a place in managing disease, but they are not a substitute for the foundation of prevention: physical activity.

For decades, medicine has searched for the perfect "polypill"—a single intervention capable of lowering blood pressure, improving cholesterol, regulating blood sugar, protecting bones, elevating mood, and extending life. That pill already exists. It is called *exercise*. And fitness professionals are the ones best equipped to prescribe it.

Physical activity functions as the true polypill: a single, side effect–free intervention that delivers wide-ranging, multifactorial benefits across nearly every system of the body.

A single exercise session can begin to trigger effects that ripple through nearly every system of the body, while long-term practice builds a shield against the leading causes of death and disability. Unlike prescription medications that affect a single pathway, exercise provides a cascade of benefits throughout the entire body. It is not enough to say that "exercise is good for us"; it is the most effective preventive health intervention ever discovered. Figure 2.1 presents the wide-ranging impact exercise has on the major systems of the body.

EXERCISE AS A HORMETIC STRESSOR

Exercise primarily benefits people because of the hormetic stress it imparts on the body. Hormesis describes a biological principle where exposure to a low or moderate dose of stress stimulates beneficial adaptation (Radak et al., 2008). Too little stress produces no effect; too much becomes harmful. The response curve is not linear but inverted U-shaped as illustrated in figure 2.2 on page 14: Inactivity and overtraining sit at either end, while the sweet spot of regular, moderate stress lies in the middle. This is where positive adaptation occurs. Much like medicine, the effects of exercise depend entirely on the dose. Insufficient exposure fails to produce a therapeutic response, while excessive dosing can overwhelm the system and lead to negative consequences such as pain and exhaustion. When applied at the right intensity, volume, and frequency, however, exercise acts as a powerful, life-enhancing intervention.

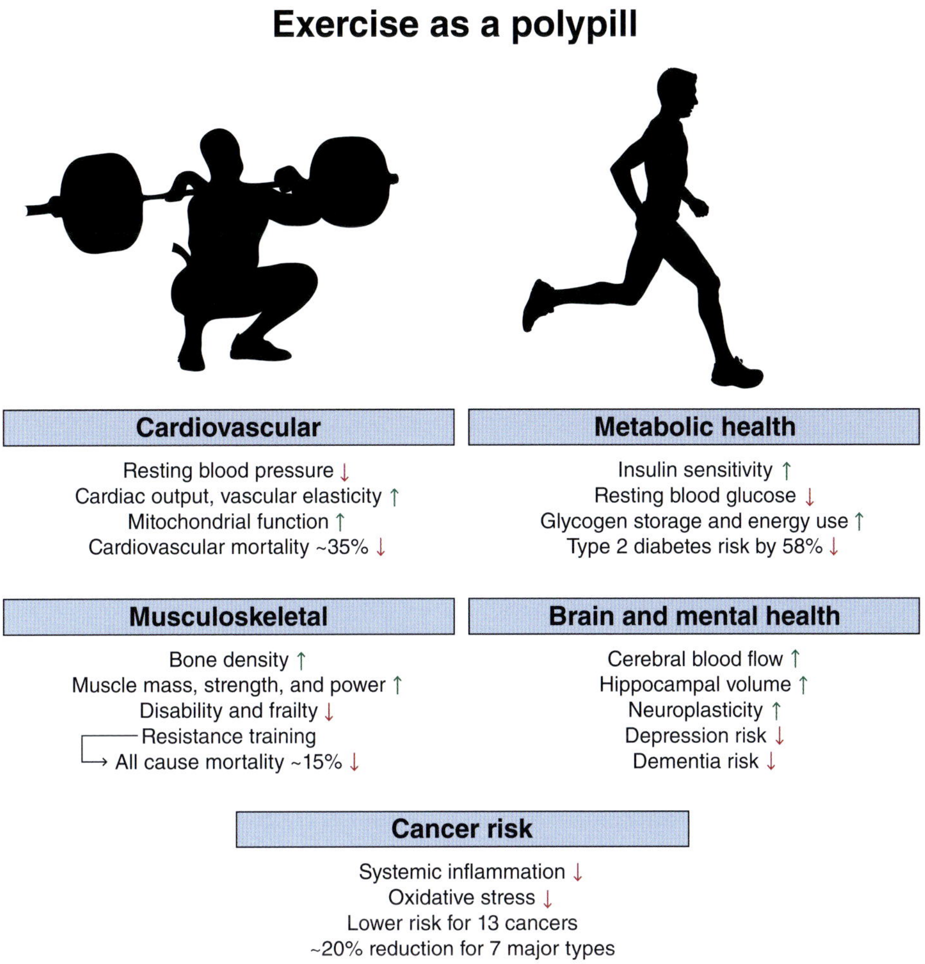

Figure 2.1 The wide-ranging impact of exercise on chronic health conditions.
Adams, 2013; Bird and Hawley, 2017; Blondell et al., 2014; Blumenthal et al., 1999; Blumenthal et al., 2007; Erickson et al., 2011; Hamer and Chida, 2009; Jensen et al., 2011; Knowler et al., 2002; Kvam et al., 2016; Moore et al., 2016; Naci and Ioannidis, 2015; Nocon et al., 2008; Netz, 2017; Noetel et al., 2024; Schuch et al., 2018; Shailendra et al., 2022.

Exercise is a perfect example of hormesis in action. Each workout temporarily disrupts homeostasis, as blood pressure rises, glycogen stores deplete, reactive oxygen species accumulate, cortisol levels spike, and connective tissues experience microscopic strain. In isolation, these look like damaging events. But when followed by recovery, they serve as powerful biological signals. The body interprets them as a call to adapt: Muscles remodel stronger, mitochondria multiply, antioxidant defenses increase, insulin sensitivity improves, and neural circuits refine. What stresses the system in the short term creates resilience in the long term. The beauty of exercise is that these adaptations are not confined

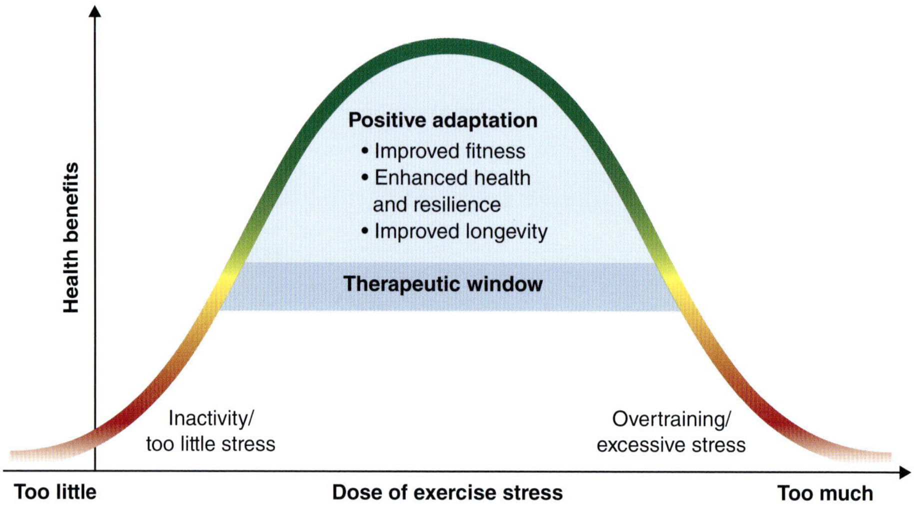

Figure 2.2 The hormetic dose-response relationship between exercise stress and health outcomes. Low levels of stress fail to stimulate adaptation, while excessive stress can be harmful. Optimal benefits occur within a moderate sweet spot of training stress, where physiological systems adapt and resilience improves.

to one system; they cascade across nearly every part of the body. However, this adaptive response is highly dependent on the dose and application of stress. When exercise is poorly programmed—whether through excessive load, volume, or frequency, or through inappropriate exercise selection—the same stressors can overwhelm the system rather than strengthen it. Instead of adaptation, the result may be persistent fatigue, elevated injury risk, chronic soreness, or diminished performance. Like any medicine, exercise is only effective when applied at the right dose. When programmed and coached appropriately, it creates a positive stress that drives adaptation and resilience. When misapplied, it can become a source of breakdown rather than progress.

THE EFFECT OF EXERCISE IN THE BODY

Of all the body's systems, the cardiovascular system may be the most profoundly shaped by exercise. Our heart and blood vessels respond remarkably to the stresses of aerobic activity. The heart grows stronger, increasing cardiac output; arteries become more elastic; resting blood pressure falls; and lipid profiles shift in a favorable direction. Over time, these adaptations translate into powerful protection for the cardiovascular system. Regular physical activity lowers the risk of cardiovascular death by roughly 35 percent and is as effective at preventing stroke-related mortality as some of the most widely prescribed drugs (Nocon et al., 2008; Naci and Ioannidis, 2015). Meta-analyses further show that consistent aerobic exercise reduces systolic blood pressure by 5 to 7 mmHg, an effect size comparable to first-line antihypertensive medications (Cornelissen and Smart, 2013).

If the cardiovascular system is the one most profoundly shaped by exercise, the musculoskeletal system is the one most visibly affected in daily life. Load a bone, and it remodels denser. Challenge a muscle, and it grows bigger and stronger. Repeated mechanical stressors fortify the tissues of our body that help us move. Muscles, bones, tendons, and joints become more resilient, protecting our independence as we age. Resistance training not only extends years free of disability but is also linked to lower mortality, reducing the risk of all-cause death by 15 percent, cardiovascular mortality by 19 percent, and cancer mortality by 14 percent, with the greatest benefit (27 percent risk reduction) seen at about 60 minutes per week (Shailendra et al., 2022).

At the same time, muscle contractions act like a sponge for glucose, improving metabolic function. Insulin works more efficiently, blood sugar stabilizes, and muscles adapt to both burn and store more glucose as glycogen, expanding the body's capacity to manage energy (Jensen et al., 2011). Even a single bout of exercise can enhance insulin sensitivity and lower blood glucose levels for up to 72 hours (Adams, 2013; Bird and Hawley, 2017). When these sessions accumulate week after week, the impact compounds. The landmark Diabetes Prevention Program found that a lifestyle intervention including just 150 minutes of weekly activity reduced the risk of progressing to type 2 diabetes by 58 percent, nearly twice the benefit of the diabetes medication metformin (Knowler et al., 2002). This demonstrates how profoundly movement can reshape metabolic health.

The brain is no less affected by exercise than the rest of the body. Aerobic activity essentially feeds the neural tissues by increasing blood flow and energy demand, and the adaptation is remarkable. Exercise stimulates the release of myokines and hormones that encourage neuroplasticity and strengthening of neural circuits. In older adults, aerobic training has been shown to increase hippocampal volume by 2 percent, essentially reversing two years of age-related decline (Erickson et al., 2011).

Beyond structure, exercise improves chemistry: Neurotransmitters and endorphins elevate mood, reduce anxiety, and sharpen focus, lowering the risk of developing depression by about 17 percent (Schuch et al., 2018), slowing cognitive decline by 35 percent (Blondell et al., 2014), and reducing the risk of dementia by nearly 30 percent (Hamer and Chida, 2009). Importantly, large randomized-controlled trials and meta-analyses now show that exercise reduces depressive symptoms as effectively as antidepressant medication, and when combined with pharmacotherapy, it often produces superior outcomes, making it both a viable alternative and a powerful adjunct in the treatment of depression (Blumenthal et al., 1999; Blumenthal et al., 2007; Netz, 2017; Schuch et al., 2016; Kvam et al., 2016; Noetel et al., 2024).

Even cancer, one of medicine's most feared diseases, can be profoundly influenced by exercise. Regular physical activity lowers systemic inflammation and oxidative stress, creating an internal environment less favorable to tumor growth. Large-scale population studies show that meeting physical activity guidelines is associated with lower risk for 13 different types of cancer, with reductions of 20 percent or more for seven of them, including esophageal, liver, lung, kidney, endometrial, gastric cardia, and myeloid leukemia (Moore et al., 2016). Few other single lifestyle behaviors offer such broad and powerful protection.

Exercise temporarily stresses the body, but in doing so, it teaches the body to adapt and improve. From heart to muscle, metabolism to mind, the evidence is overwhelming: Exercise is the closest thing we have to a true polypill for our health and longevity. But knowing *what happens in the body* is only half the story. The real challenge and opportunity lies in helping people actually do it. And this is where the fitness professional's advantage shines.

THE IMPACT OF THE FITNESS PROFESSIONAL

Exercise is an immensely powerful tool to change both the length and quality of people's lives, but behavior change is hard. For decades we have known the potential of strength training, cardiovascular exercise, and recreational activity to improve health and longevity. The challenge is not knowledge. Most people already know what they should be doing. The challenge is in taking action and sustaining it.

Unlike traditional medicine, exercise is not as painless as, "Take two of these and call me in the morning." It requires effort, consistency, and, at times, discomfort. This does not mean pain but rather the kind of discomfort that demands both physical and mental investment. Legendary strength coach Dan John captured this truth simply: "It's simple but not easy."

This is precisely where the fitness professional has massive leverage. Behavior change flourishes in the context of relationships. Trust, accountability, and frequent contact are what turn intentions into actions. Coaches must create environments where clients feel supported, challenged, and connected. In this way, fitness professionals are more than program designers; they are architects of adherence, helping people start and, more importantly, keep going.

Research supports this truth. In a study of 129 adults, McClaran (2003) found that just 10 weeks of one-on-one personal training led to significant progress in people's readiness to exercise regularly. Nearly three-quarters of participants who were not already consistent exercisers advanced to a higher level of commitment, an effect roughly twice as strong as what is typically seen in programs that rely only on handouts, incentives, or media campaigns. What made the difference was not more information but the structured support of a coach: helping clients identify benefits, overcome barriers, set goals, and plan for setbacks.

Adherence is only the beginning of the impact coaches can have on their clients. Beyond attendance, quality coaching exerts a powerful influence on the results clients can expect from exercise. Evidence shows that health club members supervised by qualified personal trainers, following structured and periodized programs, achieve significantly greater improvements in lean body mass, strength, power, and aerobic capacity than those training independently, even with similar frequency and facility access (Storer et al., 2014). The advantage was not greater motivation or effort alone but informed coaching: appropriate exercise selection, progressive overload, and the systematic manipulation of training variables applied consistently over time.

Although one-on-one personal training has been shown to have a powerful impact on behavior change and outcomes, the financial barrier—often exceeding $100 per hour—can limit access for many people seeking to improve their health. Group-led exercise programs can provide many of the same benefits as personal training at a lower cost and with the added power of community.

A meta-analysis of community-based group exercise programs found adherence rates as high as 70 percent, a level of consistency that outpaces many self-directed efforts or interventions relying on education alone (Farrance et al., 2016). These findings underscore the importance of the social environment in shaping long-term behavior change. Training alongside others enhances accountability, normalizes effort, and reinforces consistency in ways that are difficult to replicate in isolation.

Proximity and social ties are powerful shapers of behavior. Simply being in the presence of others can encourage us to show up, push a little harder, and persist a little longer. The impact of group cohesion, shared goals, and a sense of belonging creates a deeper bond that sustains motivation over the long term. When individuals feel connected to a group where healthy behaviors are the norm, adherence becomes much more likely. We tend to mirror the habits of those around us, for better or worse. Joining a group where a person's desired behavior is the normal behavior transforms consistency from an individual struggle into a collective expectation that is encouraged and celebrated.

Beyond adherence, evidence suggests that social connection itself may be a powerful determinant of long-term health and survival. In a large review of over 300,000 participants followed for 7.5 years, individuals with stronger social relationships demonstrated a 50 percent greater likelihood of survival compared to those with poor or insufficient social ties (Holt-Lundstead et al., 2010). Notably, the magnitude of this effect was comparable to well-established risk factors such as smoking cessation and exceeded the effects of obesity and physical activity.

With this in mind, coaches and gym owners should be intentional about building community into their training environments. Promoting community should not be viewed as a secondary benefit of group training but instead a core mechanism through which exercise improves both adherence and health outcomes. Group-based training lowers financial barriers while amplifying accountability, emotional support, and social connection. By fostering a close-knit, supportive environment, coaches can transform exercise from a solitary task into a sustainable lifestyle and, in doing so, influence their clients' long-term health.

FROM NOTHING TO SOMETHING

While starting an exercise program can feel intimidating and overwhelming, we as fitness professionals should take comfort in knowing that the biggest gains come right at the beginning. Going from nothing to something is where the largest health dividends are paid.

Just 10 to 15 minutes of daily activity lowers risk of early death significantly, and walking as few as 4,000 steps per day reduces all-cause mortality by nearly a third (Saint-Maurice et al., 2020). Even 10 to 59 minutes of weekly physical activity—far below the 150-minute guideline—reduces premature mortality by nearly 20 percent (Arem et al., 2015). Resistance training shows the same pattern: As little as one to two sessions per week are linked to reduced cardiovascular and cancer mortality (Momma et al., 2022).

The analysis by Arem and colleagues (2015) presented in figure 2.3 makes the dose–response relationship clear. Doing less than the guideline (under 150 minutes per week, equivalent to approximately 0.1–7.5 metabolic equivalent task hours [MET-hours], a unit that combines exercise intensity and duration) still lowered mortality by about **20 percent** compared to doing nothing. Meeting the guideline (150–300 minutes per week, 7.5–15 MET-hours) cut risk by **31 percent**, and doubling it (300–450 minutes, 15–22.5 MET-hours) lowered risk by 37 percent. Beyond that, the curve began to flatten; those exercising three to ten times the guideline still saw about a 39 percent reduction, with little additional benefit.

For clients, this knowledge is liberating: Improving one's health **does not require perfection.** Small, manageable steps matter. The role of the coach is to lower the barrier to entry, celebrate early wins, and scale gradually to ensure those first steps do not feel overwhelming.

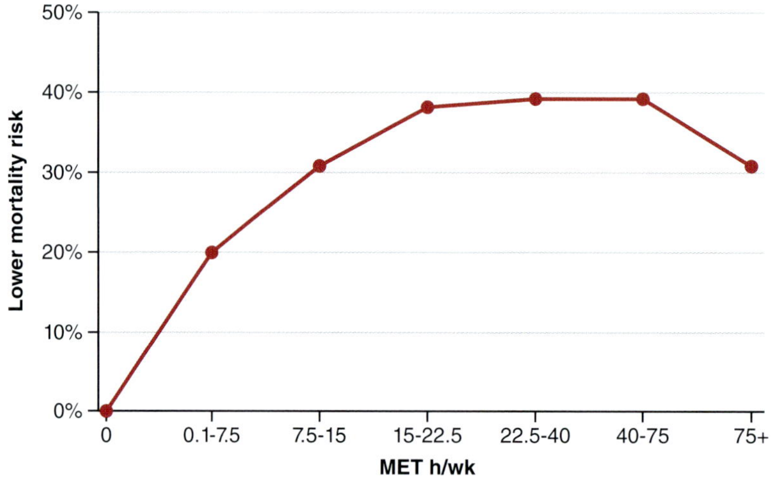

Figure 2.3 Exercise and mortality risk reduction (Arem et al., 2015).

What Is a MET-Hour?

MET-hours are a simple way researchers quantify total physical activity by combining how hard and how long someone exercises.

A MET (metabolic equivalent) represents the energy cost of resting quietly. Activities that require more effort have higher MET values. As intensity or duration increases, MET-hours accumulate more quickly, reflecting a higher overall dose of physical activity.

Examples include the following (MET values adapted from Ainsworth and colleagues [2011]):

- Walking at a moderate pace (3 METs) for 30 minutes = 1.5 MET-hours
- Jogging (7 METs) for 30 minutes = 3.5 MET-hours
- Cycling at a vigorous pace (10 METs) for 60 minutes = 10 MET-hours

Because MET-hours account for both intensity and time, they allow researchers to compare different types of activity on a common scale and examine dose–response relationships between exercise and health outcomes.

WRITING THE PRESCRIPTION

An effective plan for exercise to improve health and longevity is far simpler than many coaches and clients are led to believe. It does not require expensive equipment or endless hours in the gym. While mainstream solutions often promote one-dimensional approaches—whether it is cardio-only programs, bodybuilding splits, or flexibility routines—a well-rounded, holistic approach that integrates multiple aspects of fitness delivers the deepest impact and the most sustainable results.

Too often, strength training and cardiovascular exercise are framed as an *either-or* choice, with people asking, *"If you could only pick one, which would it be?"* The reality is far more powerful: The combination of the two produces greater benefits for health and longevity than either can on its own.

Research consistently shows this synergistic effect. An analysis of nearly 100,000 adults found that strength training alone reduced all-cause mortality risk by roughly 9 percent, aerobic activity alone by approximately 32 percent, but performing both together reduced risk by 41 percent (Gorzelitz et al., 2022).

This evidence makes clear that the benefits are not merely additive; they are synergistic. For anyone prescribing exercise as medicine, strength and cardio are not rival therapies but complementary prescriptions that amplify one another's effects.

Beyond strength and cardio, other elements of a balanced program further enhance effectiveness. Mobility and flexibility work to reduce age-related declines in movement quality and support joint health. Multiplanar movement training builds the athleticism and freedom to navigate daily life without fear of falls or disability. Power training helps slow the loss of speed and reactivity with age, qualities that are critical for independence and fall prevention. When combined, these elements create a resilient, adaptable body capable of thriving across the life span.

Each component represents a different part of the prescription; together, they form the strongest medicine for improving both health span and life span.

With the knowledge of how to program, scale, and coach these elements, fitness professionals are positioned as true frontline practitioners of preventive health. Few other professionals have the same opportunity to shape long-term outcomes as coaches and trainers.

In the chapters ahead, we will break down each element of this prescription in detail—mobility and flexibility; movement skills; power, strength, and cardiovascular training; and general physical activity—and show exactly how to deliver the world's strongest medicine to clients, one session at a time.

PART II

LOW-IMPACT MOVEMENT FOR LONGEVITY

Chapter 3

Everyday Physical Activity

Physical activity was a fundamental part of life long before the advent of gyms, treadmills, and wearable fitness trackers. People walked, carried, lifted, and worked throughout their days—not to burn calories or build muscle but to survive. Movement was an integral aspect of daily living; it was not something people scheduled or tracked but was a necessity.

For most of human history, exercise was not pursued for health or appearance. People were physically active because their environment and lifestyle required it. Activities such as hunting, gathering, farming, and building demanded movement, and in fulfilling these demands, people unknowingly maintained robust health and physical fitness.

However, as societies advanced and technology evolved, people's relationship with movement began to change. In developed countries, physical labor has been largely replaced by machines, automation, and convenience. Tasks that once required effort—such as fetching water, preparing food, traveling, and working—can now be accomplished with the press of a button or the swipe of a screen. This significant reduction in daily movement has led to increased sedentary behavior, resulting in a range of preventable health issues.

Examining cultures that rely less on technology, such as the Old Order Amish in Ontario, Canada, and hunter-gatherer groups like the Hadza tribes in northern Tanzania, provides insight into the daily physical activity people have largely lost due to modernization. On average, Amish women take about 14,196 steps each day, while Amish men average around 18,425 steps (Bassett et al., 2004). In comparison, Hadza women walk approximately 4.7 miles (7.6 km) daily, and men cover an average of 8.0 miles (12.9 km), which translates to between 10,000 and 18,000 steps per day as part of their survival (Wood et al., 2021). This includes activities such as hunting, foraging, building shelter, and playing.

Alternatively, in developed countries people work from home, drive to where they need to go, and can have all of their desires delivered to their door with the click of a button. The average American only takes about 4,700 steps per day (Althoff et al., 2017). The bottom line is that people are moving less than they have ever moved in human history, and the massive drop-off in physical activity and increase in sedentary behavior leaves people paying the price with their health.

The drop-off in daily movement shows a basic mismatch between how bodies are built to function and the way people live today. Humans are meant to move often, but current routines encourage people to sit still. Over time, this leads to reduced metabolic health, musculoskeletal resilience, cardiovascular capacity, and overall function. This chapter covers why moving less and sitting too much matter. It also shares simple, practical ways coaches can help clients move more every day, in ways that last.

SEDENTARY BEHAVIOR

Sedentary behavior refers to any activity performed while awake that requires 1.5 or fewer MET-hours, typically while sitting or reclining (Tremblay et al., 2017). This includes activities such as sitting at a desk, watching television, reading, or scrolling on phones. While some of these activities can be necessary and even restorative, the increasing prevalence of sedentary lifestyles is a cause for concern. A staggering one in four Americans spends eight or more hours sitting each day (Ussery et al., 2018).

The rise in sedentary time has contributed to a significant decline in physical activity, with nearly 75 percent of people in developed countries failing to meet the minimum recommended physical activity guidelines (Elgaddal et al., 2022). Spending more time sitting has serious implications for people's overall health. Total sedentary behavior is directly linked to increased risk of all-cause mortality as well as fatal and nonfatal cardiovascular diseases, type 2 diabetes, and metabolic syndrome (Rezende et al., 2014).

Reducing sedentary behavior should be a priority across the life span, beginning in childhood. Longitudinal, accelerometer-based data show that sedentary time increases steadily from early childhood, rising from just over 50 percent of waking hours at age 7 to nearly 75 percent by age 15 (Janssen et al., 2016). At the same time, research demonstrates a persistent decline in physical activity and key components of physical fitness, including flexibility, strength, power, and cardiorespiratory fitness, among school-age children (Itoi et al., 2015; Venckunas et al., 2017). This decline can be attributed largely to the reduction of recess and physical education classes, along with the increase in screen time for young children. As opportunities for movement diminish and screen-based activities take their place, the effects on children's physical and mental health become increasingly evident. Children who spend more time in sedentary activities are more likely to be obese, have higher blood pressure and blood lipid levels, and exhibit lower self-esteem and academic performance compared to their more active peers (Rezende et al., 2014).

While physical activity often peaks during people's younger working years, it tends to decline significantly as age advances. At the same time, older adults also begin to experience a natural loss of muscle mass, strength, power, and cardiorespiratory fitness. When combined with increasingly sedentary behavior, this decline can accelerate dramatically, leading to greater frailty, reduced independence, and a heightened risk of chronic disease. This makes the aging population particularly vulnerable to the harmful effects of inactivity.

Adults over the age of 60 reportedly spend 8 to 12 hours per day engaged in sedentary activities, accounting for about 80 percent of their awake time. With the adult population aged 60 and older projected to exceed 22 percent of the global population by 2050, it is essential for health professionals to promote physical activity and exercise while reducing sedentary behavior to improve long-term health outcomes (Rezende et al., 2014).

While regular exercise is essential for health, it does not fully counteract the harmful effects of prolonged sedentary behavior. Mounting research shows that sitting for extended periods can negatively affect metabolic and cardiovascular health—even in individuals who meet or exceed recommended physical activity guidelines. In other words, being active is not a free pass to be sedentary the rest of the day.

Recent research examining physically active young adults reveals that prolonged sitting negatively affects key cardiovascular and metabolic health markers—specifically body mass index (BMI) and the ratio of total cholesterol to high-density lipoprotein (TC/HDL)—even in early adulthood when people are generally considered healthy. While meeting current physical activity guidelines offers some advantages, it does not completely offset the negative effects of prolonged sitting. In particular, individuals in their late 20s to early 30s who sit for 8.5 hours or more each day can experience moderate cardiac risk levels, even if they adhere to basic exercise recommendations (Bruellman et al., 2024).

This underscores the importance of not just increasing participation in exercise but also reducing overall sedentary activity independent of volitional exercise. A comprehensive study of over 240,000 healthy Americans aged 50 to 70 reveals a striking link between increased sedentary behavior—such as prolonged sitting and excessive television viewing—and significantly elevated risks of all-cause mortality, cardiovascular mortality, and cancer mortality. Alarmingly, these associations hold true even after adjusting for levels of moderate to vigorous physical activity and other potential confounding factors. Specifically, individuals who spent seven or more hours per day watching television faced a staggering 61 percent higher risk of all-cause mortality, an 85 percent higher risk of cardiovascular mortality, and a 22 percent higher risk of cancer mortality compared to those who watched less than one hour daily (Matthews et al., 2012). These compelling findings strongly suggest that extended periods of sedentary behavior independently elevate mortality risk, irrespective of physical activity levels. This powerful study sends a crucial message: It is not enough to participate in regular physical activity; people must actively minimize sedentary time to effectively lower the risk of premature death from a variety of causes.

WHAT HAPPENS WHEN PEOPLE STOP MOVING?

Even the most active people can have their routines sidetracked with injury, illness, and life events that prevent them from keeping up their normal activity routines. Research shows that even relatively short stretches of inactivity and increased sedentary behavior can quickly begin to negatively affect strength, power, and cardiovascular health (Oikawa, 2019; Bowden Davies et al., 2019).

Deloading of the muscles from physical disuse leads to a decrease in muscular stimulation and protein synthesis, resulting in increased muscular atrophy, a problem that is particularly troubling for older populations that are already at risk for sarcopenia. Additionally, some studies suggest that the physical inactivity that comes from disuse also can lead to increased oxidative stress and impairment of mitochondrial function, negatively affecting muscle function, aerobic fitness, and metabolic functioning (McKendry et al., 2024).

Research on the effects of bed rest on both young and older populations reveals the profound impact that disuse can have on muscle function, particularly in the elderly. Following only 14 days of bed rest, lower body power declines by roughly 15 percent in older adults and 10 percent in younger adults. The more troubling finding, however, emerges during recovery, when older participants struggled to regain their power. Despite completing six training sessions over two weeks following their bed rest, the older participants still were unable to return to their pre–bed rest strength and power levels (Rejc et al., 2018). This highlights the difficulties older adults encounter when attempting to regain their fitness after physical setbacks, and it emphasizes the need to build a strong foundation of strength and power to aid in recovery during times of decreased activity.

NON-EXERCISE ACTIVITY THERMOGENESIS (NEAT)

The core of health and fitness routines should primarily focus on the activities people engage in at the gym. However, significant value is found in incorporating low-intensity physical activity outside of the training facility. Non-exercise activity thermogenesis, commonly referred to as *NEAT*, represents the energy people expend through all physical activities other than structured exercise. This includes the calories burned while going about daily lives—things like working, doing chores, walking, and even fidgeting. While these movements may seem small on their own, together they make up a significant portion of total daily energy expenditure.

What makes NEAT so powerful is how these seemingly minor actions add up over time. The cumulative impact of NEAT can be highly significant in influencing metabolic health and body composition. Research has shown that individuals with higher levels of NEAT tend to have lower rates of obesity and better cardiometabolic profiles (Villablanca et al., 2015). From a practical standpoint, encouraging clients to increase their baseline daily movement—whether by taking stairs, opting to walk during phone calls, or incorporating short activity breaks during sedentary periods—can lead to meaningful improvements in energy balance and health outcomes. Over time, this steady stream of low-intensity activity can help improve cardiovascular health, support weight management, and reduce the risks associated with prolonged sitting.

Daily habits can have massive impact on cumulative NEAT. Two individuals of similar size and body type can experience a variance of up to 2,000 calories in their daily NEAT due to their daily movement habits and demands of their occupations (Villablanca et al., 2015). With many professions now centered on computer-based work-from-home settings, we trainers must encourage non-exercise-based physical activity to compensate for the significant drop in movement that results from eliminating a commute to work and reducing physical activity within the workspace.

A study conducted in 2005 found that lean, sedentary individuals tend to be more active throughout the day compared to those who are sedentary and obese. The lean participants spent an average of 152 more minutes per day standing and moving than their obese counterparts. This increase in activity did not come from time spent at the gym; rather, it included simple movements such as standing, walking, and fidgeting. This additional low-intensity activity resulted in an extra calorie expenditure of approximately 350 calories per day. While this daily difference might seem small, it can accumulate significantly over time—potentially leading to a weight loss of up to 33 pounds (15 kg) over the course of a year, assuming that calorie intake remains constant (Levine et al., 2005).

What is most fascinating is that research indicates that as people increase their overall volitional physical activity, they tend to decrease their involuntary physical activity. In other words, as people begin to exercise, they tend to choose to move less in their daily lives by opting to drive instead of walking or taking the escalator instead of the stairs, effectively constraining their total energy expenditure in response to exercise (Melanson, 2017). With this in mind, people must be intentional with their physical activity choices outside of the gym if their goal is to increase energy expenditure and improve their physiological health.

Small conscious daily decisions can compound into massive changes in energy expenditure when viewed over a long period. Some simple changes include working at a standing desk, taking periodic breaks from seated work to go on a short walk, choosing the stairs rather than an elevator or escalator, walking or riding a bike to a destination rather than driving, and parking slightly farther from the destination rather than searching for the closest spot possible. Overall, the choices may seem minuscule, but when compounded, they can have a significant impact on both body weight and physiological health.

WALKING

Although walking is the most common form of physical activity, many people often discount its impact on overall health and wellness due to its low intensity. Walking, however, can serve as an extremely effective low-barrier option for people to begin exercising and fill the gaps between training sessions in a gym with increased physical activity.

With the advent of fitness wearables, step counts have become a popular means to track overall physical activity—and with good reason. Researchers have been able to identify direct correlations between overall step counts with numerous long-term health outcomes.

Modest increases in daily step count can have a massive impact on both life span and cardiovascular health. Even with minimal walking, small and progressive increases can have major implications on health span and life span. Starting at about 2,000 steps per day, every additional 1,000 steps taken confers a 15 percent reduction in all-cause mortality (Stens et al., 2023). The images in figure 3.1 show the relationship between daily step count and all-cause mortality and incidences of both fatal and nonfatal cardiovascular disease.

Sedentary adults who increased their step count by 3,000 steps per day, the equivalent of roughly 30 minutes of walking, experience significant reduction in both systolic and diastolic blood pressure (Lefferts et al., 2023). Walking between 7,000 and 13,000 steps per days can reduce cardiovascular mortality by 49 percent (Banach et al., 2023).

The value of walking as a form of preventive health practice extends beyond hearts to brains, highlighting the interconnectedness of cardiovascular and cognitive health. Researchers have discovered that walking up to 9,800 steps per day can reduce risk for developing dementia by up to 50 percent. And the walking pace seems to amplify the effect. If participants walked with purpose, at a rate of 40 steps per minute, it reduced the risk by another 57 percent (Del Pozo Cruz et al., 2022).

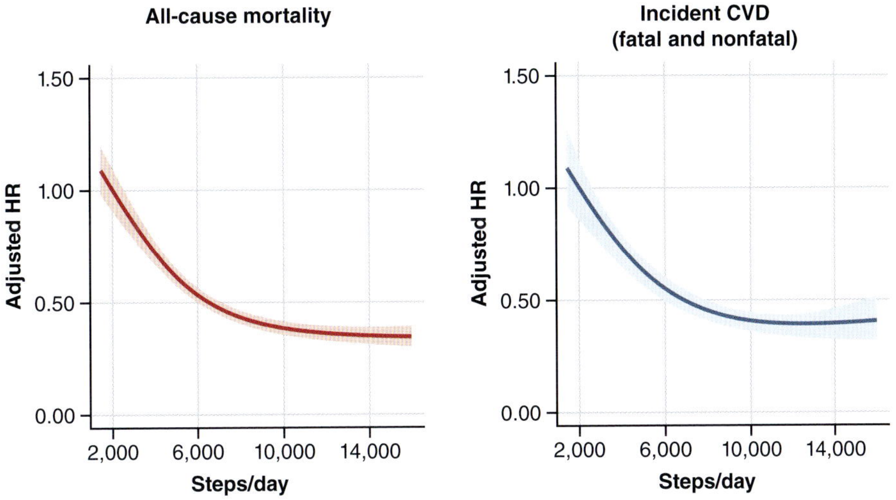

Figure 3.1 Relationship between daily step count and all-cause mortality and cardiovascular disease.

Reprinted by permission from N.A. Stens, E.A. Bakker, A. Mañas, et al., "Relationship of Daily Step Counts to All-Cause Mortality and Cardiovascular Events," *Journal of the American College of Cardiology* 82, no. 15 (2023): 1483–94, permission conveyed through Copyright Clearance Center, Inc.

As coaches, we should encourage our clients to incorporate daily walking into their weekly routines as a form of low-intensity exercise, in addition to their formal strength training and cardiovascular workouts. With the rise of fitness wearables and smartphones that track steps, clients can easily monitor their progress.

To help clients increase their daily steps, it is important to meet them where they are and suggest small, gradual increases to their step counts. For example, asking clients to boost their daily steps from 4,000 to 10,000 all at once is likely to lead to failure, because large changes in behavior are often unsustainable. Instead, we can recommend that they add one or two short walking sessions throughout the day. This approach helps establish a habit, laying a foundation for further improvement. Incorporating two 10-minute walking periods into their workday can effectively break up sedentary time and increase their daily step count by up to 2,000 steps, which can lead to a 30 percent reduction in mortality risk.

MINIMUM EFFECTIVE DOSE AND EXERCISE SNACKS

The common all-or-nothing mindset around exercise often causes people to abandon their fitness routines entirely when they cannot stick to a consistent schedule or when life gets in the way. Although people may go through periods of time when their schedules make it challenging to commit to a full workout, it is important to strive to find ways to incorporate physical activity into the day even if the duration or intensity may not be as high as normally performed. With lack of time and access to exercise facilities being the most common reasons people cite for failing to participate in physical activity, coaches should look for nontraditional means of exercise to encourage increased physical activity for their clients.

Emerging research on minimum effective dose training has shown that even short, nontraditional bouts of exercise can produce meaningful health benefits. The concept of the minimum effective dose refers to the smallest amount of exercise required to produce a desired physiological benefit. The term *exercise snacks* was first popularized by Howard Hartley in 2007 and has since been used in the scientific literature to describe brief, vigorous bouts of physical activity performed intermittently throughout the day to improve cardiometabolic health (Hartley, 2007; Islam et al., 2022).

Minimum effective dose training offers a time-efficient approach to maintaining or even improving cardiovascular fitness, muscular strength, and metabolic health. These short, targeted sessions often lasting 10 minutes or less have been shown to significantly enhance $\dot{V}O_2max$, muscular strength, blood pressure regulation, and blood glucose control when performed regularly (Islam et al., 2022).

Moreover, these brief sessions can serve as a practical strategy for encouraging exercise adoption among those struggling to maintain a regular exercise habit due to poor fitness or time constraints. A consistent commitment to short exercise sessions creates an opportunity for non-exercisers to develop a lifelong commitment to fitness that can grow over time.

Exercise snacks provide a convenient and accessible way to engage in physical activity, making them especially appealing for individuals with low fitness levels, time constraints, or inconsistent schedules. The brief, manageable nature of exercise snacks lowers the psychological and logistical barriers that often prevent people from maintaining a regular routine. As a result, they serve as a practical gateway to long-term exercise adherence, allowing non-exercisers to build confidence and consistency over time.

Numerous studies have demonstrated the effectiveness and tolerability of exercise snack interventions (Fyfe et al., 2022). Protocols as brief as one to two minutes per session have been shown to improve functional outcomes, cardiovascular performance, and muscular strength (Islam et al., 2022). A systematic review published in 2025 reported adherence rates of 92 percent or higher across both supervised and unsupervised interventions, even among participants with chronic conditions or sedentary lifestyles (Brown et al., 2025). These high adherence rates highlight the practicality of exercise snacks as a sustainable fitness strategy. Importantly, their flexibility makes them ideal for maintaining physical activity during travel or periods of schedule disruption, offering a reliable fallback to support consistent movement in everyday life.

EXERCISE SNACK PROGRAMMING

The effectiveness of exercise snacks can be attributed largely to their high intensity. These brief, vigorous bouts of physical activity can be effective at jump-starting physiological processes to stimulate protein synthesis, enhance mitochondrial health, improve blood glucose, and elevate aerobic fitness. The following exercise snack protocols have been shown through research to improve measures of functionality, muscle strength, and cardiovascular fitness.

Sprint Interval Training

Sprint interval training (SIT) is a time-efficient form of high-intensity exercise that involves brief, maximal, all-out efforts separated by longer recovery periods. Unlike traditional forms of cardiovascular exercise, SIT relies on very short bouts of supramaximal work to drive meaningful adaptation, including improvements in cardiovascular fitness, mitochondrial function, and metabolic health (Gibala et al., 2012).

Short, high-intensity cycling sprints have been demonstrated to be a highly effective method for improving cardiovascular fitness and peak cycling performance. In particular, performing three 20-second all-out sprints with three minutes of rest between efforts, three times per week, led to significant improvements in $\dot{V}O_2max$, peak power output, and time trial performance (Little et al., 2019). The appeal of this approach lies in its efficiency: It delivers measurable cardiovascular benefits with just 60 seconds of total work and 9 minutes per session, making it a practical and time-efficient training strategy. Figure 3.2 provides a visual representation of the 3 × 20-second cycling sprint interval protocol.

3 × 20-Second Sprint Interval Protocol Session Format

- 2-minute light pedaling warm-up
- 3 × 20-second all-out cycling sprints
- 3-minute passive rest between each sprint

Total session duration: 9 minutes per session

Frequency: 3 sessions per week

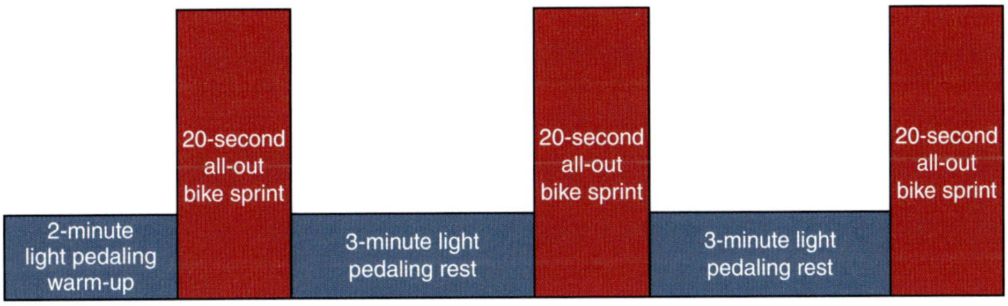

Figure 3.2 3 × 20-second sprint interval protocol.

Stair Climbing

All-out stair climbing has been shown to serve as an effective, equipment-free exercise snack strategy that enhances cardiovascular fitness and lower-body strength. The practicality and adaptability of this routine is particularly suitable for workplace settings, where time and resources may be limited.

A study published in *Applied Physiology, Nutrition, and Metabolism* demonstrated that sedentary young adults who performed three daily bouts of vigorous stair climbing (60 steps per bout) over six weeks experienced significant improvements in their $\dot{V}O_2$max and lower body power (Jenkins et al., 2019).

The specific protocol used by researchers was as follows:

Frequency: 3 times per day, 3 days per week

Duration: Each session includes climbing a 3-flight stairwell (about 60 steps) as quickly as possible, taking approximately 20 to 30 seconds.

Intensity: Sprint up the stairs as fast as possible.

Rest intervals: Allow 1 to 4 hours between each climbing session within the same day.

Bodyweight Exercise Circuit

Short, simple bodyweight routines can provide a surprisingly powerful stimulus for maintaining muscle mass, strength, and functional capacity. Even brief circuits have been shown to stimulate muscle protein synthesis and improve functional outcomes such as sit-to-stand performance (Fyfe et al., 2022; Moore et al., 2022; Brandt et al., 2024). Because these routines require no equipment and minimal time commitment, they offer a practical and accessible strategy for preserving physical function during periods of reduced activity, making them especially valuable in the fight against sarcopenia.

The following modified bodyweight exercise circuit blends elements from the protocols used in the previously referenced studies, combining the most practical and effective components into a single, streamlined approach.

Frequency: 1 time per day, 3 to 5 days per week

Duration: Alternating 30 seconds of work and 30 seconds of rest for 2-3 rounds for a total of 5-15 minutes

Intensity: Complete as many full range-of-motion repetitions as possible in the given time.

Routine (complete 2-3 rounds)

- *Bodyweight squat:* 30 seconds
- *Rest:* 30 seconds
- *Single-leg deadlift:* 15 seconds each leg
- *Rest:* 30 seconds
- *Push-up (or incline push-up):* 30 seconds

- *Rest:* 30 seconds
- *Lateral squats:* 30 seconds (alternating sides)
- *Rest:* 30 seconds
- *Calf raise:* 15 seconds each leg
- *Rest intervals:* 1 minute between rounds

RECREATIONAL PHYSICAL ACTIVITY

Engaging in recreational physical activity, such as participating in amateur sport events, is an excellent way to improve overall fitness outside of traditional gym environments. After completing their high school or collegiate athletic careers, many adults stop participating in sports such as basketball, soccer, hockey, and tennis. Instead, they often turn to formal fitness activities, such as weightlifting and running. While resistance training and structured cardiovascular exercise are essential components of a balanced workout program, participating in recreational sports can offer additional benefits that go beyond typical exercise routines.

Recreational sports provide a competitive, unstructured, and variable environment that promotes the development of cardiovascular health, power, agility, and neuromuscular coordination in ways that traditional exercise cannot replicate. Research on master's-level athletes consistently shows that they achieve elite levels of health and performance compared to their non-sport-competing peers.

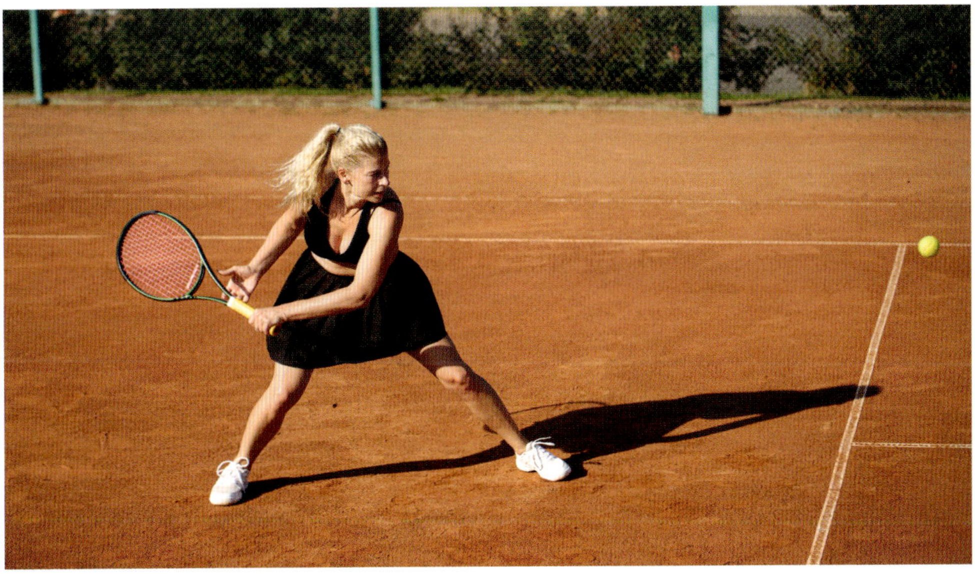

Sergey Mironov/Moment/Getty Images

Recreational sports provide a unique avenue for adults to accumulate more total physical activity in a variable, dynamic, and mentally engaging environment.

Case Study: Luis

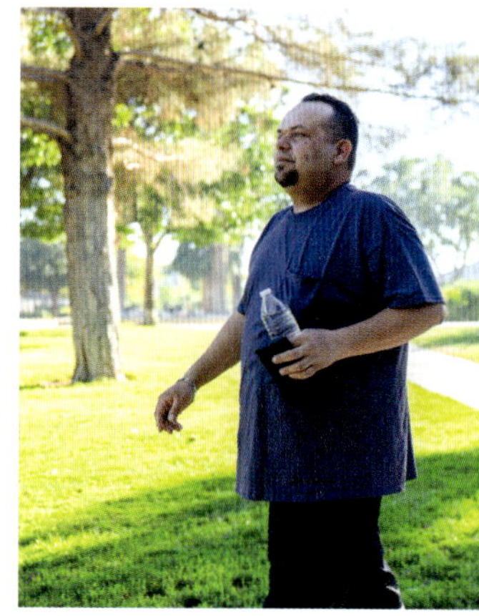
LPETTET/iStock/Getty Images

Luis is a 42-year-old man who works from home. Although he consistently participates in a two-day-per-week strength and cardiovascular training program, he still fails to meet the minimum exercise guidelines. Due to his desk-bound job, he spends most of his day sedentary, achieving less than 4,000 steps daily.

To address this, we established a gym routine and created a plan to incorporate exercise snacks and walking to increase his overall physical activity and reduce sedentary behavior. Together, we aimed to develop a realistic plan that Luis could commit to consistently, with the goal of building a lasting habit over time.

We agreed on the following activities:

- *Walking:* 30 minutes per day, which can be broken into multiple sessions or completed in one session, five days per week on days he is not going to the gym
- *Exercise snacks:* One set of 15 squats and 15 push-ups, performed three times throughout the day on days he is not at the gym
- *Stretching:* One set of stretches, including the 90/90 hip stretch, Spiderman stretch, active lumbar flexion and extension stretch, and band-assisted leg lower stretch (see chapter 4), performed once daily, seven days a week to break up his sedentary periods

After Luis established a walking habit, we gradually increased both the total duration and intensity of his walks to enhance his cardiovascular health. We also increased the amount of exercise he performed during his exercise snacks. This approach allowed us to progressively boost Luis's total physical activity over a three-year period.

At the beginning, his average daily step count, as recorded on his activity monitor, was 3,800 steps. After the first six months, we raised this average to over 5,000 steps per day. By 18 months, we had increased his daily average to over 6,400 steps, and by the end of three years, he was averaging over 8,000 steps per day. Over these three years, we successfully increased his step count by more than 100 percent.

This progress helped him approach the optimal level for reducing the risk of all-cause mortality and cardiovascular disease based on his total step count. Through this modest and gradual strategy, we effectively established lasting habits and improved his overall physical activity over time.

Furthermore, the enjoyment and social aspects of recreational sports lead to higher levels of adherence and satisfaction than structured exercise. Participation in team sports has been shown to enhance mental health and social outcomes in adults (Soundy et al., 2015; Eather et al., 2023). This improvement can be attributed largely to how involvement in sports fosters a sense of personal identity and belonging, as well as social connections with teammates. This experience differs significantly from structured resistance and cardiovascular training, which often are performed in isolation.

Everyday physical activity such as walking, standing, and simply moving more throughout the day forms the foundation of long-term health. It fills the gaps between workouts, offsets the effects of prolonged sitting, and lowers the barrier to consistent movement. But while daily activity is essential, it is not sufficient on its own.

To preserve strength, mobility, power, and cardiovascular capacity throughout the aging process, people must also engage in purposeful, well-designed exercise.

The chapters that follow shift the focus from how much we move to how we train, beginning with mobility and preparation, and progressing toward a structured approach to strength, power, and conditioning. Together, daily movement and intentional training form the complete prescription for health, function, and longevity.

Chapter 4

Mobility and Flexibility

It is no secret that our bodies tend to get stiffer as we age. When we are young, stretching is usually an afterthought, if we think about it at all. We can roll out of bed, jump into a game, or sit through a long car ride without a second thought. But as the years go by, things change. Joints get cranky. Muscles feel tighter. And loosening up before exercise starts to feel less optional and more essential.

For many people, the value of flexibility training does not become apparent until they actually need it. But flexibility and mobility work is not just for those trying to reclaim what they have lost; it is for anyone who wants to move well, feel good, and stay active at every age.

The truth is that mobility starts to decline earlier than most people realize. By the time people hit their 30s, subtle changes in connective tissue begin to take place. Tissues stiffen, elasticity decreases, and the cumulative effects of sitting more and moving less start to show up in posture and movement patterns. These changes are part biological and part behavioral, driven by both the aging process itself and the simple fact that many people stop moving the way they used to.

As stiffness increases and mobility decreases, movement patterns shift. This can lead to more stress on the joints, less efficient movement, and a general sense of discomfort that creeps in slowly but steadily. The good news is that consistent mobility and flexibility training can counteract many of these effects and prevent them from getting worse.

CONNECTIVE TISSUE HEALTH AND AGING

As we enter middle age, the natural maintenance and quality of connective tissues begin to decline, and this is further exacerbated by inactivity. With aging, the connective tissue that surrounds and supports muscles, known as the *extracellular matrix*, undergoes several changes. These include an increase in stiff collagen, a decrease in stretchy elastic fibers, and a reduction in lubricating substances that facilitate the sliding of tissues (Fede et al., 2022). Consequently, the tissue becomes less flexible and less able to adapt to stress. This stiffness hampers the smooth sliding and movement of muscles, ultimately diminishing their ability to contract and function effectively.

In addition to changes in connective tissue, joints also undergo transformations during the aging process. The joint capsules gradually thicken and become stiffer, while both the composition and volume of synovial fluid—the lubricant within joints—decrease (Marucci and Reggiani, 2020). These alterations contribute to increased stiffness and a reduced range of motion.

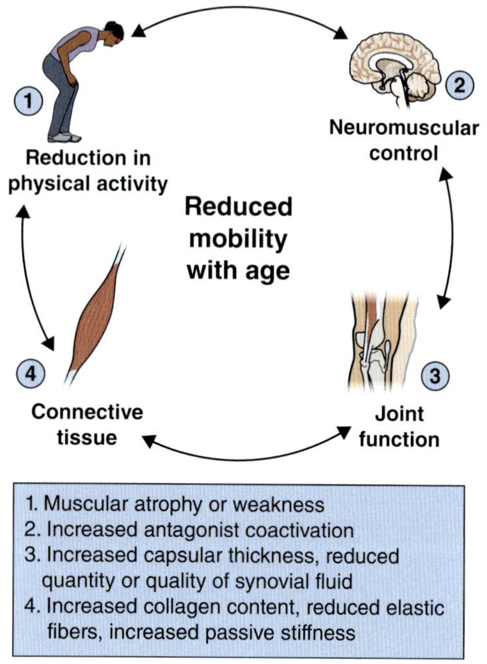

Figure 4.1 Effects of aging on mobility.

Aging also affects how the nervous system controls muscle activity, directly affecting joint mobility. Specifically, antagonist coactivation often increases, where the muscles opposing a movement (such as the hamstrings during knee extension) become excessively active (Marucci and Reggiani, 2020 ; Kubota et al., 2023). This change is a compensatory strategy employed by the nervous system to enhance joint stability in response to decreased muscle strength that accompanies aging and inactivity. However, this heightened coactivation can lead to reduced movement efficiency and a restriction in the range of motion at the joints. Over time, these changes, shown in figure 4.1, partially explain why many people experience a loss of mobility as they grow older.

MOBILITY AND DAILY LIFE

During the aging process, progressive stiffness in the joints and connective tissues can significantly reduce mobility, which in turn affects quality of life. What starts as minor tightness can eventually make basic tasks—such getting dressed, bathing, or standing up from a chair—feel difficult or even painful. These physical limitations often lead to a cycle of reduced movement, decreased independence, and declining overall fitness, all of which can shorten health span and life span.

Movement is essential for maintaining health and function. The ability to stay active largely depends on how well joints can move into the proper positions to absorb and adapt to the forces of daily life and training. When joint mobility becomes limited—whether due to inactivity, increased physical stress, or age-related changes—the connective tissues around those joints often become neurologically tense and mechanically stiff. This reduces the joint's range of motion and compromises the quality of movement. If this lack of mobility is not addressed, it can lead to joint wear and tear, connective tissue injuries, and compensatory movement patterns that place additional stress on other areas of the body. This is particularly problematic due to the principle of regional interdependence that can affect the body, which indicates that the function of one joint is closely linked to the joints above and below it. When one area loses mobility, the body often compensates by moving less efficiently elsewhere, raising the risk of injury and reinforcing poor movement habits.

Maintaining adequate mobility in all joints is crucial to ensure the body can move freely through its full range of motion without overloading the joints or surrounding tissues. In short, preserving mobility throughout aging is not just about stretching; it is about protecting independence, reducing the risk of injury, and being able to do the things you love for as long as possible. The good news is that the impact of many of the age-related changes already mentioned can be reduced and significantly mitigated by regularly stretching, staying physically active, and moving the joints through a full range of motion—whether through mobility drills or strength training with free weights.

Throughout the aging process, people need to devote more time to focused mobility work. While younger individuals may get away with doing less, as adults advance in age, they should dedicate more time—both during training and outside of the gym—to maintaining mobility in order to counteract the effects of aging on the connective tissues.

FOAM ROLLING

To help clients move and feel their best, each training session should begin with a brief foam rolling routine. This practice can help reduce resting muscle tone and sensitivity, setting the stage for more effective mobility work and higher-quality movement during training. Foam rolling has become a fundamental activity in fitness facilities over the past two decades, yet debate still persists among coaches and researchers regarding how exactly it works and how effective it truly is. While some early proponents claimed foam rolling could physically break up adhesions or release fascia, the evidence has shifted away from these structural explanations.

Current research suggests that the primary mechanisms behind foam rolling are neurological and sensory in nature. By applying mechanical pressure to soft tissues, foam rolling stimulates nerve endings in the fascia and muscle. This input appears to reduce muscle tone, decrease peripheral sensitivity, and improve tolerance to stretch, resulting in temporary increases in joint range of motion and flexibility, even after as little as one minute of rolling (Beardsley and Škarabot, 2015).

In addition to the physiological effects, psychological benefits also play a role. Foam rolling can reduce sensations of stiffness and soreness, which may help clients feel more prepared and willing to train. This subjective sense of readiness is especially important for clients who are sore, fatigued, or hesitant to push themselves.

When properly integrated, foam rolling acts as a useful primer by preparing the nervous system, improving range of motion, and creating a more comfortable and confident starting point for the work that follows, particularly stretching, dynamic warm-ups, and loaded movement.

Begin by having the client spend 5 to 10 minutes on the major muscle groups with a foam roller. Encourage slow and deliberate movement focusing on areas of muscular tightness or soreness.

Cue the client to breathe deeply and relax into the roller. This helps reduce resting muscle tone and promotes a more effective release of tension. The goal is not to smash tissues but to send calming input to the nervous system. Remind the client that discomfort is okay but that pain is not the objective.

Focus on large muscle groups that are commonly tight or sore from training, such as the quads, glutes, hamstrings, calves, and lats. Tailor the routine to the individual's needs and movement limitations. Foam rolling acts as a bridge between rest and activity, creating a neurological window of increased flexibility and a decreased sensation of tightness, allowing the client to both move more freely and feel better during the workout that follows, making its impact valuable from both a physiological and psychological perspective.

With the general principles established, the following exercises will help coaches apply foam rolling where it matters most. Each drill targets areas that are commonly affected by tightness and limit movement quality. Coaches should prioritize the regions that align with the client's restrictions and training demands, using foam rolling as a brief, purposeful reset before moving on to dynamic warm-ups and loaded work.

GLUTEUS MAXIMUS AND HIP ROTATOR MUSCLES

Benefits

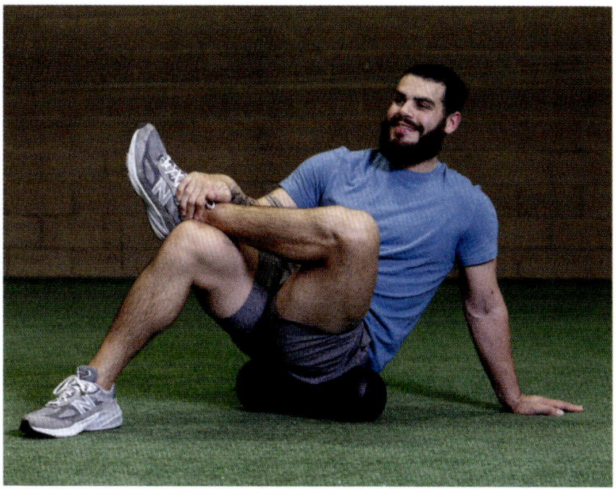

Foam rolling the glutes and deep hip rotators such as the piriformis is especially effective for clients with limited hip mobility that affects their ability to squat or hinge. Targeting the lateral and posterior hip musculature can help improve hip range of motion, alleviate muscular tension, and reduce discomfort associated with lumbar or sacral region pain.

Instructions for the Client

1. Sit on the foam roller so it is positioned horizontally beneath your glutes.
2. Cross one ankle over the opposite knee to place the target hip in slight external rotation.
3. Shift your weight toward the glute of the crossed leg to focus pressure on that side.
4. Slowly roll back and forth along the glute and lateral hip, from just below the iliac crest down toward the top of the hamstrings, circling around the head of the femur.
5. Pause and spend extra time on any tender or tight spots, maintaining steady breathing.
6. Repeat on the other side.

QUADRICEPS AND HIP FLEXORS

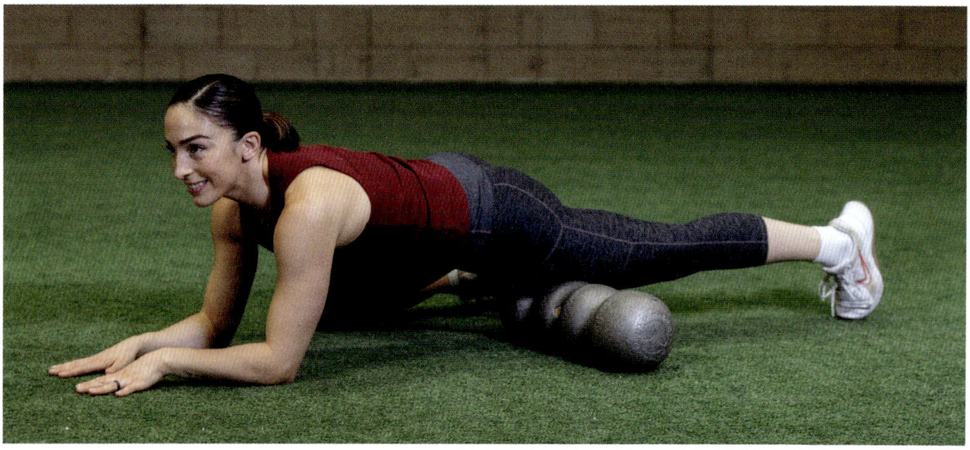

Benefits

Foam rolling the quadriceps and hip flexors can be highly effective for clients with limited hip extension or knee flexion due to tightness in the iliacus, rectus femoris, and surrounding quadriceps musculature. Targeting these areas can improve mobility at the hip and knee joints and reduce discomfort during knee-dominant exercises, such as squats and lunges.

Instructions for the Client

1. Begin by lying face down with a foam roller positioned under the front of one thigh.
2. To target the quadriceps, slowly roll up and down the front of the thigh, moving from the hip (proximal attachment) to just above the kneecap (distal attachment). Shift slightly side to side to emphasize the medial (inner) and lateral (outer) quadriceps.
3. To target the hip flexor region (particularly the iliacus and proximal rectus femoris),
    - position the roller near the front of the hip, just inside the bony ridge of the anterior iliac crest;
    - gently rock or roll in small motions, focusing pressure just below the hip bone without crossing into the abdominal area; and
    - relax your body and breathe deeply to allow the tissues to release.
4. Switch sides and repeat the same sequence on the opposite leg.

ADDUCTOR MUSCLE GROUP

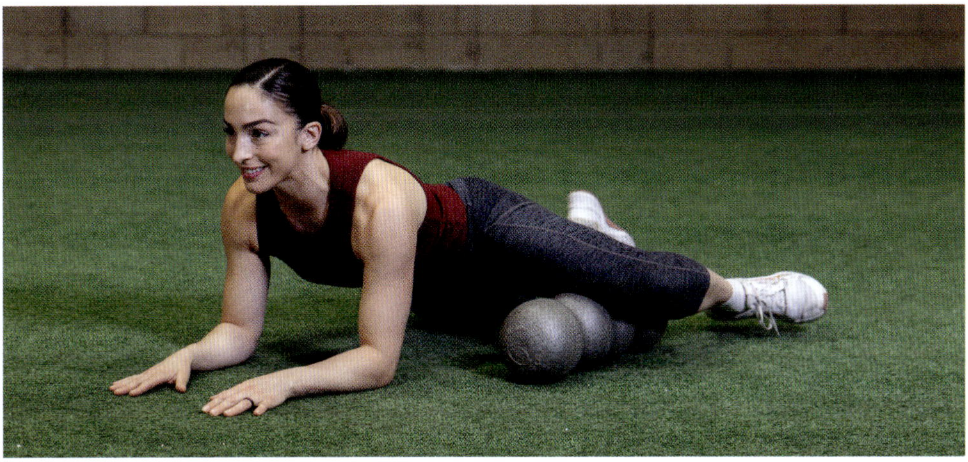

Benefits

The adductors are a commonly overlooked muscle group that plays a critical role in hip stability, mobility, and force production across all planes of motion. Because the adductor muscle group crosses both the hip and knee joints and contributes to movements like squatting, lunging, and directional change, tightness in this area can significantly restrict function. Foam rolling the adductors can improve hip mobility, alleviate groin tightness, and reduce compensatory movement patterns caused by restriction in this region.

Instructions for the Client

1. Lie face down with a foam roller placed parallel to your torso, positioned at your side.
2. Bring one leg out to the side in an abducted position, bending the knee to approximately 90 degrees, so the inner thigh rests on the roller.
3. Slowly roll along the adductor muscle group, working from just above the knee (distal attachments including the vastus medialis and pes anserine) up toward the proximal origin near the pubic bone. Shift your weight and angle to emphasize different parts of the adductors, including the posterior adductor magnus and medial thigh.
4. Maintain relaxed breathing and spend extra time on areas that feel especially tight or tender.
5. Repeat on the other side.

LUMBAR MUSCLES

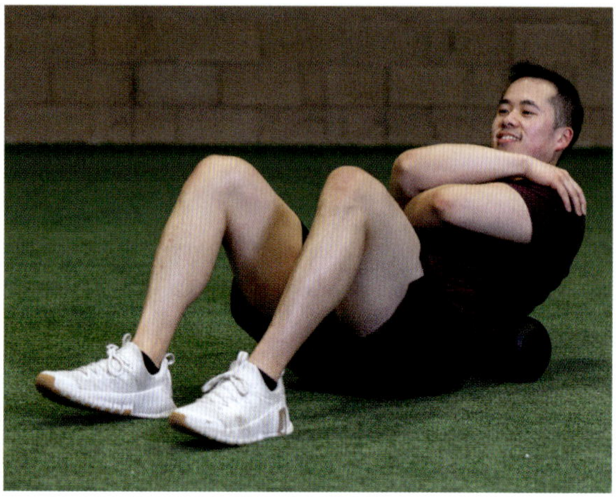

Benefits

Foam rolling the muscles of the lower back—particularly the lumbar paraspinals and quadratus lumborum (QL)—can help reduce resting muscle tone, relieve stiffness, and enhance mobility in the lumbar spine. This is especially beneficial for individuals who experience discomfort or restriction during lumbar flexion. By improving tissue tone and promoting relaxation in these regions, clients may experience better movement quality and reduced low back tension.

Instructions for the Client

1. Lie supine with knees bent and feet flat on the floor. Position the foam roller horizontally beneath your lower back, just above the sacrum.
2. Do the following to target the lumbar paraspinals:
   - Shift your weight slightly to one side so that pressure is focused along one side of the spine, avoiding rolling directly on the spine itself.
   - Slowly roll from the sacrum up toward the lower thoracic spine, focusing on the muscles that run along the spine.
   - Keep your core gently engaged and movements controlled.
   - Repeat on the opposite side.
3. Do the following to target the quadratus lumborum (QL):
   - Shift to a side-lying position with your elbow on the floor for support.
   - Position the foam roller between the top of the pelvis's iliac crest and the bottom of the rib cage, just behind the side of the torso.
   - Gently rock your body forward and backward or side to side to allow the roller to work into the QL.
   - Breathe deeply and relax into the roller to promote tissue release.
   - Repeat on the opposite side.

THORACIC SPINE

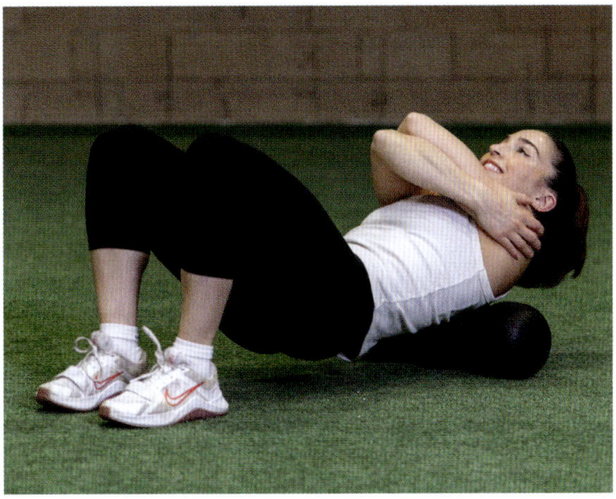

Benefits

Foam rolling the thoracic spine serves a dual purpose: It reduces excessive resting tone in the thoracic paraspinals, lower trapezius, and rhomboids while also promoting mobility of the thoracic vertebrae and vertebrocostal joints, where the ribs articulate with the spine. The downward pressure of the roller into the rib cage can help facilitate joint mobilization and improve thoracic extension, rotation, and rib excursion, which are critical for both shoulder and spinal function.

Instructions for the Client

1. Lie supine with the knees bent and the feet flat on the floor. Position the foam roller horizontally across your mid to upper back, just above the bottom of the rib cage.
2. Do the following to roll the thoracic musculature:
   - Slowly roll up and down along the thoracic portion of the spine, stopping just below the base of the neck, avoiding rolling the cervical spine.
   - When moving upward toward the shoulder blades, wrap your arms in a self-hug to move the scapulae out of the way and expose the rhomboids and lower traps.
   - Shift your body slightly side to side to explore both sides of the spine, avoiding direct pressure on the vertebrae themselves.
3. Do the following to enhance thoracic and rib joint mobility:
   - When pausing on tender or stiff areas, take deep, diaphragmatic breaths—in through the nose and out through the mouth.
   - This deep breathing, combined with the roller's pressure, helps mobilize the vertebrocostal joints and improve thoracic expansion.
   - Repeat for 30 to 60 seconds, adjusting position slightly to cover the full length of the thoracic spine.

LATS, SERRATUS ANTERIOR, AND POSTERIOR SHOULDER MUSCLES

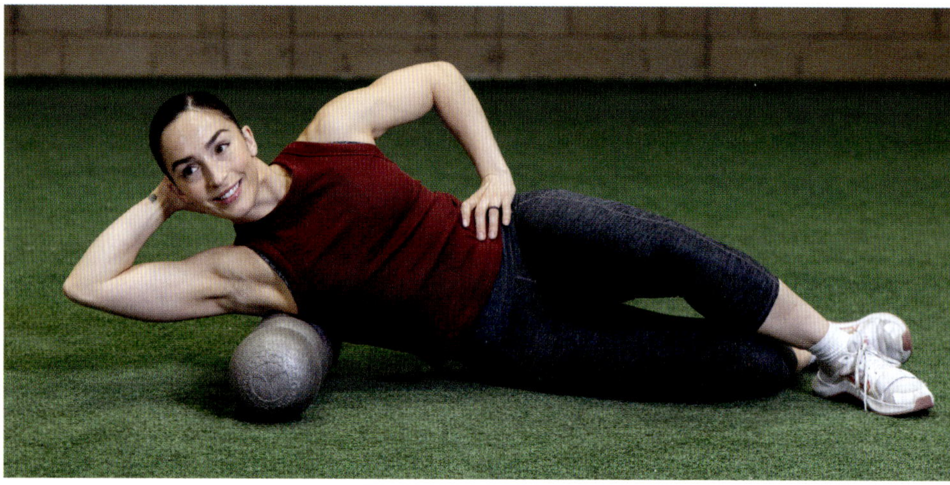

Benefits

The latissimus dorsi, serratus anterior, and posterior shoulder muscles—including the teres minor and infraspinatus—are frequently restricted in individuals with limited shoulder mobility or shoulder-related pain. These areas are especially important to address when clients struggle with movements like overhead reaching or internal rotation. Foam rolling in this region can provide noticeable relief from shoulder tension; reduce pain; and lead to significant improvements in shoulder flexion, overhead motion, and rotator cuff function.

Instructions for the Client

1. Lie on your side with the foam roller placed horizontally beneath your lateral torso, just below the armpit of your bottom arm.
2. Do the following to roll the lats and serratus anterior:
    - Begin rolling slowly from the armpit down toward the bottom of the rib cage, targeting the length of the latissimus dorsi.
    - To emphasize the serratus anterior and anterior portion of the lats, gently rotate the torso forward, allowing the foam roller to apply pressure to the outer and slightly front-facing portion of the rib cage.
    - Move slowly forward and backward over this area, keeping your breathing relaxed.

3. Do the following to roll the posterior shoulder:
   - Bend your top arm and place your hand behind your head to open the posterior shoulder area.
   - Shift the roller behind the armpit to target the posterior deltoid, teres minor, and infraspinatus.
   - Slowly roll horizontally, forward and backward, applying pressure along the back of the shoulder joint.
4. Repeat on the opposite side.

LOWER LEG MUSCLES

Benefits

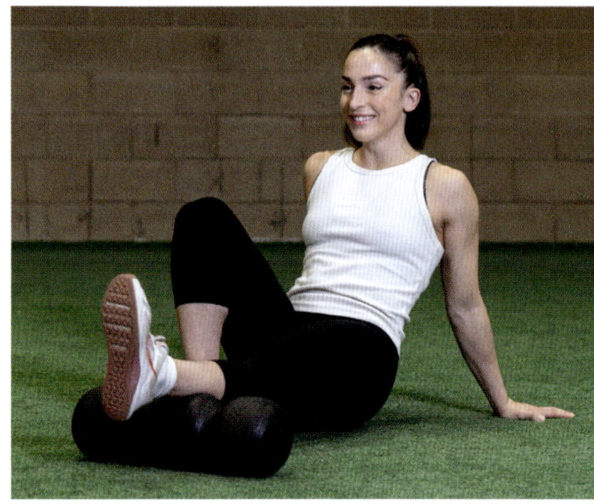

The muscles of the lower leg—including the gastrocnemius, soleus, posterior tibialis, and peroneus longus—play critical roles in ankle stability, foot control, and shock absorption during running, jumping, and daily movement. Tightness or restriction in these muscles can lead to reduced ankle mobility, compromised foot mechanics, and increased risk of pain or overuse injury. Foam rolling this region can improve ankle range of motion, reduce postactivity soreness, and enhance overall lower leg function.

Instructions for the Client

1. Sit on the ground with one leg extended and the opposite leg bent, foot flat on the floor for support. Position the foam roller horizontally beneath the calf of the extended leg, just below the knee joint.
2. Do the following to roll the calf muscles (gastrocnemius and soleus):
   - Lift your hips slightly off the ground using your hands, and slowly roll from just below the back of the knee down toward the Achilles tendon.
   - Use small, controlled movements and pause on any areas of tension or tenderness.
3. Do the following to target the posterior tibialis:
   - Internally rotate the leg so the medial side of the lower leg makes contact with the roller.
   - Apply gentle pressure along the inside of the calf, just behind the tibia, working from mid-calf to above the ankle.
4. Do the following to target the peroneus longus:
   - Externally rotate the leg to expose the lateral side of the calf.
   - Roll along the outside of the lower leg, following the line of the fibula, from just below the knee down toward the lateral ankle.
5. Repeat on the opposite leg.

STRETCHING AND ACTIVE MOBILITY WORK

Following foam rolling, clients should engage in a brief, full-body active mobility routine. Stretching before exercise plays a valuable role in preparing the body for movement. It helps reduce the sensation of tightness, increases available joint range of motion, and allows clients to move more freely and train through greater ranges—ultimately supporting better movement quality and strength development.

While stretching is often associated with preworkout preparation, it offers benefits at any time—before training, after training, or even on rest days. The simple act of accumulating time in stretched positions can contribute to improved flexibility over time. That said, active mobility work is particularly effective before a workout, offering both acute and chronic benefits.

- ***Acute benefits of stretching:*** When performed before a workout, stretching and mobility work can modulate the stretch reflex, reduce resting neurological tension in the connective tissues, and improve the sensation of mobility. This not only enhances movement quality during the workout but also can help clients feel more comfortable and confident in their bodies as they train.
- ***Chronic benefits of stretching:*** With consistent practice, active stretching can lead to long-term changes in tissue extensibility, joint mechanics, and overall movement efficiency. While the nervous system adapts quickly to mobility work, structural changes in connective tissue take more time and require repeated exposure. Over the long term, this consistency can lead to lasting improvements in flexibility and movement capacity.

In short, stretching is always valuable, but placing it at the front end of a workout provides a unique opportunity to prepare the body, enhance performance, and reinforce better movement patterns session after session.

How to Stretch

To get the most out of a stretching routine, it is important to follow a few key principles that enhance its overall effectiveness. Stretching is not just about passively holding positions; it should be looked at as an active process that requires intention, control, and time to produce meaningful improvements in mobility.

1. ***Breathe:*** Stretching can be uncomfortable, which often leads clients to unconsciously hold their breath. Encourage deep, controlled breathing—inhale through the nose, exhale through the mouth—to promote relaxation and reduce excess tension. This helps the nervous system stay calm, allowing for more effective mobility work.
2. ***Muscle activity:*** To make stretching more effective, incorporate active contractions of the muscles surrounding the target joint. This creates isometric strength and control at end ranges, enhances the neurological effects of

stretching, and builds usable strength in deep positions—ultimately reducing the risk of strain-related injuries.

3. ***Time under tension:*** For meaningful results, aim to accumulate at least one minute of total time under tension per stretch. This can be done continuously or in shorter intervals. Consistent exposure to stretch positions is key to creating lasting improvements in mobility.

A Note on Stretching Discomfort

One of the most important things for clients to understand is that effective stretching should be slightly uncomfortable but never painful. A good stretch produces what I would refer to as "pleasurable discomfort"—an intense, manageable sensation through the target tissue. It should feel like a sustained force through the muscle or connective tissue without sharpness, pinching, or pain.

This discomfort is necessary to generate enough mechanical force to influence the connective tissues and nervous system, both of which play a key role in improving mobility. However, it is critical to distinguish between productive discomfort and harmful pain.

A key guideline for safe and effective stretching is to pay attention to where the stretch is felt; discomfort should be felt on the open, or obtuse, angle of the joint. This typically indicates tension through the intended muscle or connective tissue. For example, in a 90/90 hip stretch targeting external rotation, the stretch should be felt in the glute or deep hip rotators of the front (bottom) leg, as shown in figure 4.2.

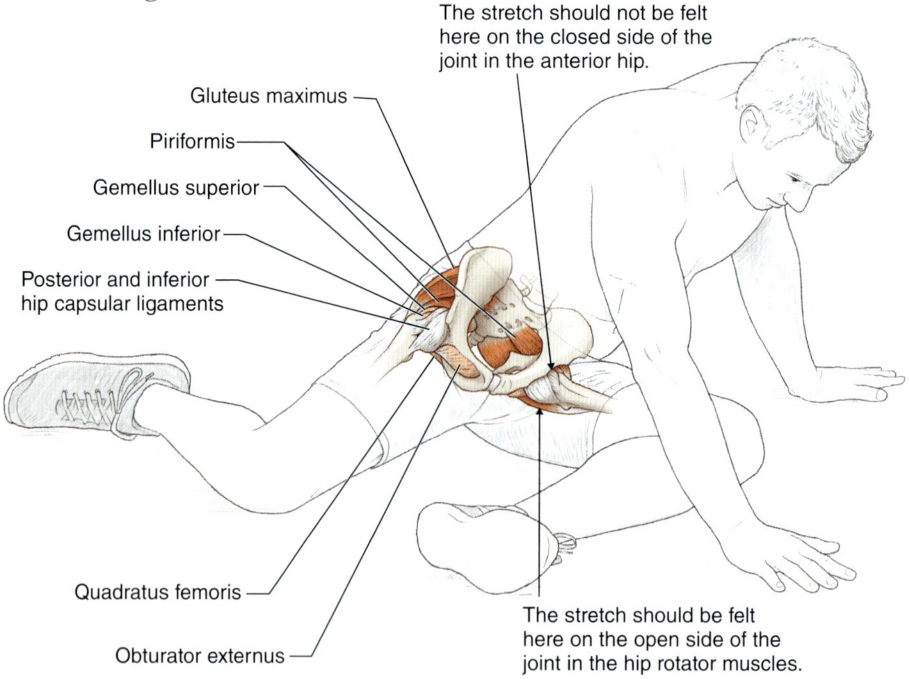

Figure 4.2 During the 90/90 hip external rotation stretch, the client should experience the stretch sensation on the open side of the joint in the hip rotator muscles.

The client should not feel discomfort on the closing, or acute, angle of the joint. Sensations such as pinching, sharpness, or tightness on the compressed side often suggest joint impingement, not a muscle stretch. This means force is being directed into the joint capsule or bony structures—something that should be avoided.

The simple question "Where do you feel this?" can make or break a stretching session. If a client reports feeling the stretch in the wrong place, modify the position, adjust the alignment, or choose a different exercise to ensure the stretch is both effective and safe.

ACTIVE MOBILITY DRILLS

The following active mobility drills can be performed at the beginning of a workout following foam rolling, as recovery after a workout, or on off days to aid in recovery from exercise.

Mobility of the hip joint and the flexibility of the surrounding musculature are essential for pain-free, unrestricted movement in daily life. The abilities to squat, bend forward, move laterally, or perform dynamic athletic tasks all depend on the hips' capacity to flex, extend, abduct, and rotate through a full, functional range of motion.

However, prolonged sitting and sedentary lifestyles often contribute to a loss of hip mobility over time. As these restrictions accumulate, they can lead to discomfort and limitations during activities of daily living. Regular mobility training helps restore range of motion, improve joint health, and enhance overall movement quality.

90/90 HIP STRETCH (HIP EXTERNAL AND INTERNAL ROTATION)

Benefits

The 90/90 hip stretch is a powerful tool for improving hip rotation range of motion on both sides of the joint—external rotation in the front leg and internal rotation in the back leg. This position allows clients to train both simultaneously, making it a staple in any hip mobility routine.

Instructions for the Client

1. Sit on the ground with both hips, knees, and ankles positioned at 90-degree angles, with one leg in front in external rotation and one leg behind in internal rotation.
2. Do the following to perform external rotation focus (front leg):
   - Starting in the 90/90 position, place hands on the floor on either side of your front leg for support.
   - Actively contract the glute on the front leg and press the leg down into the floor.
   - Keeping a tall spine, use your hip flexors to gently pull your torso forward over the front leg.
   - Hold for 60 seconds while breathing deeply, then switch sides.

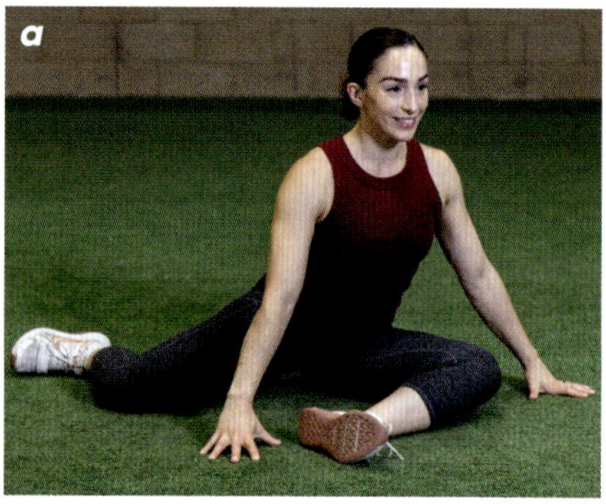

3. Do the following to perform internal rotation focus (rear leg):
   - Begin in the same 90/90 position with the front leg in external rotation and the rear leg in internal rotation.
   - Sit up tall and position your hands on either side of your hips for support.
   - Actively press both legs into the floor to engage the surrounding musculature.
   - Slowly rotate your torso toward the rear leg, focusing on feeling a stretch through the musculature of the lateral hip.
   - Hold for 60 seconds, then switch sides.

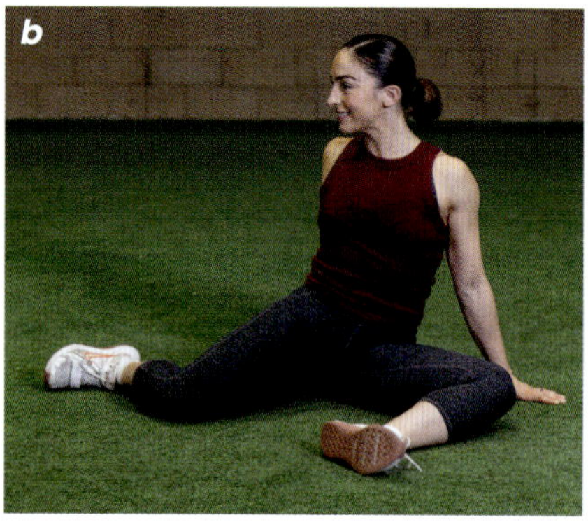

SPIDERMAN STRETCH (HIP FLEXION AND HIP EXTENSION)

Benefits

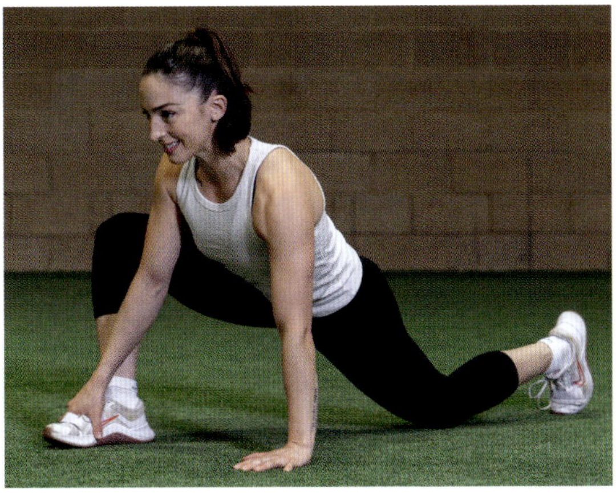

The Spiderman stretch is a highly effective mobility exercise that targets both hips simultaneously, improving hip flexion in the front leg and hip extension in the rear leg. This is especially valuable for clients who spend much of their day sitting, which often leads to tight hip flexors and reduced hip extension mobility.

Instructions for the Client

1. Start in a high plank position, with your hands under your shoulders and your body in a straight line from head to heels.
2. Step your right foot forward, placing it just outside your right hand. Lower your left knee to the floor. Place your right hand on your right foot.
3. Drive your right elbow toward the inside of your right knee while simultaneously pressing the knee back into the elbow to create an isometric contraction by engaging your adductors.
4. Press your rear hip down toward the floor, actively engaging the glute on the back leg to move the hip into extension.
5. Maintain deep, relaxed breathing while holding the stretch for 60 seconds.
6. Return to the starting position and repeat on the opposite side.

ADDUCTOR ROCKING STRETCH (HIP ABDUCTION)

Benefits

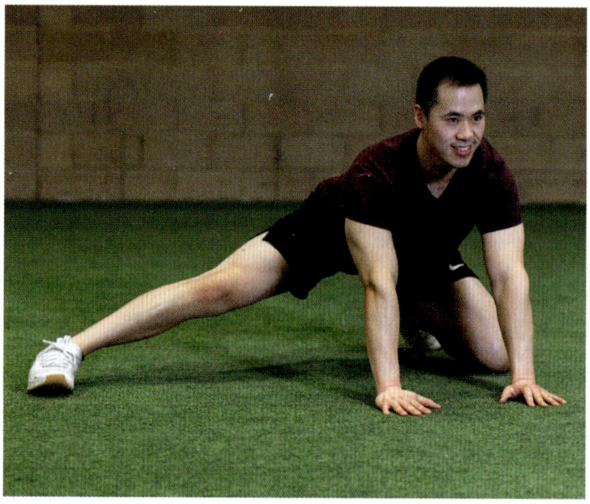

Straight-leg adductor rocking helps improve tissue extensibility into hip abduction—a range of motion often limited by prolonged sitting and a lack of lateral movement in daily life. Restoring mobility in this area can reduce inner thigh and groin tightness while improving the ability to move sideways during everyday tasks such as playing recreational sports, getting up off the floor, or stepping over obstacles.

Instructions for the Client

1. Start in an all-fours position, with both knees on the floor and your hands placed directly under your shoulders.
2. Extend your right leg out to the side, keeping the knee straight and the foot flat on the ground.
3. Maintain a neutral spine and begin to rock your hips backward, as if sitting toward the heel. A stretch should be felt along the inner thigh of the extended leg.
4. Throughout the stretch, actively press your foot into the ground to engage the adductors and create an isometric contraction while maintaining the stretch.
5. Rock forward to return to the start position and repeat for the prescribed repetitions, then switch sides.

WALL QUAD STRETCH (KNEE FLEXION AND HIP EXTENSION)

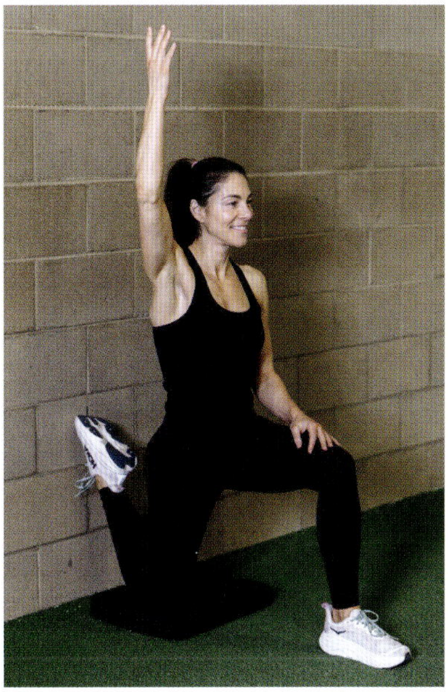

Benefits

Limited flexibility in the quadriceps can restrict knee flexion and contribute to chronic knee discomfort, particularly during daily activities such as walking, kneeling, or climbing stairs. This stretch helps restore tissue extensibility in the quadriceps and hip flexors, which in turn can improve motion and reduce excess pressure at the knee joint.

Instructions for the Client

1. Begin in a half-kneeling position with your back facing a wall.
2. Wedge your right knee up against the base of the wall, with your shin vertical and your foot resting flat against the wall to the rear. Use a pad or mat under your knee for comfort if needed.
3. Step your left leg forward so the knee is bent at 90 degrees and the foot is flat on the floor in front.
4. Sit up tall, extending through your hips and spine to create a straight line from your back knee up to your head. Reach the arm on the same side as your back leg overhead to further encourage full-body extension.
5. Tuck your pelvis slightly into a posterior tilt and engage your abdominal muscles.
6. While holding the stretch, focus on diaphragmatic breathing—inhaling through the nose and exhaling fully through the mouth.
7. Hold for 60 seconds, then switch sides.

WIDE SPLIT THORACIC ROTATION (THORACIC ROTATION AND EXTENSION)

Benefits

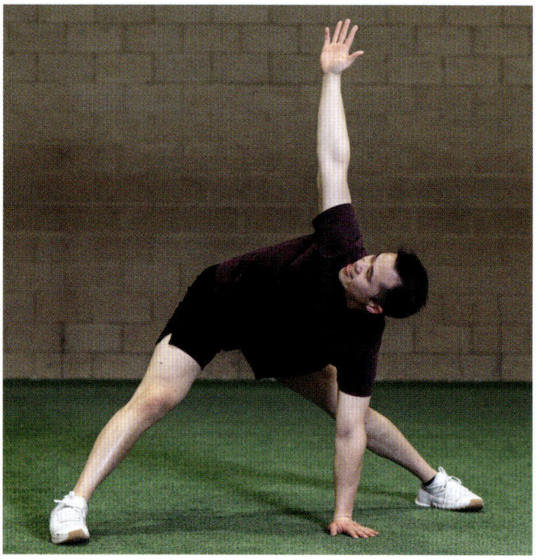

The ability to rotate and extend through the thoracic spine is essential for efficient overhead and rotational movement patterns, whether reaching, lifting, or twisting. Prolonged sitting, such as working at a desk, can lead to stiffness in the thoracic spine, reducing shoulder mobility and causing compensatory motion through the lower back. Thoracic mobility drills like this one help counteract this stiffness, restore upper back movement, and prepare the body for shoulder and rotation-focused exercises.

Instructions for the Client

1. Stand in a wide stance with your feet flat on the floor and knees straight.
2. Hinge forward at the hips, pushing your hips back and placing both palms flat on the floor beneath your shoulders.
3. Rotate your torso to the right, looking over your right shoulder while reaching your right arm toward the ceiling. At the same time, press your left hand firmly into the floor to create stability and enhance the rotation.
4. Return to center and repeat on the left side, alternating back and forth.
5. Perform for the prescribed number of controlled repetitions on each side.

SHOULDER ARTICULAR ROTATIONS (SHOULDER CIRCUMDUCTION)

Benefits

Shoulder articular rotations help develop strength and control at end range through full shoulder circumduction. They can be performed with a flexion bias (moving forward and overhead) or an extension bias (moving backward behind the body), depending on the target range of motion. Practicing these regularly supports the health of the shoulder capsule and helps maintain active mobility critical for reaching, lifting, and moving the arm freely in all directions.

Instructions for the Client

Flexion-Focused Rotation

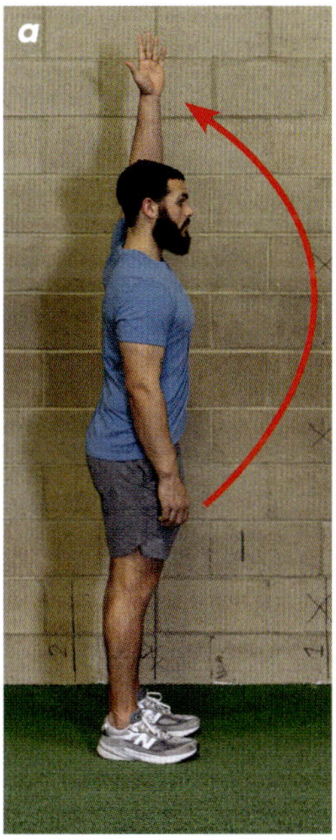

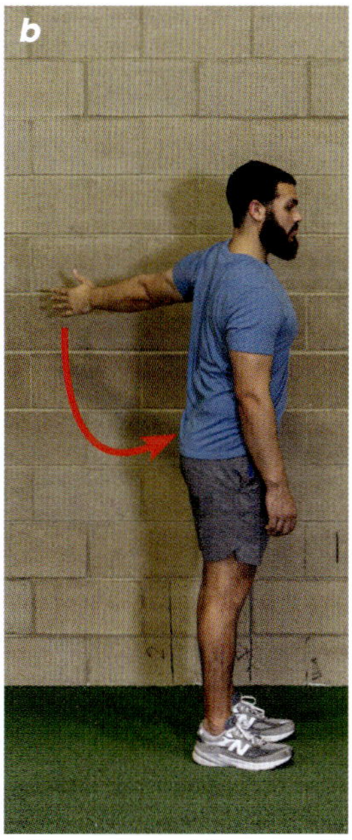

1. Stand about 1 foot (30 cm) in front of a wall, with the side of your shoulder facing the wall.
2. With your arm fully straight, supinated (palm forward), and externally rotated, slowly begin to flex the shoulder, lifting your arm in front and overhead as far as possible without arching your back or rotating your torso.
3. At your overhead end range, begin to internally rotate and pronate the arm, turning the palm backward, and continue the motion in a circular arc behind your body, finishing with the arm down by your side.
4. Perform 5 slow, controlled repetitions, maintaining muscular tension and staying tall through your spine. Then switch sides.

SHOULDER ARTICULAR ROTATIONS (SHOULDER CIRCUMDUCTION) *(continued)*

Extension-Focused Rotation

1. Start with your arm straight and positioned at your side, fully internally rotated and pronated (palm facing behind the body or toward the body).
2. Begin to extend your shoulder, slowly reaching your arm behind your body as far as possible without leaning forward or rotating your chest.
3. At full extension, externally rotate and supinate the arm (turn the palm forward), and continue the arc up and overhead, returning to the start position in reverse.
4. Maintain full-body tension and avoid any compensatory motion through the spine or ribs.
5. Perform 5 controlled repetitions, then switch sides.

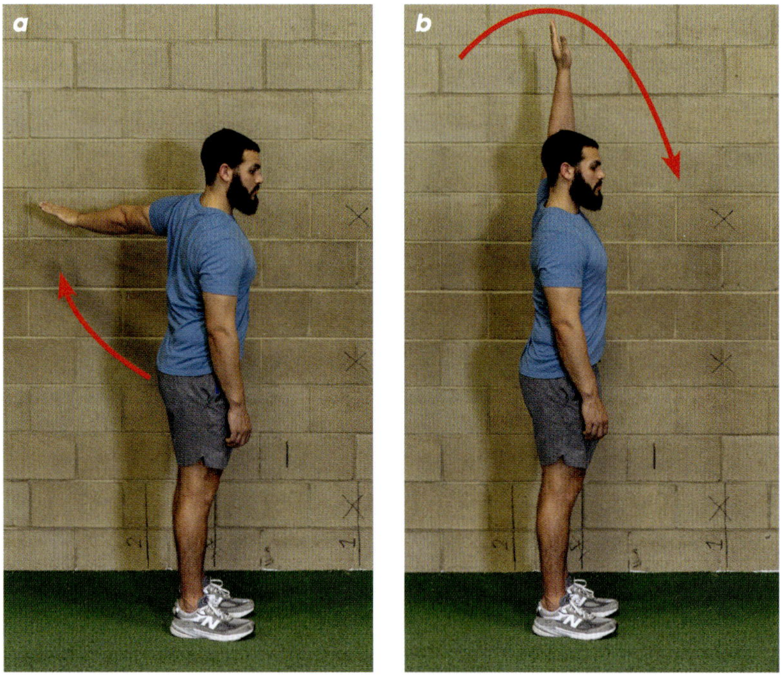

WALL ANKLE MOBILITY (ANKLE DORSIFLEXION)

Benefits

Adequate ankle dorsiflexion is essential not only for athletes—who rely on it for sprinting, cutting, and decelerating—but also for anyone performing day-to-day activities such as walking, squatting, or climbing stairs. Limited mobility at the ankle can disrupt lower body mechanics and lead to compensations at the knee, hip, or lower back. Over time, this may contribute to issues like Achilles tendon irritation, plantar fascia strain, or chronic joint stiffness.

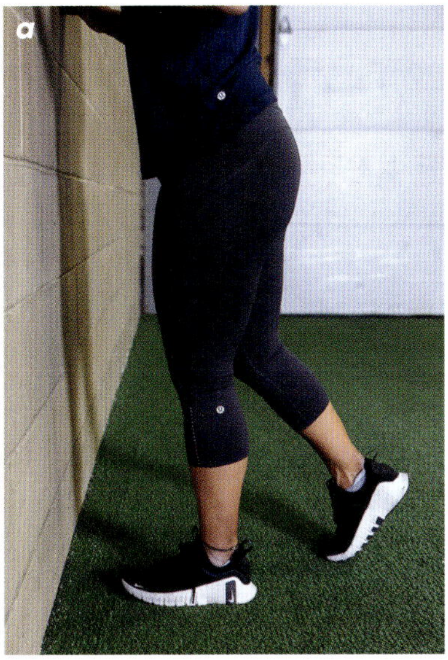

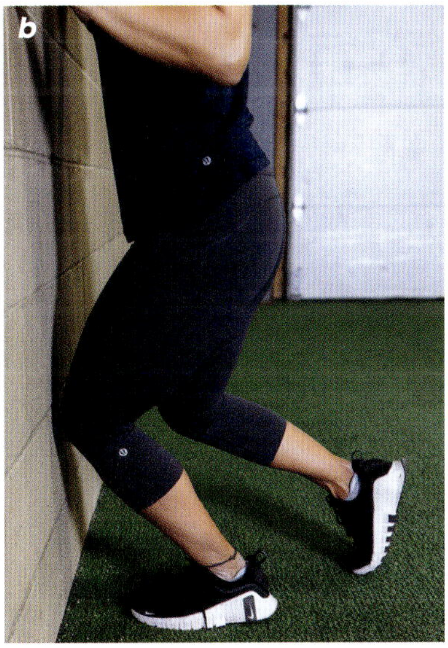

Instructions for the Client

1. Stand about 1 foot (30 cm) in front of a wall, with your palms pressed firmly against the wall for support.
2. Step one foot back with a staggered stance, placing about 90 percent of body weight on the front leg.
3. Drive your front knee forward, aiming to move it over the middle of the foot and past the toes without lifting your heel.
4. At end range, actively pull the front foot into dorsiflexion by contracting the anterior tibialis muscle on the front of the shin.
5. Hold for 5 to 10 seconds, then return to the start and repeat for the prescribed number of repetitions.
6. Switch legs and repeat on the opposite side.

ACTIVE CERVICAL ROTATIONS (CERVICAL MOBILITY)

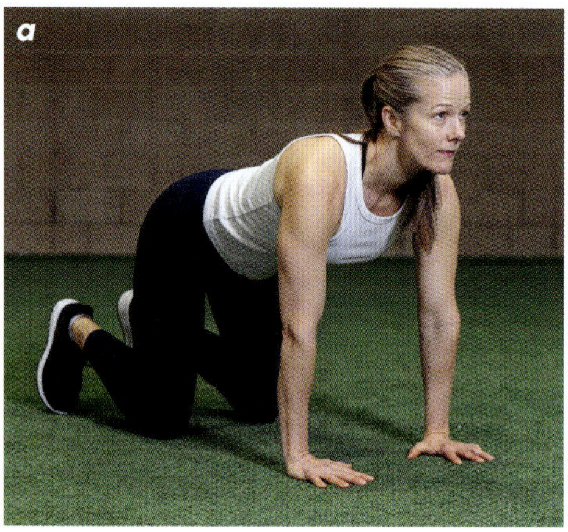

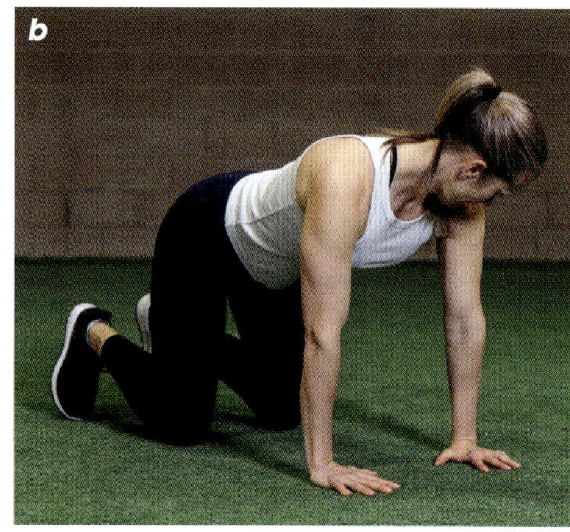

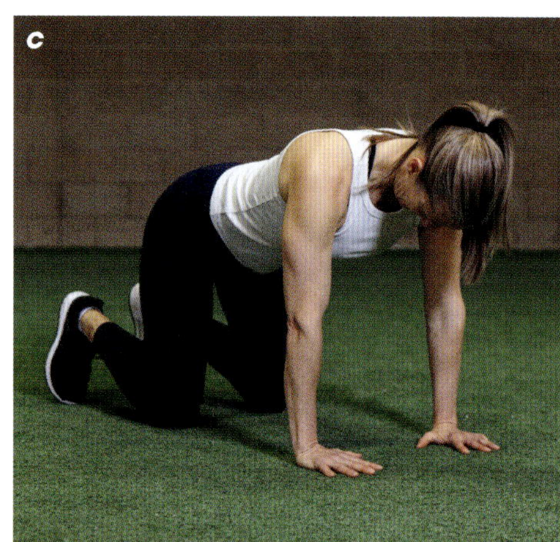

Benefits

Cervical spine stiffness is a common issue, especially for individuals who spend long hours sitting with a forward head posture. Over time, this restriction can contribute to neck pain, headaches, and difficulty with upper body movement or training. Active cervical rotations help restore mobility and motor control in the neck by encouraging smooth, controlled motion through the entire range. Practicing this drill regularly can help reduce tension, improve posture, and support more efficient upper body mechanics.

Instructions for the Client

1. Begin in an all-fours position, with your hands under your shoulders and knees under your hips.
2. Brace your upper back and shoulder muscles to create a stable base and limit compensation through the torso.
3. Start by extending your neck, slowly looking up toward the ceiling.
4. Begin a controlled circular motion by turning your head to one side and bringing your chin toward your shoulder, then down across your collarbone toward your chest.
5. Continue rotating until your chin reaches the opposite shoulder, then lift your head back into extension to complete the circle.
6. Maintain active muscular engagement in the neck throughout the motion; this is not passive movement.
7. Complete the prescribed number of slow, controlled repetitions, then repeat in the opposite direction.

ACTIVE LUMBAR FLEXION AND EXTENSION (LUMBAR MOBILITY)

Benefits

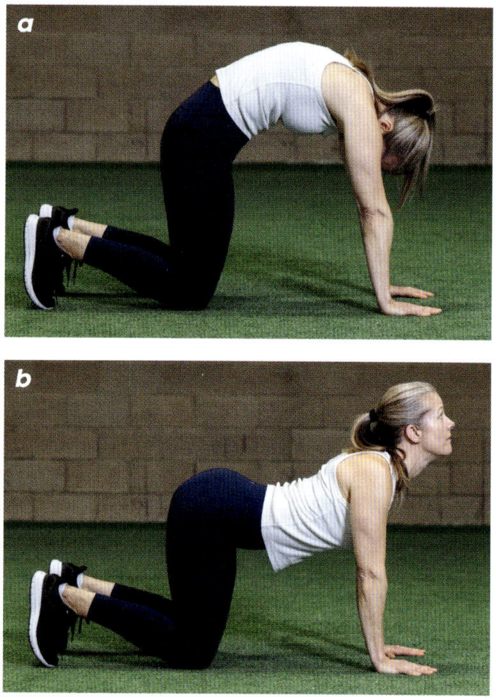

Limited mobility and poor motor control through the lumbar spine are common, particularly in individuals who spend long periods sitting or who avoid spinal movement due to fear of pain or stiffness. Over time, this lack of motion can contribute to reduced spinal awareness, increased rigidity, and compensatory movement strategies during daily activities and training.

Active lumbar flexion and extension help restore segmental movement, improve spinal awareness, and reintroduce controlled motion through the lumbar spine. By actively moving through flexion and extension, this drill encourages coordination between the pelvis and spine while gently loading spinal tissues in a safe, controlled manner.

Instructions for the Client

1. Begin in an all-fours position, with your hands under your shoulders and knees under your hips.
2. The spine is in a neutral position, with your head in line with your torso.
3. Initiate the movement by slowly rounding your lower back, tucking your pelvis under while flexing through the lumbar spine up toward the ceiling. Allow your head and upper back to follow naturally.
4. Pause briefly at the end of the flexed position, maintaining active control rather than relaxing into the stretch.
5. Reverse the motion by anteriorly tilting the pelvis and gently extending through the lumbar spine, allowing the chest to open and the head to lift.
6. Move slowly and deliberately between flexion and extension, focusing on smooth, controlled motion through the spine.
7. Breathe naturally throughout the drill and avoid forcing the range of motion.
8. Complete the prescribed number of repetitions.

Case Study: Stephen

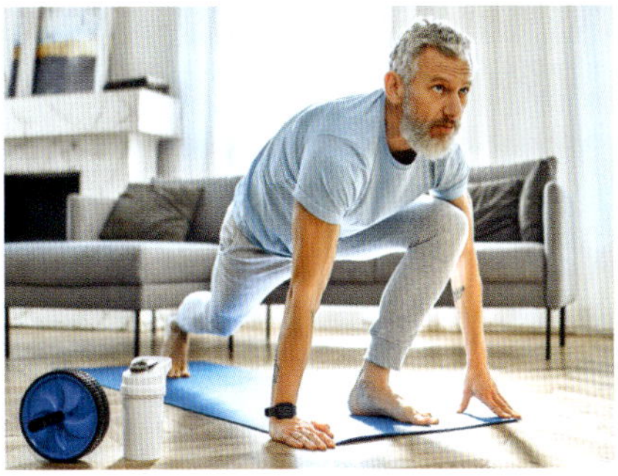
Valerii Apetroaiei/iStock/Getty Images

Stephen is a 56-year-old man who works a desk-based job and spends most of his day seated at a computer and on phone calls. He consistently participates in strength training two to three days per week and enjoys playing tennis and golf recreationally in his free time.

Over the past several years, Stephen began to notice increasing stiffness and soreness, particularly during and after exercise and recreational activities. He often struggled to loosen up during training sessions and frequently experienced discomfort in the days following more intense workouts. Due to his busy schedule, he routinely skipped any form of mobility work, often jumping directly into strength training without foam rolling or stretching. Outside of the gym, he performed no structured movement or mobility work.

When we began working together, our primary goal was to improve Stephen's movement quality and reduce postexercise stiffness without significantly increasing his total training time. To accomplish this, we designed a three-day-per-week strength training program that included a brief, targeted mobility sequence prior to each session. In addition, we created a simple at-home mobility routine for his non-training days to improve range of motion in the hips, thoracic spine, and shoulders, which are key areas for both golf and tennis.

Stephen's pretraining and off-day mobility routine included the following:

- *Full-body foam rolling:* 5 minutes
- *90/90 hip stretch:* 1 minute per side
- *Spiderman stretch:* 1 minute per side
- *Wide-split thoracic rotation:* 10 reps per side
- *Shoulder articular rotations:* 10 reps in each direction
- *Active lumbar flexion and extension:* 10 reps

(continued)

Case Study: Stephen *(continued)*

After consistently performing mobility work before training sessions and on his days outside of the gym, Stephen reported noticeable improvements in both his range of motion and overall comfort. He experienced improved rotational ability during his golf swing, felt looser during strength training sessions, and reported significantly less stiffness and soreness following exercise.

By integrating brief, consistent mobility work into his existing routine, we were able to improve how Stephen moved, trained, and recovered while supporting his long-term participation in both exercise and recreational sport.

Improving and maintaining joint mobility and tissue flexibility is foundational to staying pain-free and active during the aging process, but flexibility alone does not make people resilient. Range of motion only matters if it can be controlled and expressed dynamically in daily life and in training. This is where the active warm-up becomes essential. Dynamic, multidirectional movement serves as a bridge between restoring movement and expressing strength and power, preparing tissues while reinforcing coordination and motor control. The chapter that follows outlines a comprehensive, progressive warm-up strategy designed to prepare the body for higher-intensity work and support long-term performance.

Chapter 5

The Warm-Up

Warming up the body before exercise is often the section of the workout that many people choose to skip in favor of saving time, believing that there is little to no value to be gained from movements that are not loaded heavily or performed at high intensity. However, in addition to creating the physiological conditions for a safer and more effective environment for exercise, the warm-up also can serve as an opportunity for assessment, motor learning, and overall physical development.

The warm-up allows clients to begin priming their bodies for the demands of exercise, helping to put them in a better internal environment both psychologically and physiologically. For the coach, the warm-up can allow an opportunity for daily assessment and observation, helping to shape future sessions based on visual and subjective feedback from clients.

THE IMPORTANCE AND PURPOSE OF A WARM-UP

Participating in an adequate warm-up period is essential to ensuring a training session that is both safe and optimally physiologically effective. Clients and trainers alike often cite time availability as the primary reason for skipping a warm-up, but this concern is often misguided and short sighted. Much value is to be gained from participating in a brief warm-up before engaging in intense exercise, so much so that it should not be seen as an accessory to exercise but a part of the complete exercise plan.

A well-rounded and complete active warm-up should not require more than 10 minutes of time while conferring many benefits that will affect not only the current training session but will help to enhance the overall physiological and cognitive development of the individual.

Increasing Body Temperature and Priming the Central Nervous System

The primary goal of a warm-up is to elevate both internal and external body temperature, creating a physiological environment better suited for exercise. As body temperature rises, a series of internal and external adaptations is triggered that helps the body transition from rest to movement. A well-structured warm-up not only enhances performance but also reduces injury risk, making it a vital component of any training session.

Internally, a rise in core temperature enhances enzyme activity and accelerates energy-producing reactions. This makes metabolic processes more efficient, particularly those involved in aerobic energy production. Simultaneously, the heart rate increases and blood vessels dilate, improving circulation and delivering more oxygen and nutrients (e.g., glucose and fatty acids) to working muscles (Bishop, 2003).

Peripherally, increased tissue temperature improves flexibility, joint mobility, and soft tissue extensibility. This reduces the sensation of stiffness and lowers resistance to movement, allowing clients to move more freely and with less risk of injury (Bishop, 2003).

Neurologically, warm-ups elevate central nervous system activity, increasing its excitability. This heightened neural readiness enhances muscle recruitment, coordination, and the speed and force of muscular contractions, ultimately setting the stage for more effective, powerful training.

It is common for fitness professionals to begin a session by having clients walk on a treadmill or pedal a stationary bike for a few minutes. While this type of warm-up does increase body temperature and blood flow, it falls short of preparing the body and brain for the demands of a full training session. This classic approach lacks the movement variability, coordination challenges, and sensory stimulation needed to truly prepare clients for dynamic activity. A well-designed warm-up should do more than just elevate heart rate; it should provide a neurologically enriching environment that sharpens motor control, reinforces movement patterns, and stimulates the nervous system.

When implemented thoughtfully, the warm-up becomes a powerful opportunity to improve movement quality, build physical literacy, and enhance readiness—not just physically but cognitively as well. In the following section, we will explore how incorporating multidirectional movement, pattern practice, and cross-body coordination can transform the warm-up into one of the most valuable components of a training session.

Developing, Maintaining and Rediscovering Movement Skills

One of the most overlooked aspects of the warm-up is its value in improving skill acquisition and motor development. For many clients, especially beginners, the warm-up provides a daily opportunity to practice and refine foundational movement patterns in a low-load, low-stress environment.

Because the intensity is low and injury risk is minimal, the warm-up is an ideal setting for movement exploration, coordination work, and building neuromuscular control. Coaches should view this time not just as a physiological ramp-up but as a chance to groove essential patterns such as squatting, hinging, lunging, and pushing using body weight or lightly loaded drills performed with precision and intent. It also serves as a daily assessment tool, giving coaches a chance to visually evaluate how a client is moving, identify any compensations, and adjust the day's plan accordingly. At the same time, it gives clients space to check in with their own bodies and gauge how they are feeling physically and mentally before training begins.

This approach helps reinforce movement quality, improve mobility, and lay the foundation for future loading or higher-speed training. Think of it as daily movement hygiene: Clients warm up their joints through full ranges of motion while rehearsing patterns they will use later in the session. Over time, these drills can be progressed by adding load, increasing speed, introducing deceleration, or incorporating different planes of motion.

In addition to reinforcing foundational patterns, the warm-up is also the perfect time to reintroduce multiplanar movement skills, especially for adults who may have lost them over time. As people age, their movement variety tends to shrink. People not only move less, but they move in fewer ways, typically in the same sagittal plane over and over again. Over time, this lack of variability contributes to decreased proprioception, stiffer joints, and reduced neuromuscular control across all planes of motion. The result is a body that is less adaptable, less resilient, and more prone to injury in unpredictable environments. Think about the way children move: They skip, hop, crawl, roll, and change direction fluidly without hesitation. Fast forward a few decades, and many adults struggle to skip or shuffle, not due to injury but simply because they have stopped practicing those movements.

The warm-up offers a unique, low-risk opportunity to reintroduce these skills. Drills such as skipping, shuffling, backpedaling, crawling, and ladder patterns help reawaken proprioception and recondition the nervous system to control the body in multiple directions. They also increase body temperature, improve coordination, and prepare clients for more dynamic activity, making them a perfect addition to any warm-up.

While heavy or loaded multiplanar exercises may not always be appropriate, using the warm-up to restore basic movement variability can help adults build a more resilient, athletic body—one that is better equipped to handle the dynamic nature of both sport and life.

Using Movement to Stay Sharp: The Connection Between Brain and Body

Beyond the physical benefits, reintroducing multiplanar movement during the warm-up also offers powerful cognitive rewards. Movements that involve coordination across the midline, such as skipping, crawling, and ladder drills, do not just challenge the body; they challenge the brain.

These types of dynamic, cross-body movements require contralateral coordination, where opposite limbs must work together in rhythm. This stimulates the corpus callosum, the bundle of nerve fibers that connects the left and right hemispheres of the brain. Strengthening this connection can enhance communication between both sides of the brain, which is critical for coordination, balance, and complex motor learning.

Research also suggests that coordinated muscular activity, especially novel or cognitively demanding movement, can promote the release of neurotrophic factors such as dopamine and brain-derived neurotrophic factor (BDNF). These chemicals support the growth of new neurons, strengthen existing neural connections, and improve overall brain plasticity (Hannaford, 2005).

In other words, a warm-up that includes multiplanar and cross-body movement does not just prepare clients physically; it helps keep their brains sharp. Consistently challenging the nervous system with coordinated, full body actions can support both physical resilience and long-term cognitive health.

STRUCTURING A WARM-UP

The warm-up period should occur after completing mobility exercises such as foam rolling and stretching, as explained in chapter 4, and before higher intensity activities such as power training, strength training, and cardiovascular work. The intensity of the exercise program should ramp up from low-intensity activities to high-intensity activities that progressively increase the metabolic and neurological demand of the workout.

When designing the warm-up it is recommended to progressively move from isolated movements that focus on single-joint motions to integrated movements that incorporate full body, multijoint movements. Similarly, it is recommended to progress the warm-up from static to dynamic activities, moving from in-place activities toward more dynamic multiplanar movements. Following this natural progression allows clients to warm up the body progressively by first warming up the joint in isolation and then integrating into full body dynamic movements. Figure 5.1 demonstrates how to progressively ramp up the activities used in the warm-up for optimal effectiveness.

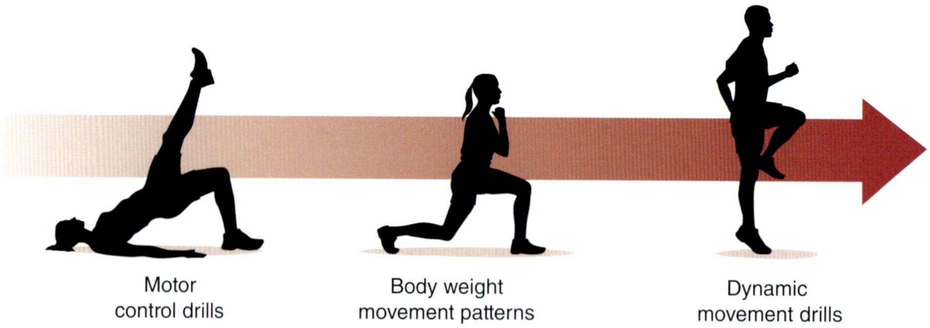

Figure 5.1 A recommended warm-up progression moves from isolated, single-joint movements and advances toward dynamic, full body patterns as intensity and complexity increase.

MOTOR CONTROL DRILLS

Movement preparation drills serve as a bridge between mobility work and the more demanding strength and power exercises in a training session. Their primary goal is to teach clients how to move the right joints, with the right muscles, at the right time, establishing efficient movement patterns under low-load, low-speed conditions before progressing to more intense work.

These drills enhance motor control, which is the neuromuscular ability to coordinate and sequence movement effectively. Movement preparatory drills provide the opportunity to groove these patterns with intention and control, reinforcing proper joint alignment and muscle activation in a safe, low-stress environment following mobility work.

Many athletes exhibit compensatory movement strategies, such as using lumbar extension to make up for poor hip mobility or core stability, that not only reduce performance but also increase the risk of overuse injuries and joint dysfunction. By retraining movement patterns early in the session, athletes can gradually replace inefficient habits with more effective ones, reducing the likelihood of injury and improving long-term durability.

For the best results, movement preparation drills should be strategically selected to mirror the movement patterns and joint actions used in the upcoming strength and power work. When low-threshold drills are meaningfully connected to high-threshold outputs, they set the stage for more efficient, safer, and more effective performance under load and speed. As clients develop proficiency with these isolated drills and demonstrate improved control and coordination, they often reach a point of diminishing returns. At that stage, it becomes more effective to transition toward integrated, full body movement patterns that better reflect the demands of the training session. These dynamic drills not only continue to reinforce quality movement but also offer greater specificity and a more comprehensive warm-up effect.

BILATERAL HIP LIFT

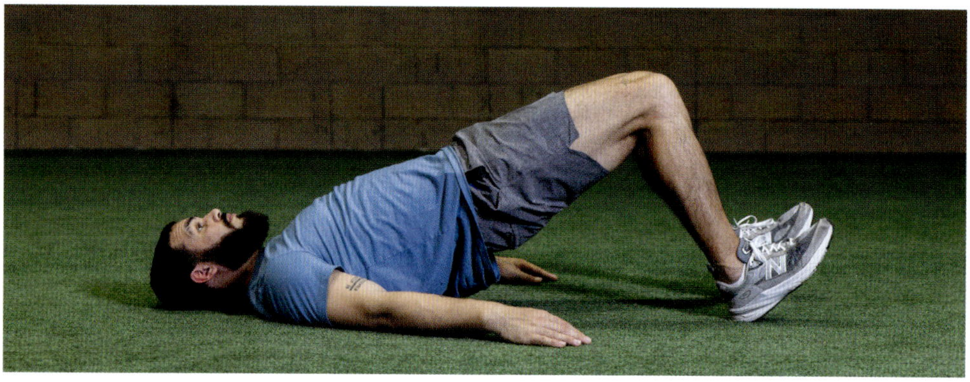

Benefits

The bilateral hip lift exercise is designed to warm up the posterior chain muscles and improve the ability to differentiate between hip extension and the extension of the spine and pelvis. Clients often compensate for insufficient hip extension and core strength by excessively arching their lower backs. This inefficient movement strategy can hinder a client's ability to perform a proper hip hinge and may increase the risk of back pain. By teaching clients to engage their abdominal muscles and drive extension through their glutes, we can help them achieve full hip extension without over-relying on the lumbar spine.

Instructions for the Client

1. Begin by lying in a supine position with your knees bent and your heels on the ground. Lift your toes off the floor while maintaining contact through your heels.
2. Inhale deeply through the nose and exhale through the mouth while actively bracing your abdominals by drawing your ribs downward.
3. As you brace your abs, lift your hips up by pushing your whole foot forcefully into the ground.
4. Bridge up until you fully extend your hips, creating a straight line from your knees to your shoulders. Be sure not to overextend your spine and pelvis.
5. Return back to the starting position and repeat for the prescribed repetitions.

Variation

Progression: Single-Leg Hip Lift

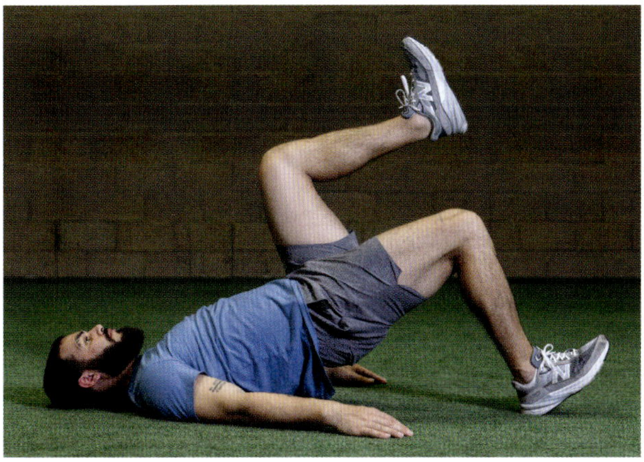

The single-leg hip lift is a progression from the standard bilateral hip lift to increase difficulty. This unilateral variation requires greater hip strength to achieve hip extension and places additional demands on the abdominal muscles to control spine and pelvic alignment.

This variation uses the same setup as the bilateral hip lift but becomes unilateral by flexing one knee toward the chest while the opposite foot remains planted on the ground. Coaches should cue a level pelvis, avoid lumbar extension or rotation, and maintain light abdominal tension throughout. The range of motion and intent remain unchanged; only the support base differs.

SHOULDER FLOOR SLIDE

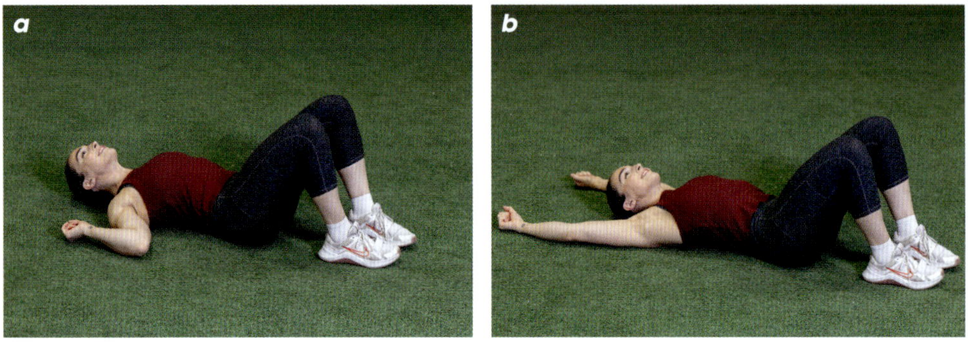

Benefits

The shoulder floor slide will enhance mobility in both the glenohumeral and the scapulothoracic joints while teaching clients to control the thorax during shoulder flexion. Athletes with limited shoulder mobility and poor control of their torsos in the sagittal plane often compensate by extending their trunks rather than achieving proper shoulder flexion. This compensation can increase the risk of shoulder impingement and cause pain in the neck and shoulders due to improper movement patterns. This drill teaches clients to achieve shoulder flexion and external rotation of the humerus, as well as upward rotation of the scapula, while maintaining rib cage depression and internal rotation. Improvement in this exercise will enhance trunk and shoulder mechanics during overhead movements, such as throwing, overhead presses, and pull-ups.

Instructions for the Client

1. Lie flat on your back with your knees bent and feet flat on the floor. Position your shoulders in a horizontally abducted and externally rotated posture, with your hands aligned with your head and your arms forming a W shape on the floor beside you.
2. Slightly tilt your pelvis posteriorly so that your spine lies flat against the floor.
3. Before starting the exercise, inhale through your nose. Exhale through your mouth while sliding your arms overhead as far as possible, ensuring that the backs of your hands and elbows maintain contact with the ground.
4. Inhale while returning your elbows to the starting position. Throughout the entire exercise, keep your lumbar spine in contact with the ground.
5. Return to the starting position and repeat for the recommended number of repetitions.

Variation

Progression: Shoulder Wall Slide

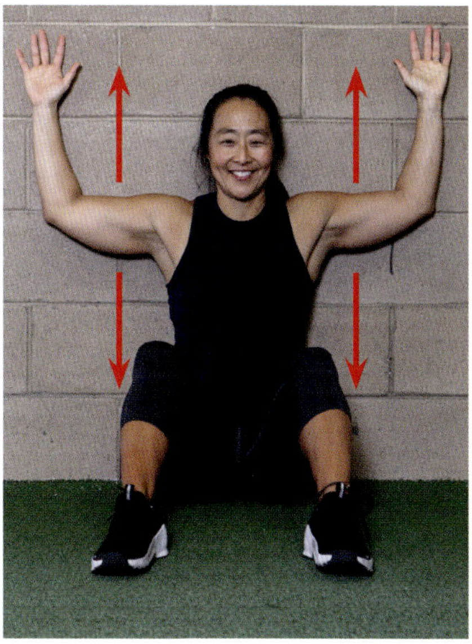

The shoulder wall slide is a progression of the floor slide, presenting a greater challenge due to the vertical orientation of the torso. As the client progresses from a supine to an upright position, it becomes essential to stabilize the spine in the sagittal plane without the support of the ground. In the vertical position, gravity no longer assists the upper back and posterior shoulder musculature in maintaining contact with the wall, increasing the demands on postural control and shoulder mobility.

SUPINE BAND HIP FLEXION

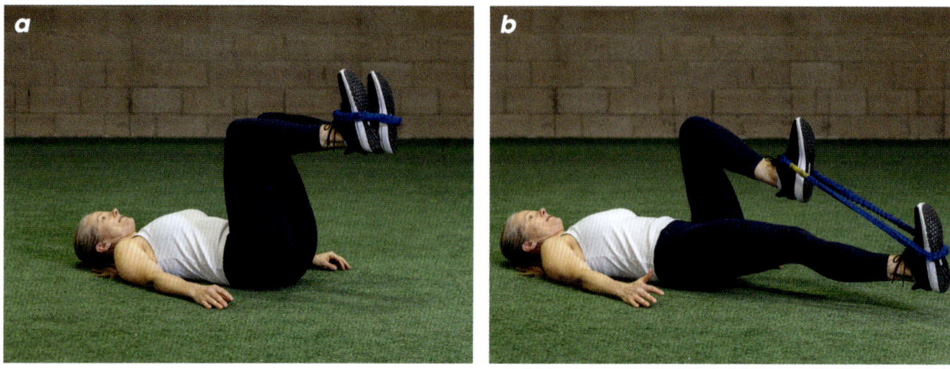

Benefits

The aim of this drill is to strengthen the hip flexor muscles, particularly the psoas and iliacus, while also enhancing stability in the pelvis and lower back. This exercise focuses on controlling pelvic position during active hip flexion. It emphasizes the active engagement of the psoas and iliacus muscles to flex and extend the hips effectively.

Instructions for the Client

1. Begin in a supine position with both knees bent and drawn toward your chest at an angle greater than 90 degrees. Place a light band around the arches of your feet.
2. Inhale through your nose to prepare for the exercise. As you exhale through your mouth, slowly extend one leg straight while keeping the opposite hip fully flexed, resisting the tension in the band.
3. Inhale again as you return your knee to the starting position. Repeat the movement on the opposite side.

Variation

Progression: Prone Hip Flexion

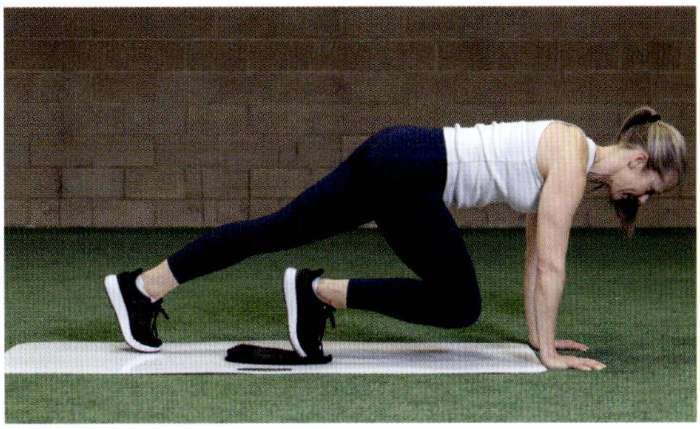

The prone hip flexion drill is a progression of the supine band hip flexion exercise performed from a high plank position to increase difficulty. In this variation, band resistance is removed and a slider is placed under the working foot to assist the toe dragging along the floor. The goal shifts away from isolated hip flexor strength toward controlling the trunk and pelvis during active hip flexion. This position places greater demands on the anterior core and pelvic stabilizers, because the client must maintain spinal and pelvic alignment without support from the floor.

BAND-ASSISTED LEG LOWER

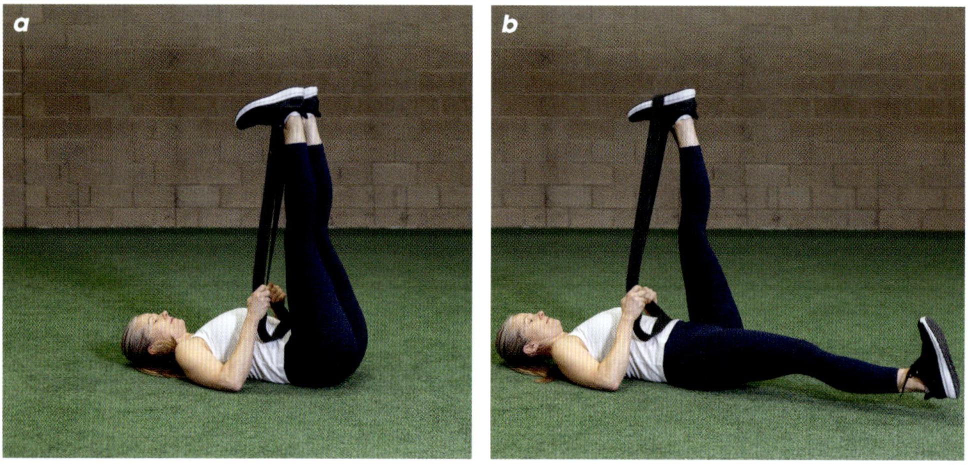

Benefits

The leg-lowering progression is designed to improve the opposing movements of hip flexion and extension. Being able to flex and extend the hips simultaneously through a full range of motion is crucial for running and hinging without compensating through the spine and pelvis.

Instructions for the Client

1. Lie on your back with your knees straight and a resistance band in your hands, positioned around the arch of one foot.
2. Flex your hips to raise both your legs as high as possible while keeping your knees straight.
3. Inhale through your nose before starting the exercise. Exhale through your mouth as you slowly lower the leg without the band toward the ground, ensuring that the knee remains straight.
4. Keep the leg with the band completely still and straight throughout the movement. Inhale as you bring the other leg back to the top position. Complete all prescribed repetitions, and repeat the exercise on the opposite side.

Variation

Progression: Unassisted Leg Lower

In this progression, the leg lower is performed without band assistance, shifting the emphasis from an assisted mobility drill to an active trunk-stability exercise to increase difficulty. The top leg is held in isometric straight-leg hip flexion while the opposite leg slowly extends toward the floor. This significantly increases the demands on the anterior trunk and pelvic musculature, because the client must maintain pelvic position and lumbar control throughout the movement.

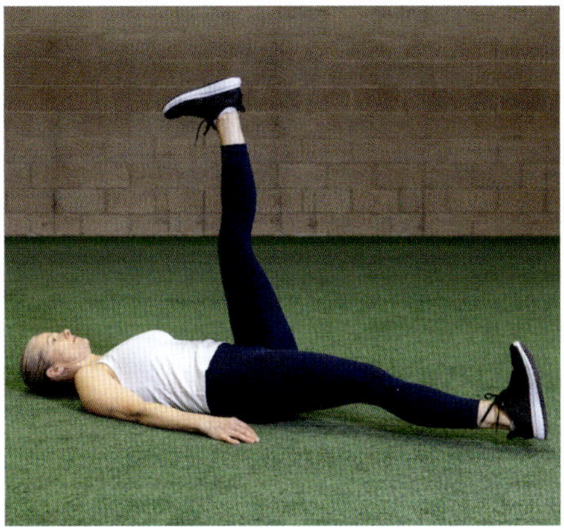

PATTERN PRACTICE

After executing motor control movement preparation drills, the client should proceed to practicing fundamental movement patterns. Performing basic movement patterns on a daily basis provides repetitive motor learning, improves mobility, and prepares the body for upcoming training sessions.

Since the average trainee visits the gym only twice per week, it is essential that each training session includes all fundamental movement patterns. Because most clients are not regularly squatting, hinging, lunging, pushing, or pulling through full ranges of motion outside the gym, it becomes the coach's responsibility to provide consistent exposure to these patterns during formal training sessions—most commonly during the warm-up or as part of the strength program.

This approach acts as a form of basic movement hygiene, helping clients develop and maintain essential movement skills such as squatting, lunging, hinging, and pushing. It also serves to effectively prepare the body for those same patterns, allowing for heavier loads or higher speeds later in the training session. In addition, basic bodyweight exercises can function as mobility work by loading the joints through full ranges of motion, improving capsular mobility and tissue extensibility under load, and ultimately enhancing overall movement quality.

The following exercise progressions can be used as part of a comprehensive warm-up program to develop basic motor patterns, improve mobility, and prepare the body for higher-intensity activities later in the session. Warm-up activities should be performed with body weight or light loads and progressed over time to prevent boredom, introduce movement variability, and challenge the nervous system. Progressions may include adding light external load, increasing movement speed, or incorporating multiple planes of motion to further challenge stability and motor control.

SQUAT PRESS-OUT

Benefits

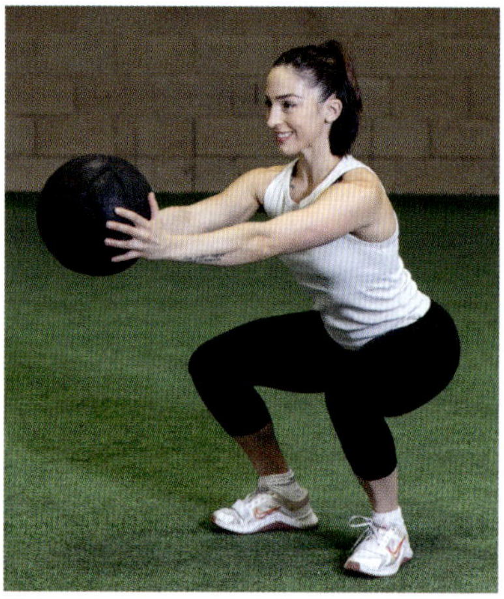

The squat press-out reinforces proper squat mechanics by encouraging an upright torso and improved trunk engagement. The forward press of a light weight or medicine ball provides a counterbalance, making it an effective teaching tool for beginners. This exercise works well as a lower body warm-up for strength and power activities, such as jumping, while also giving coaches a simple way to assess a client's squat pattern, mobility, and control.

Instructions for the Client

1. Begin standing with your feet shoulder-width apart or slightly wider, toes pointing straight ahead or slightly outward. Hold a light weight or medicine ball close to your chest with both hands.
2. Brace your abdominals and create tension through the lower body by lightly screwing your feet into the floor.
3. Initiate the squat by sitting down and back. As you descend, slowly press the weight or medicine ball forward, keeping your arms extended at approximately chest height.
4. Maintain an upright torso as you lower under control until your thighs are parallel to the floor or you reach your deepest comfortable squat position.
5. Reverse the motion by driving through your feet to stand up while pulling the weight or medicine ball back toward your chest. Repeat for the prescribed number of repetitions.

Variations

Progression 1: Light Zercher Squat

This exercise adds variety to the squat pattern while increasing the demand on trunk stability. The client holds a medicine ball or sandbag close to the body in the crooks of the elbows, promoting a tall posture and creating full body tension. The load placement challenges the core to maintain stiffness throughout the squat, making it a useful progression from the squat press-out.

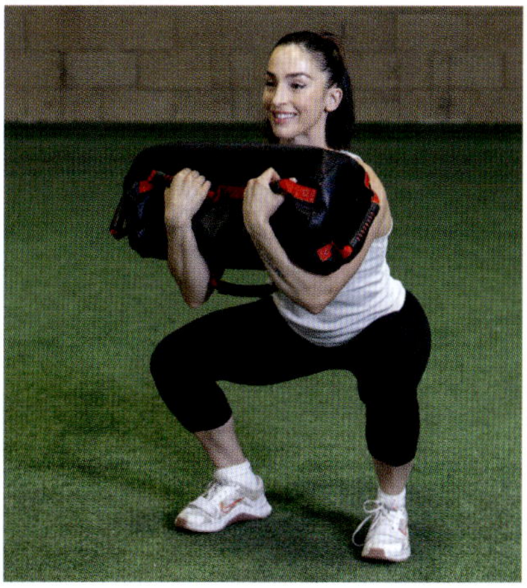

Progression 2: Sandbag Offset-Loaded Squat

As a progression, the offset-loaded squat introduces an asymmetrical challenge to enhance core stability and postural control. The client holds a sandbag over one shoulder or a kettlebell in a single-arm rack position, creating an unbalanced load to resist during the squat. This exercise reinforces bracing, improves lateral stability, and provides increased movement variability in the squat pattern.

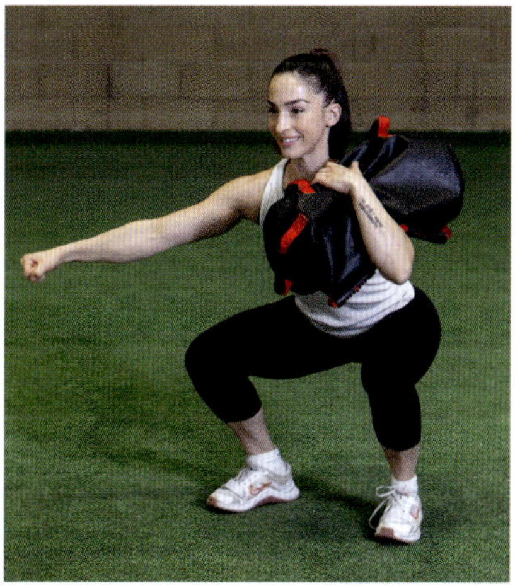

SPLIT SQUAT

Benefits

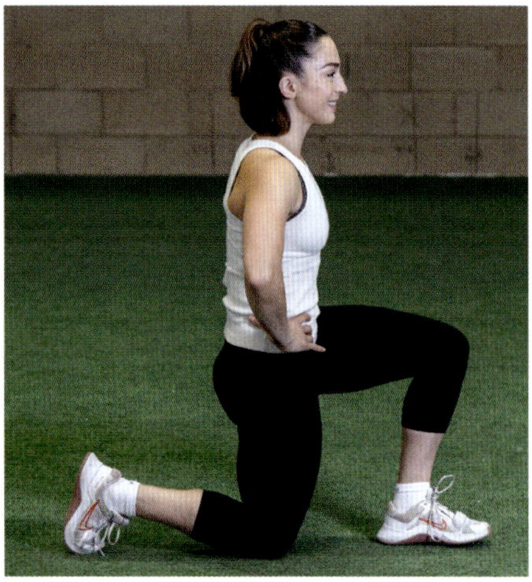

The bodyweight split squat develops split-stance control, balance, and lower body stability. It prepares the hips, knees, and ankles for unilateral training while reinforcing proper lower body alignment. This exercise also allows the coach to assess a client's hip mobility, coordination, and baseline strength, making it a useful tool for identifying an appropriate entry point for lower body progressions.

Instructions for the Client

1. Begin standing tall and step one foot forward and one foot back into a split stance, with the front foot flat on the ground and the back toe dug in the ground and heel slightly elevated.
2. Maintain an upright posture and brace your abdominals to keep the trunk stable throughout the movement.
3. Lower your body under control by bending both knees, allowing the back knee to move toward the floor while keeping most of your weight through the front foot.
4. Descend until the front thigh is approximately parallel to the floor or until you reach your deepest comfortable position while maintaining balance and alignment.
5. Drive through the front foot to return to the starting position. Complete the prescribed number of repetitions, then switch sides.

Variations

Progression 1: Reverse Lunge

The reverse lunge is a natural progression from the split squat, introducing more dynamic movement in a split stance. By stepping backward into each repetition, the client develops greater motor control, balance, and coordination. This variation also challenges eccentric strength and stability, making it an effective warm-up drill for unilateral lower body training.

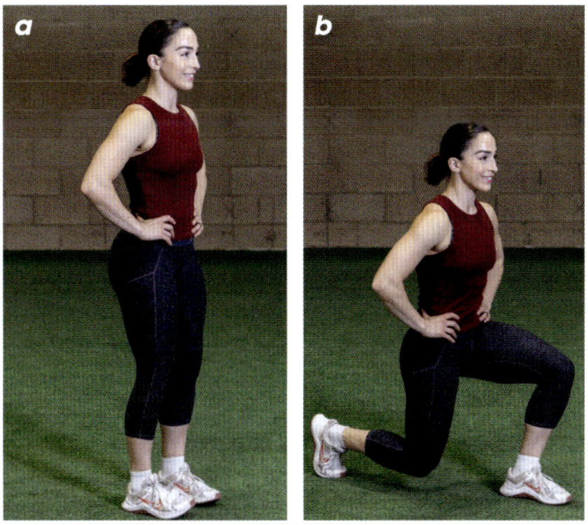

Progression 2: Forward Lunge

The forward lunge adds a deceleration component to the split-stance pattern. By stepping forward and then pushing back to the starting position, the client must control and reverse forward momentum, placing greater demand on eccentric strength and joint stability. This makes it a valuable warm-up drill for building control and resilience in lower body movement.

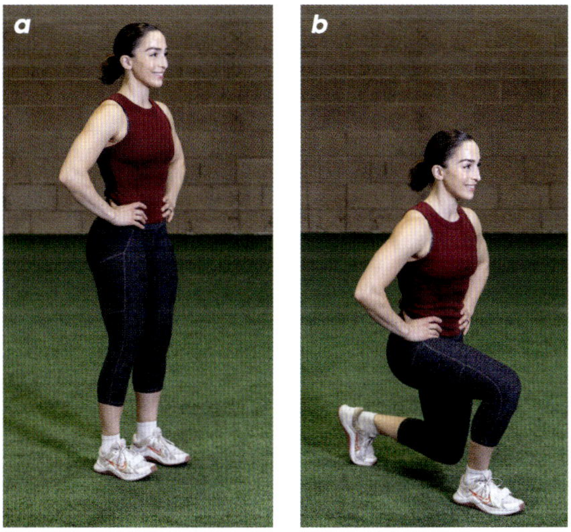

LATERAL SQUAT

Benefits

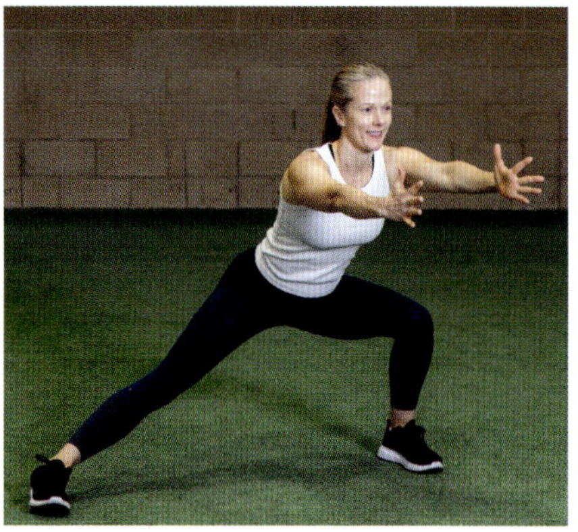

The lateral squat is a valuable warm-up drill for assessing and improving hip mobility in the frontal plane. By shifting laterally and sitting back into the hips, the exercise encourages controlled depth and range of motion. This movement helps open the adductor musculature and hips while reinforcing lower body mobility and stability outside the sagittal plane.

Instructions for the Client

1. Stand with your feet wider than shoulder-width apart and your toes pointed straight ahead or slightly outward.
2. Shift your body weight laterally toward one side while sitting back into the hips of the working leg. Reach your arms straight out in front of your torso to help you sit your hips back and maintain an upright torso position.
3. Keep your working foot flat on the floor while maintaining a neutral spine. Your opposite leg should remain straight with your foot planted on the floor.
4. Push through your working foot to return to the starting position, then repeat on the opposite side.
5. Continue alternating sides for the prescribed number of repetitions.

Variations

Progression 1: Lateral Lunge

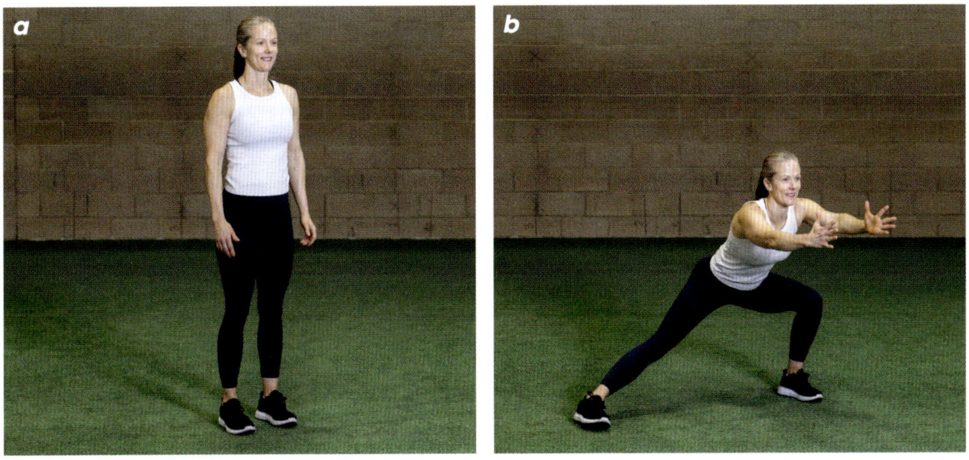

The lateral lunge builds on the lateral squat by adding dynamic movement and greater deceleration demands. The client steps out and loads into one side, controlling their momentum and stabilizing through the hip, knee, and ankle. This variation improves frontal plane strength, mobility, and coordination.

Progression 2: Diagonal Lunge

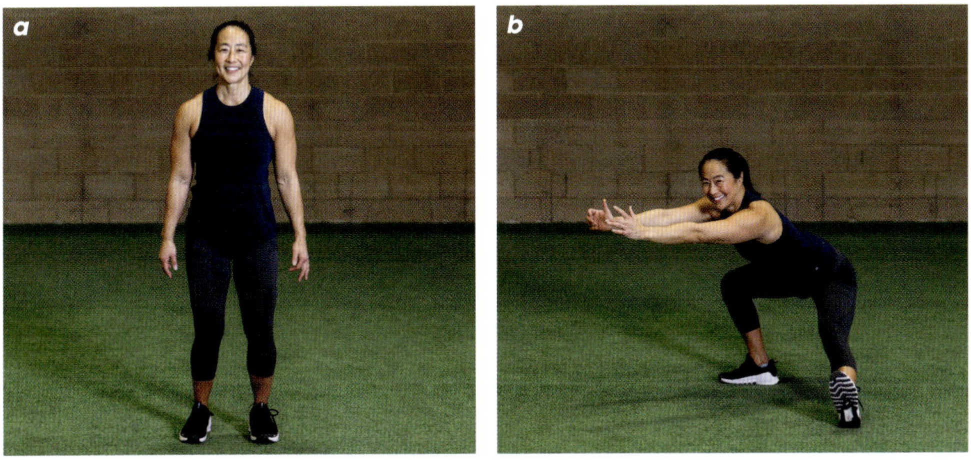

The diagonal lunge introduces a multiplanar challenge by having the client step backward at a 45-degree angle from the midline. This movement targets hip mobility and stability while reinforcing control through rotation and lateral loading. It is an effective way to prepare the lower body for complex movement patterns encountered in sport and daily life.

CHEST-LOADED BILATERAL HIP HINGE

Benefits

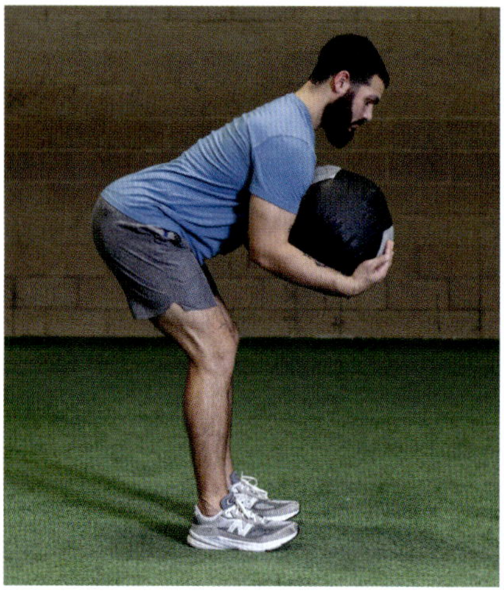

The chest-loaded bilateral hip hinge serves as both a teaching and assessment tool for developing proper hinge mechanics and warming up the posterior chain. Holding a light weight or medicine ball at the chest provides a counterbalance that encourages an effective hip shift backward. This movement allows the coach to evaluate hip mobility, spinal control, and overall movement quality—key indicators of readiness for more advanced hip-dominant strength exercises.

Instructions for the Client

1. Begin standing tall with your feet hip- to shoulder-width apart, holding a light weight or medicine ball close to your chest.
2. Brace your abdominals and maintain a neutral spine as you prepare to hinge at the hips.
3. Initiate the movement by pushing the hips backward while keeping a slight bend in the knees and the chest tall.
4. Lower the torso under control until you feel tension in the hamstrings or reach your deepest comfortable hinge position without losing spinal alignment.
5. Drive the hips forward to return to the starting position, maintaining trunk control throughout. Repeat for the prescribed number of repetitions.

Variations

Progression 1: Reaching Single-Leg Deadlift

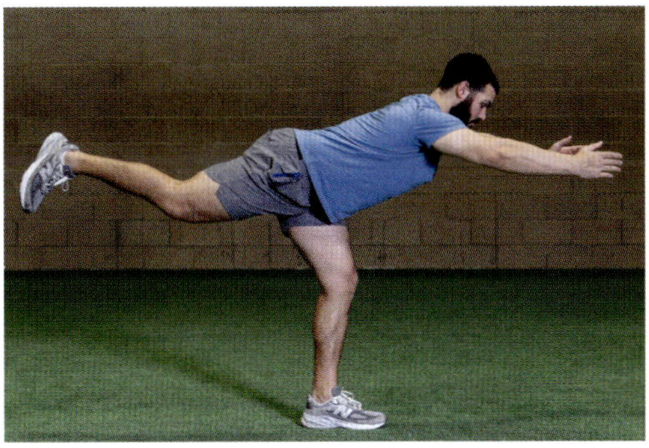

The reaching single-leg deadlift is a progression of the hip hinge pattern that challenges balance, proprioception, and multiplanar hip stability. The client should reach forward while hinging on one leg to engage the posterior chain musculature and develop stability through the hips, core, and ankle. This dynamic warm-up drill reinforces single-leg stability and prepares the body for unilateral strength work.

Progression 2: Triplanar Reaching Single-Leg Deadlift

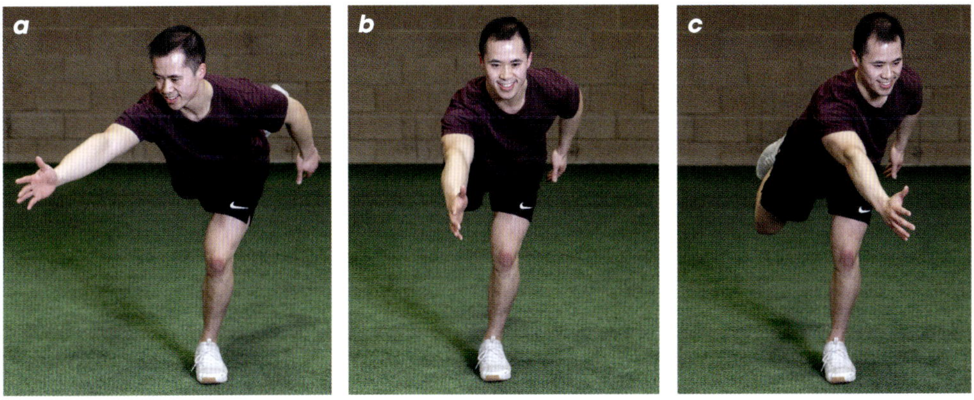

This progression of the single-leg deadlift introduces a multidirectional reaching pattern to further challenge balance and hip stability. The client performs the hinge while reaching across the body medially, straight ahead, and laterally, increasing the demand on the foot, ankle, and hip to stabilize through multiple planes. This variation is an excellent way to build proprioception, control, and resilience in the lower body.

PATTERN PRACTICE

PUSH-UP

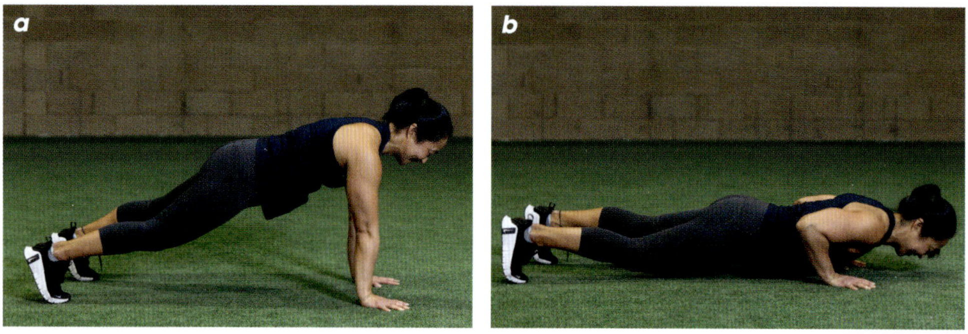

Benefits

The push-up is an effective warm-up drill for the trunk and upper body while allowing the coach to assess baseline upper body strength and stability. The exercise reinforces core control and shoulder stability prior to upper body training. If a client is unable to perform a full push-up from the floor, the movement can be regressed easily to an incline position using a bench or box placed under the hands.

Instructions for the Client

1. Begin in a prone position with your hands placed slightly wider than shoulder width and your body forming a straight line from head to heels.
2. Brace your abdominals and glutes to maintain a rigid trunk and neutral spine throughout the movement.
3. Lower your body under control by bending the elbows, keeping them at a comfortable angle relative to the torso.
4. Descend until your chest is just above the floor or your hands while maintaining full body tension.
5. Press forcefully through the hands to return to the starting position, keeping the body aligned. Repeat for the prescribed number of repetitions.

Variations

Progression 1: Push-Up to Downward Dog

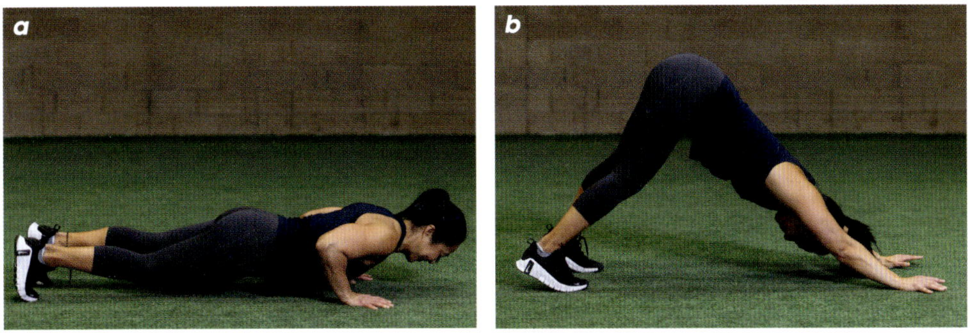

This variation progresses the standard push-up by incorporating a downward dog position between each repetition. After pressing up, the client shifts into downward dog, driving the hips upward and reaching the heels toward the floor. This movement increases strength and stability demands on the trunk and shoulders while also providing a dynamic stretch for the posterior chain, including the hamstrings, calves, and lats.

Progression 2: Push-Up to Single-Arm Downward Dog

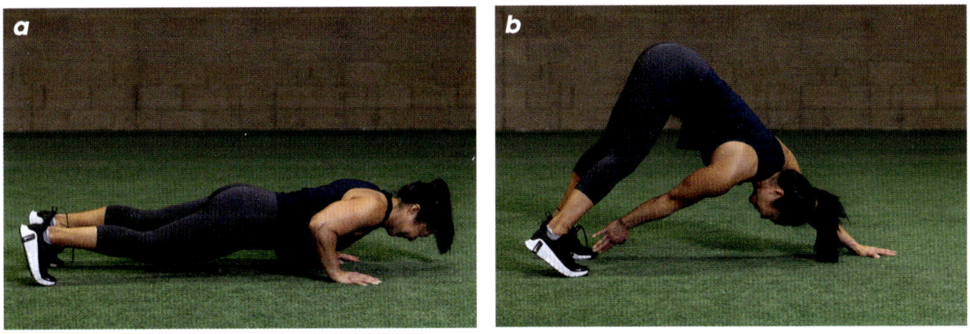

This advanced variation increases both the strength and mobility demands on the shoulder complex. After performing a push-up with feet set slightly wider for stability, the client reaches one hand across to touch the toes of the opposite foot while shifting into a downward dog position. This movement enhances shoulder stability, thoracic mobility, and posterior chain flexibility, making it a dynamic and challenging warm-up drill.

COMPONENTS OF A DYNAMIC WARM-UP

After rehearsing fundamental movement patterns should come more dynamic locomotion drills. Multidirectional movement skills such as skipping, crawling, shuffling, and backpedaling not only improve athletic performance but also enhance resilience, enabling clients to move more dynamically and reducing the risk of falls and lower body injuries. Incorporating multidirectional movement drills such as skipping or ladder drills regularly can help enhance the nervous system and overall body awareness. Additionally, these warm-up drills can serve as a bridge to low-impact power exercises for clients who may not be prepared for traditional plyometrics such as hopping, jumping, and bounding. The following drills should all be performed for 10-20 yards (meters) each.

BEAR CRAWL

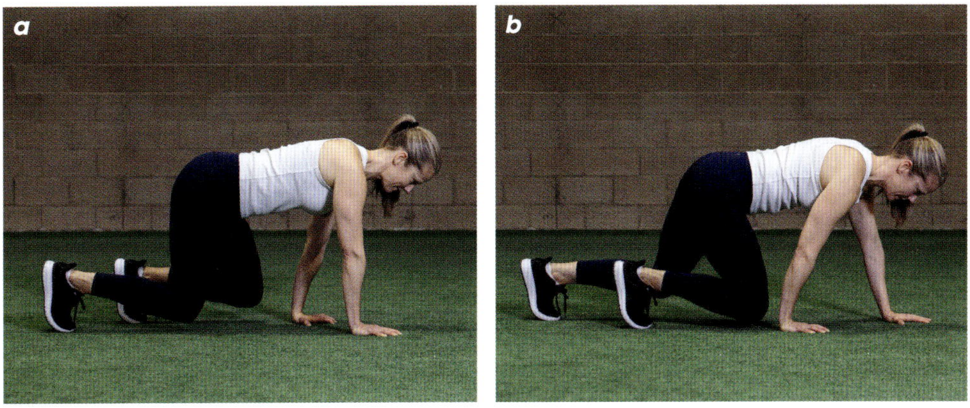

Benefits

The bear crawl is a versatile drill used to warm up the upper body, activate the core, and reinforce contralateral coordination. It is particularly effective for developing shoulder stability, trunk control, and total body coordination.

Instructions for the Client

1. Begin in a quadruped position with your hands directly under your shoulders and your knees under your hips.
2. Brace your abdominals and gently lift your knees 1 to 2 inches (2.5-5 cm) off the ground, keeping the spine in a flat, neutral position.
3. Move forward by taking small, controlled steps, advancing the opposite hand and foot at the same time.
4. Keep your hips low and your trunk still, minimizing rotation or excessive shifting side to side.
5. Continue crawling forward under control for the prescribed distance.

LATERAL CRAWL

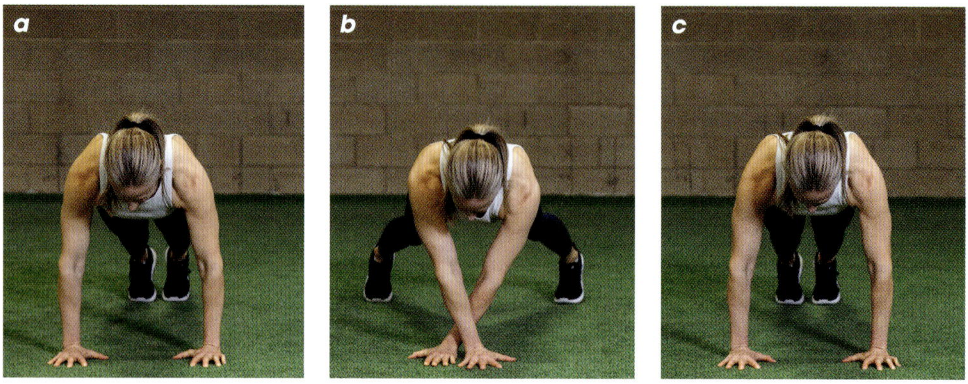

Benefits

The lateral crawl drill is an effective warm-up exercise for the trunk, shoulders, and scapulothoracic musculature while promoting contralateral coordination and core stability. This movement serves as an excellent preparatory exercise for upper body training.

Instructions for the Client

1. Begin in a stable push-up position with your hands directly under your shoulders, feet together, and spine in a neutral alignment.
2. Brace your abdominals and create full body tension to maintain trunk stability.
3. When moving to the left, initiate the movement by stepping simultaneously with your right hand and left leg, allowing the hands to briefly cross as you move sideways.
4. After each step, reset into a solid push-up position before beginning the next repetition.
5. Keep the movement slow, controlled, and deliberate, maintaining core engagement throughout while avoiding sagging at the hips or excessive arching of the lower back.

FORWARD A-SKIP

Benefits

The A-skip is a foundational drill used to develop contralateral coordination, rhythm, and the fundamental mechanics of running. It also serves as a low-impact power exercise, making it a great option for individuals who may struggle with higher-intensity plyometric activities.

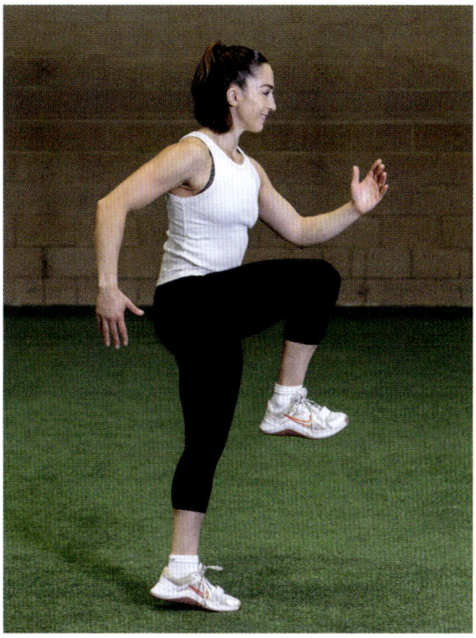

Instructions for the Client

1. Begin standing tall with your feet approximately shoulder-width apart and your posture upright.
2. Initiate the drill by driving one knee upward to approximately hip height while maintaining coordinated arm action with the opposite arm moving forward.
3. Actively flex the hip, knee, and ankle of the swinging leg, keeping the foot dorsiflexed.
4. As the lifted leg returns to the ground, immediately switch sides by driving the opposite knee upward to continue the skipping rhythm.
5. Bounce lightly and reactively off the forefoot of the stance leg to propel the movement forward while maintaining rhythm and posture. Perform for the prescribed distance.

LATERAL A-SKIP

Benefits

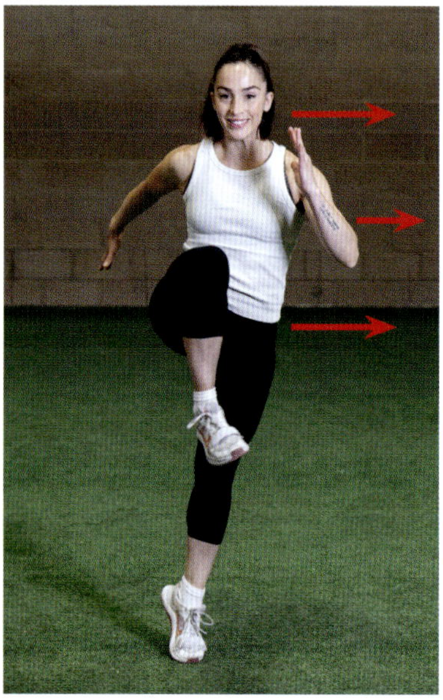

The lateral A-skip is a variation of the traditional A-skip that introduces movement in the frontal plane. It is an effective drill for warming up the hip abductors, improving lateral coordination, and developing frontal-plane power and rhythm.

Instructions for the Client

1. Begin by skipping in place to establish a steady rhythm and reinforce proper mechanics, including hip flexion, dorsiflexion, and contralateral arm swing.
2. Initiate lateral movement by pushing off the stance leg and actively abducting the hip to drive yourself sideways.
3. Maintain an upright posture with coordinated arm action while staying light and reactive on the forefoot.
4. Focus on crisp, rhythmic steps and smooth lateral transitions with each skip for the prescribed distance.

HIGH KNEE RUN

Benefits

The high knee run is a dynamic drill used to activate the hip flexors, reinforce efficient running mechanics, and promote quick ground contact. It is commonly included in warm-ups to prepare the lower body for sprinting or explosive movement.

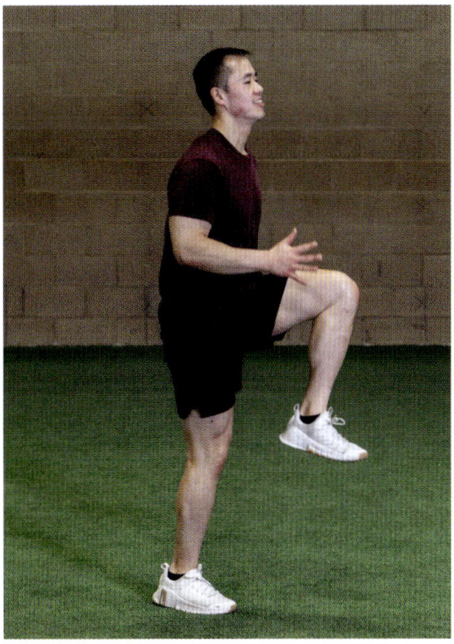

Instructions for the Client

1. Begin standing tall with an upright posture and arms positioned to allow a coordinated, contralateral arm swing.
2. Drive the knees rapidly upward to approximately hip height or slightly above while maintaining a tall trunk position.
3. Focus on short, quick steps with minimal ground contact time, striking through the forefoot.
4. Stay light and reactive with each step, maintaining rhythm and arm–leg coordination.
5. Perform for the prescribed distance.

HEEL TO BUTT

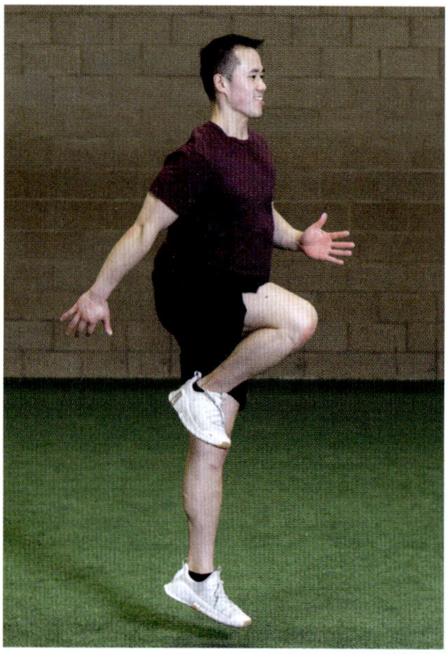

Benefits

The heel to butt drill is used to activate the hamstrings and reinforce key mechanics for top-speed running. It promotes coordination; rhythm; and fast, efficient ground contact while warming up the posterior chain.

Instructions for the Client

1. Begin standing tall with an upright posture and coordinated, contralateral arm swing.
2. Actively flex the knee to bring the heel toward the glutes while simultaneously driving the thigh upward through active hip flexion.
3. Focus on using the hamstrings to control the motion rather than allowing the leg to swing passively.
4. Stay light on the forefoot with quick, elastic ground contacts as you alternate legs.
5. Maintain rhythm, posture, and coordination throughout the drill for the prescribed distance or time.

LATERAL SHUFFLE

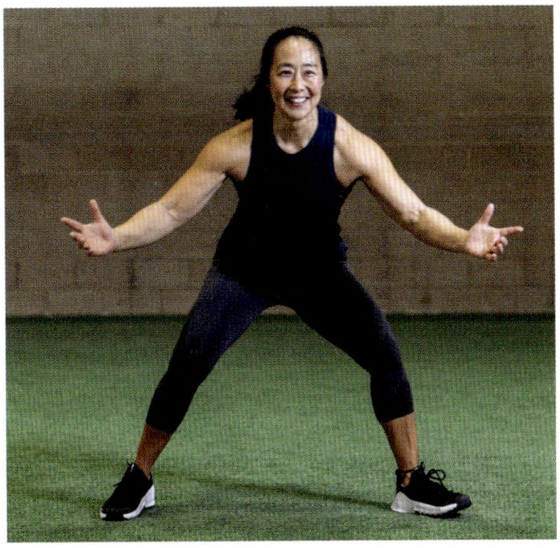

Benefits

The lateral shuffle is an effective drill for developing coordination and movement efficiency in the frontal plane. It reinforces the ability to decelerate and reaccelerate laterally while building foundational movement capacity for cutting, change-of-direction tasks, and sport-specific lateral actions.

Instructions for the Client

1. Begin in a low athletic stance with your feet slightly wider than shoulder-width apart and your toes pointing straight ahead.
2. Keep your chest tall, hips low, and shoulders level throughout the movement.
3. Initiate the shuffle by pushing forcefully off the trail leg to move laterally.
4. Maintain a consistent distance between your feet to preserve a strong base of support, avoiding heel contact or letting the feet come together.
5. Stay low, light, and reactive with each step for the prescribed distance.

CARIOCA

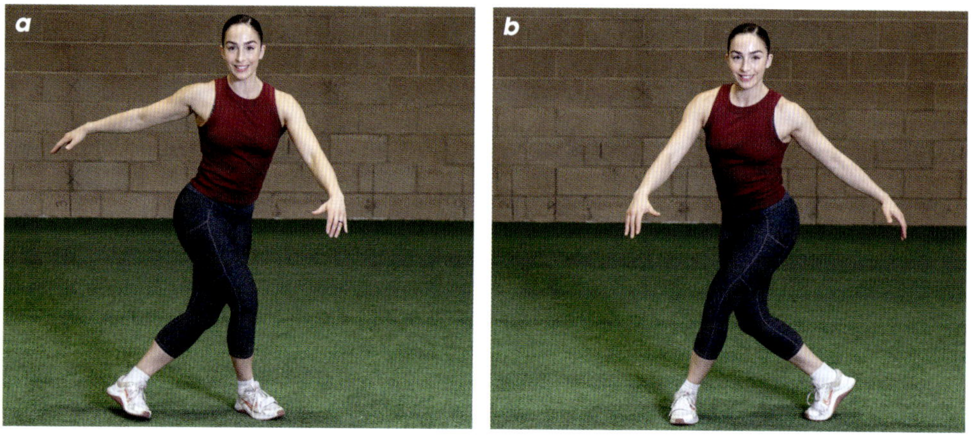

Benefits

The carioca drill develops coordination between opposing trunk and hip rotation while improving lower body footwork and rhythm. It is especially valuable for enhancing full body coordination, balance, and mobility, making it an effective option for older clients or anyone working to improve multiplanar movement skills.

Instructions for the Client

1. Begin in an athletic stance facing forward with a slight bend in the knees and an upright posture.
2. Move laterally by stepping one foot across the front of the body.
3. Quickly bring the opposite foot behind the body, continuing in a weaving pattern as you move sideways.
4. Allow the hips and trunk to rotate naturally in opposition to the legs while keeping the arms relaxed and swinging rhythmically.
5. Focus on smooth, controlled steps rather than speed, staying light on your feet and maintaining clear, intentional foot placement to avoid tripping. Perform for the prescribed distance.

BACKPEDAL

Benefits

The backpedal drill is used to warm up the hamstrings, hips, and quads and improve coordination, control, and movement efficiency while traveling in reverse. It can be especially useful for helping older clients regain competency and confidence in multiplanar coordination.

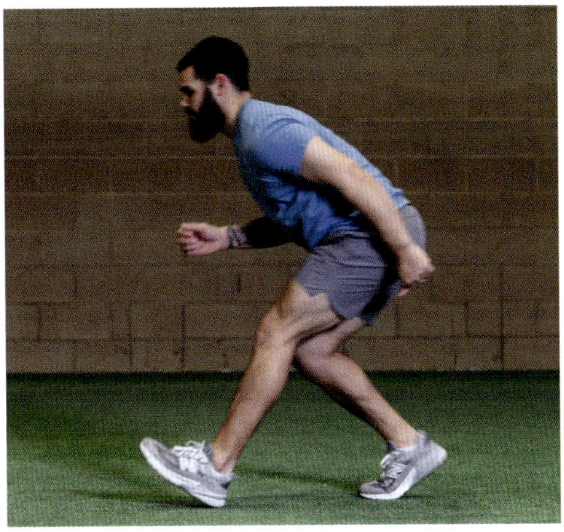

Instructions for the Client

1. Begin in an athletic stance with the knees slightly bent, hips pushed back, and chest tall.
2. Initiate backward movement by actively extending the knee and driving through the heel of the pushing leg.
3. Keep the feet in front of the body as you move, emphasizing strong, deliberate pushes with each step.
4. Maintain balance, a controlled arm swing, and a steady, rhythmic cadence throughout the drill.
5. For beginners, perform the movement slowly and under control to build coordination and avoid loss of balance or falling backward. Perform for the prescribed distance.

LADDER DRILLS

Agility ladder drills can serve as an effective and engaging alternative to traditional warm-up methods, especially for general population clients. These drills improve footwork, coordination, and change-of-direction ability while also promoting balance, rhythm, and spatial awareness. Because ladder drills involve dynamic, low-impact movement across multiple planes of motion, they provide a valuable opportunity to develop movement literacy without excessive joint stress.

For clients who may lack athletic backgrounds or who need to improve general motor control, agility ladder drills offer a safe and scalable way to reintroduce multiplanar movement. They also help stimulate the nervous system, increase heart rate, and activate key muscle groups, making them an effective bridge between mobility work and more intense strength or power training.

I recommend alternating between the active warm-up drills outlined earlier and ladder drills throughout the training week. This approach adds movement variety, prevents monotony, and allows clients to build competence across a broad range of patterns, ultimately enhancing overall movement quality and physical preparedness.

1-2 STICK

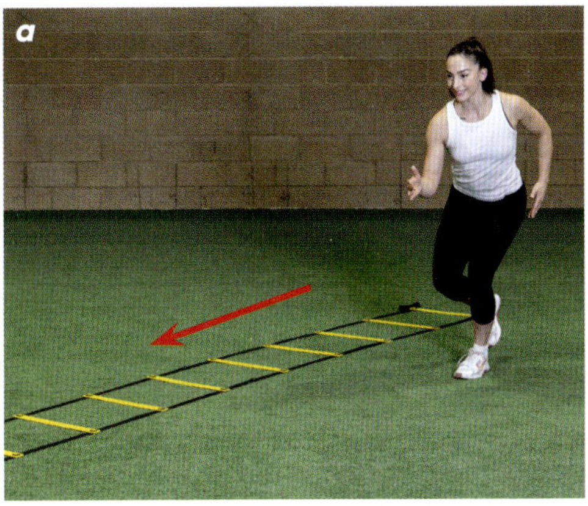

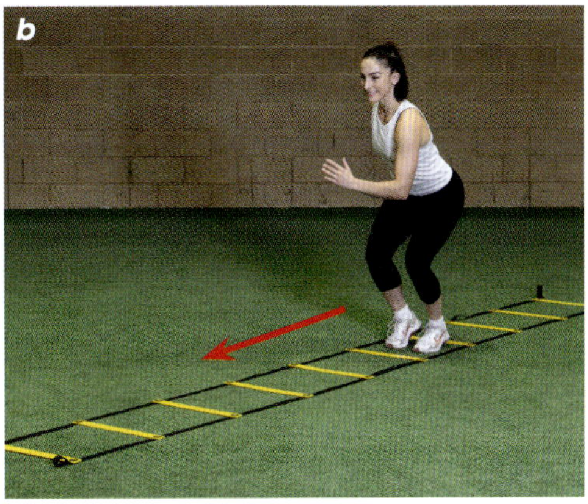

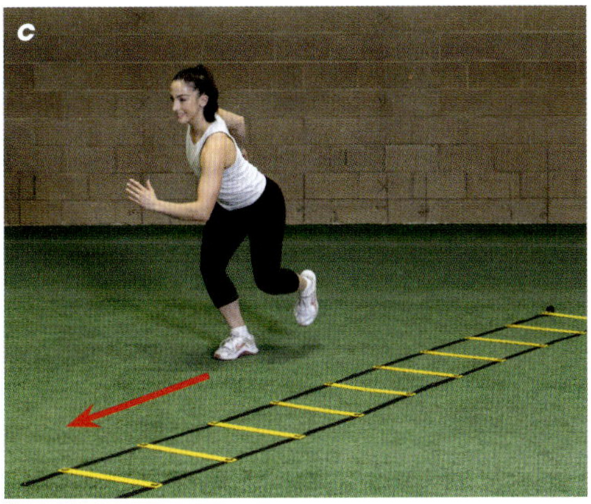

Benefits

The 1-2 stick ladder drill develops frontal-plane movement skills, single-leg stability, and balance. It reinforces controlled foot placement, lateral deceleration, and the ability to stabilize on one leg, making it an effective drill for building coordination and lower body control.

Instructions for the Client

1. Begin standing to the side of the ladder in an athletic stance.
2. Step both feet into the first box of the ladder.
3. Step both feet out to the opposite side of the ladder, finishing in a stable single-leg athletic position on the outside leg.
4. Pause briefly to reinforce balance, posture, and control before continuing.
5. Progress forward down the length of the ladder using the same side-to-side pattern.
6. After reaching the end, repeat the drill in reverse while moving backward through the ladder.

CROSS IN FRONT

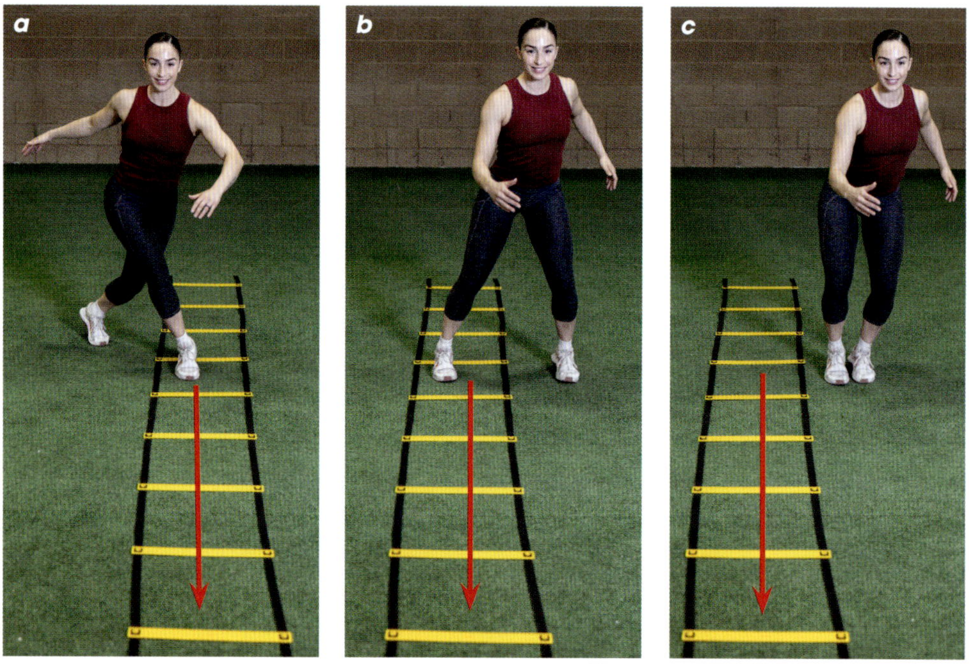

Benefits

The cross in front ladder drill develops multiplanar movement skills and foot coordination. It is especially valuable for fall prevention and athletic movement training, because it challenges balance, hip rotation, and controlled foot placement during lateral movement.

Instructions for the Client

1. Begin standing to the side of the agility ladder in an athletic stance.
2. Cross the outside leg in front of your body by rotating the hips and stepping into the first box of the ladder.
3. Step the inside leg across to the far side of the ladder, followed by the outside foot.
4. Continue this crossing pattern as you move down the length of the ladder, alternating sides with each sequence.
5. For an added challenge, repeat the drill in reverse by moving backward through the ladder to further enhance coordination and control.

CROSS BEHIND

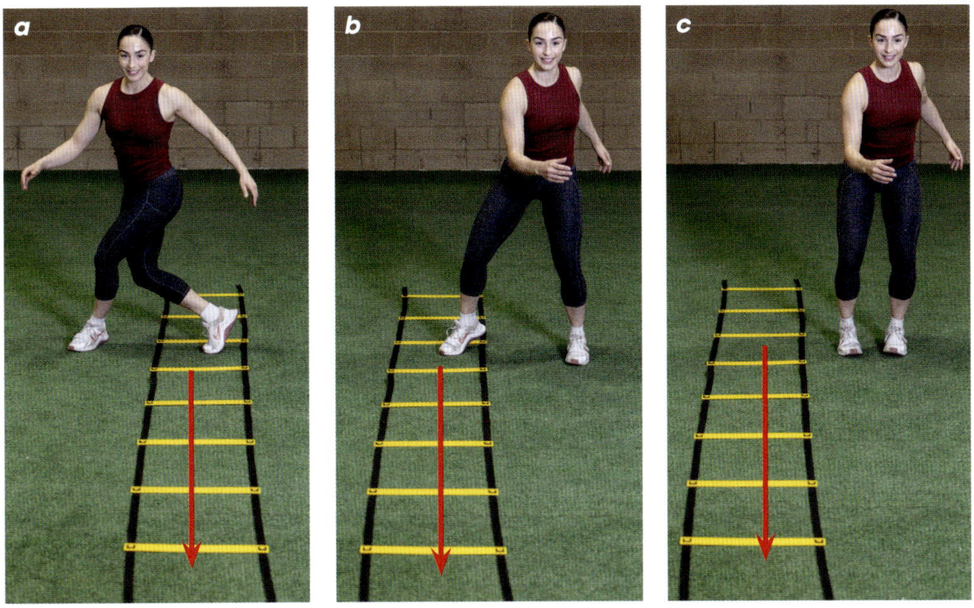

Benefits

The cross behind ladder drill develops multiplanar coordination, hip mobility, and controlled foot placement. As a variation of the cross in front drill, it places a greater rotational and balance demand on the lower body, making it useful for improving movement awareness, coordination, and fall-prevention capacity.

Instructions for the Client

1. Begin standing to the side of the agility ladder in an athletic stance.
2. Rotate the hips and step the outside leg behind your body into the first box of the ladder.
3. Step the inside leg across, then bring the outside leg to the opposite side of the ladder.
4. Continue this crossing-behind pattern as you move down the ladder, alternating sides with each sequence.
5. To increase the coordination and complexity of the drill, repeat it in reverse by moving backward through the ladder.

IN-IN-OUT-OUT FORWARD/BACKWARD

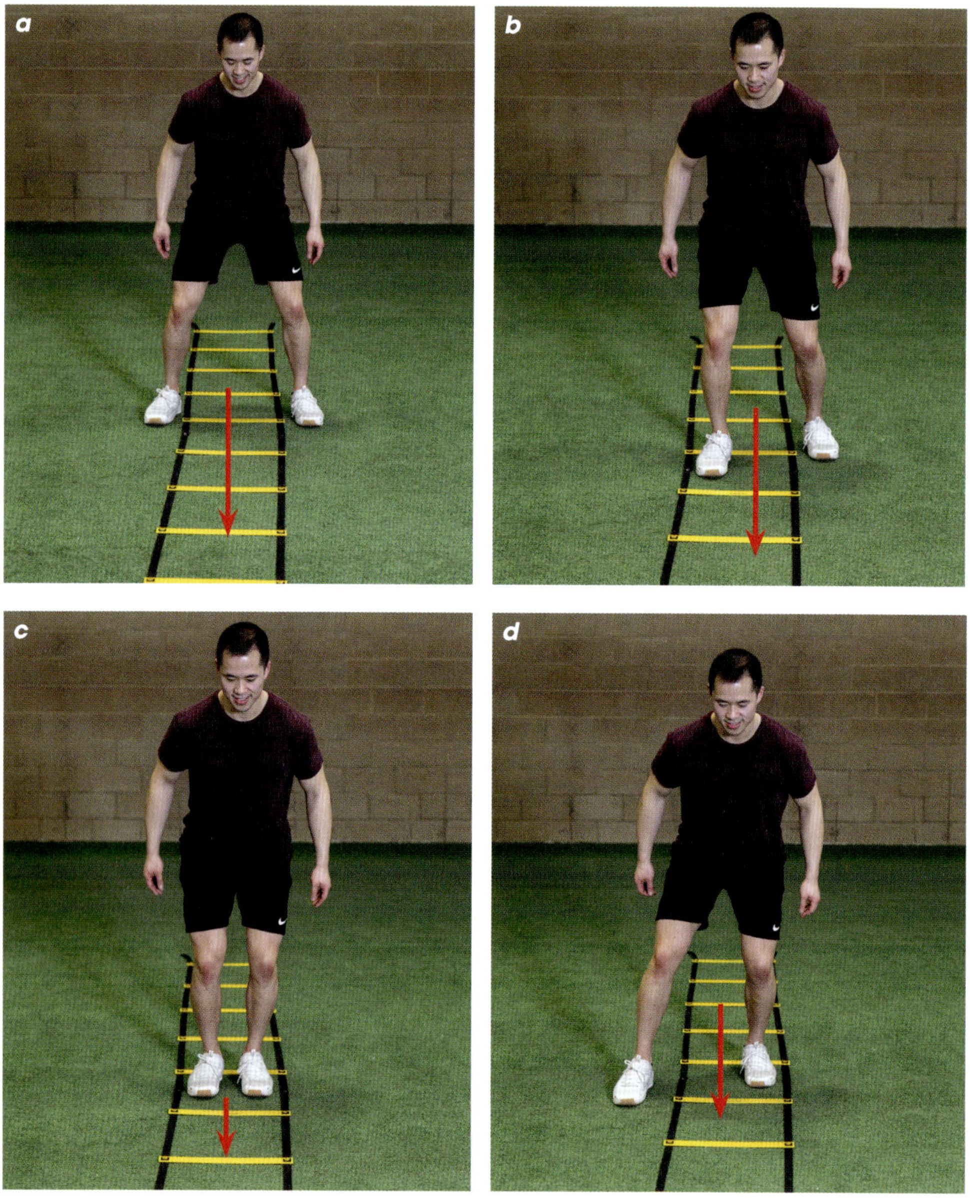

Benefits

The in-in-out-out ladder forward/backward drill develops rhythm, footwork coordination, and timing. It reinforces precise foot placement and body control while moving through space, making it a foundational drill for improving agility and movement efficiency.

Instructions for the Client

1. Begin by straddling the first box of the ladder with your feet positioned on either side and your body facing forward.
2. Step both feet into the first box one at a time in an "in-in" pattern.
3. Step both feet out to the sides in an "out-out" pattern as you move forward to the next box.
4. Maintain a steady pace, low athletic posture, and coordinated arm action as you progress through the ladder.
5. To increase the challenge, repeat the drill in reverse by moving backward through the ladder while maintaining control and rhythm.

IN-IN-OUT-OUT SIDEWAYS

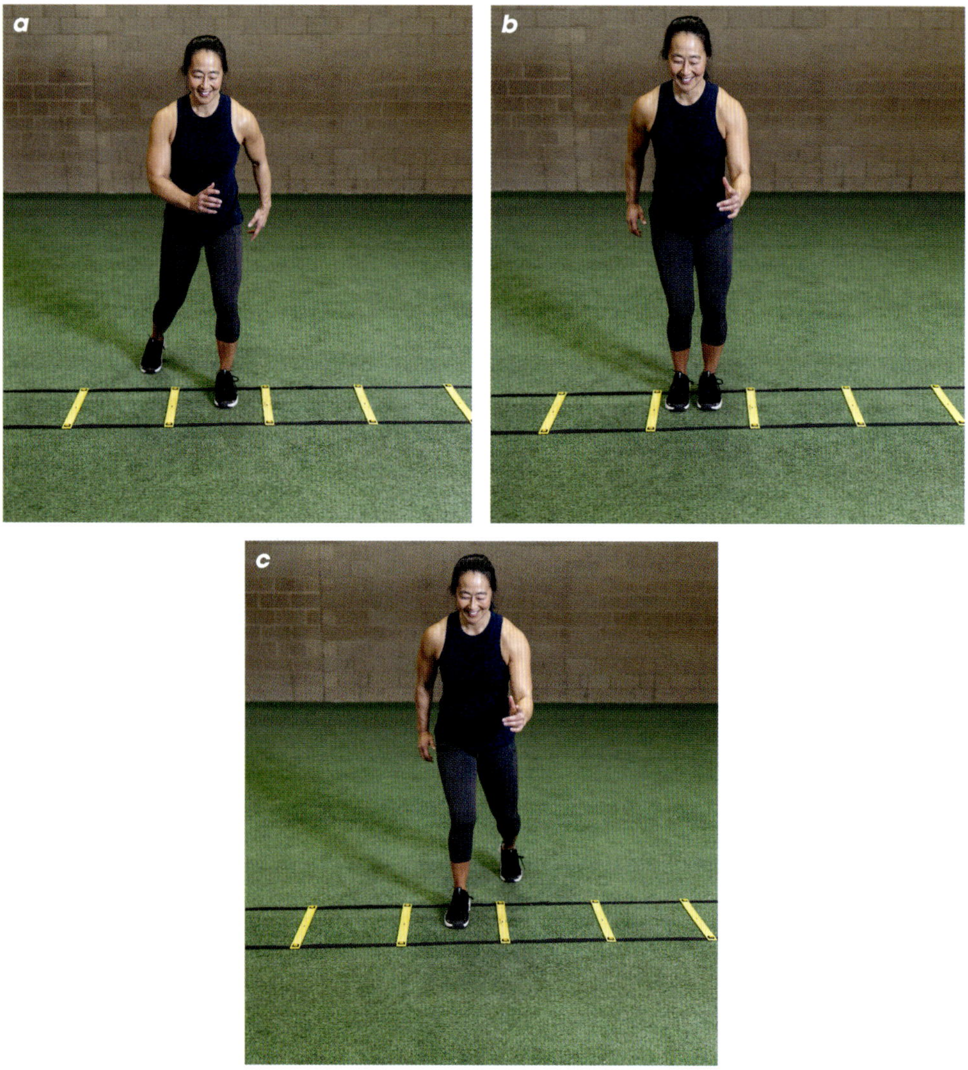

Benefits

The in-in-out-out sideways ladder drill develops footwork coordination while reinforcing lateral movement, rhythm, and body control. It is an effective progression for building frontal-plane agility and consistent movement timing.

Instructions for the Client

1. Begin standing to the side of the ladder, facing forward, with the ladder positioned directly in front of you.
2. Step into the first box with the lead foot, followed by the trail foot in an "in-in" pattern.
3. Step out to the side with the lead foot, followed by the trail foot in an "out-out" pattern.
4. Continue this sequence down the length of the ladder while maintaining an athletic stance and consistent tempo.
5. Repeat the drill in the opposite direction to ensure balanced development on both sides.

The active warm-up, while essential for readiness, skill development, and injury risk reduction, serves primarily as a primer for the most important components of physical development.

Once joints are prepared, movement patterns are integrated, and the nervous system is engaged, the remainder of the training session should be devoted to developing the physical qualities that matter most: power, strength, and cardiovascular capacity.

From this point forward, the focus of this book shifts from preparation to training, outlining the why and how of developing lifelong physical capacity.

PART III

ESSENTIAL EXERCISES FOR LONGEVITY

Chapter 6

Power Training

One of the unavoidable realities of aging is that we gradually slow down. This likely does not come as a surprise; we have all watched our favorite athletes lose a step as they enter the twilight of their careers. Even at the highest levels of training and competition, no one is immune to the effects of time.

What is most surprising, though, is when this decline begins. It is not in one's 60s or 70s as many believe but often as early as age 30 (Lexell et al., 1988). As people move beyond their 20s, the ability of the brain and nervous system to send signals quickly to the muscles and for the muscles to respond with rapid, powerful contractions starts to diminish (Hunter et al., 2016). This decline in power is driven by a combination of natural aging processes and the tendency of people to participate in reduced amounts and intensities of exercise and physical activity as they age.

One key factor is the loss of type II muscle fibers, the fast-twitch fibers responsible for explosive, high-force movements. During the aging process, these fibers decrease in number and size and are often replaced by slower, more endurance-oriented type I fibers (Deschenes et al., 2004; Brunner et al., 2007). At the same time, the neurological connection between the brain and muscles weakens. This includes a reduction in the number of spinal motor neurons, along with slower firing rates and less efficient signaling from the central nervous system (Klass et al., 2008; Aagaard et al., 2010). The result is a delayed and less forceful muscular response.

Finally, age-related changes in tendon structure also play a role. Tendons lose their natural stiffness and elasticity, reducing their ability to act as spring-like power amplifiers during quick, explosive movements (Stenroth et al., 2012; Fukashiro et al., 2006). This not only affects athletic performance but also everyday tasks that require quick movements, leaving people more susceptible to injury.

This decline in neuromuscular power is subtle at first, but over time it becomes one of the most significant factors in decreased physical performance and increased injury risk.

Fortunately, appropriately prescribed power training exercise can significantly reduce the rate of decline of muscular power that comes with age. Power training methods are often associated with athletic performance training, leading them to be overlooked and even intentionally avoided by average gymgoers who often view these methods as risky or unnecessary in their training programs. Unfortunately, the average coach and training client often do not realize how essential and effective power training is for the adult population.

As people age, a lack of exercise can make them vulnerable to sarcopenia, a condition characterized by the loss of muscle mass and strength. Even more concerning is that muscular power—the ability to exert force quickly—declines at nearly twice the rate of muscular strength and mass. Freitas and colleagues (2024) introduced the term *powerpenia* to describe the specific age-related loss of muscular power, distinguishing it from sarcopenia, which primarily focuses on declines in muscle mass and strength. Figure 6.1 demonstrates the onset and rate of decline of muscle power, strength, and mass with age.

Longitudinal studies indicate that muscular strength typically decreases by about 1 to 2 percent each year. In contrast, muscular power, particularly in untrained individuals, can drop by as much as 3.5 percent annually (Marsh et al., 2009). This rapid decline in power can severely impact the ability to engage in recreational activities, carry out daily living tasks, maintain balance, and enjoy overall quality of life during the aging process.

In a cross-sectional analysis of over 3,000 adults aged 65 and older, Dos Santos and colleagues (2017) found that while low muscle mass alone was associated with a 1.6-times increased risk of losing physical independence, the combination

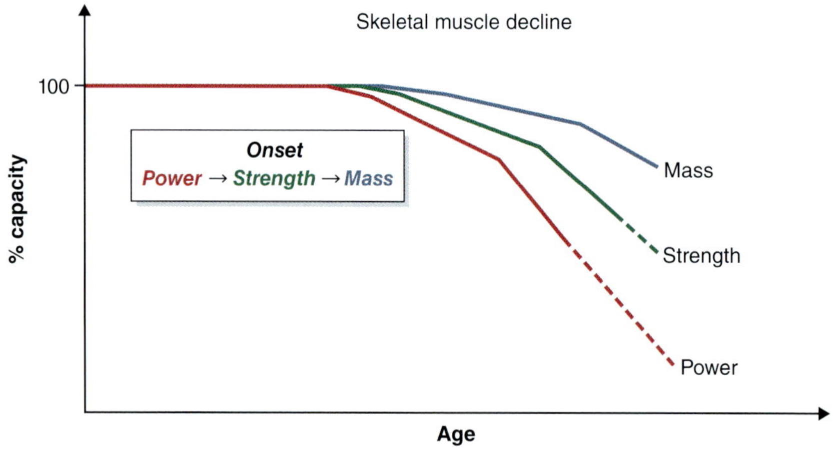

Figure 6.1 The onset and rate of decline of muscle power, strength, and mass with age.

of low muscle mass and poor muscle function—as measured by a 30-second sit-to-stand test—raised that risk dramatically to 12.3 times by the age of 90. This distinction highlights a critical point: Maintaining neuromuscular function—the ability to generate force quickly, efficiently, and with coordination—is far more predictive of long-term independence than muscle mass alone.

Recent research reinforces this point even further, showing that muscular power may be one of the strongest predictors of survival. In a study with nearly 4,000 men and women aged 46-75, those with the lowest levels of muscular power had a five- to sevenfold greater risk of mortality compared with those with the highest levels—an effect far stronger than that seen with muscular strength (Araújo, et al. 2005). In other words, it is not just how much force you can produce, but how quickly you can produce it that matters most.

To preserve this neuromuscular power as we age, it is not enough to simply stay active. Walking and general physical activity provide meaningful health benefits, but they do not deliver the focused, high-force stimulus required to maintain power output.

In a longitudinal study of adults aged 70 to 85, researchers compared healthy, high-functioning older adults with peers who had mobility limitations and followed them for nearly three years. Despite clear differences in physical function, both groups experienced nearly identical declines in lower body power over time (Reid et al., 2014). Notably, the healthy older adults maintained muscle mass and strength throughout the study yet still lost power, highlighting that preserving muscle mass alone is not sufficient to protect against age-related, neurological declines in power.

What aging adults need is not just movement—they need a structured training program that includes targeted strength and power exercises designed to keep the nervous system fast, responsive, and resilient.

ACCIDENTAL FALL RISK

Maintaining lower body power is a critical factor in staying upright, mobile, and independent in aging adults, and reducing the risk of falling becomes critically important because one in four adults over the age of 65 experiences a fall each year (Kakara et al., 2023). Accidental falls are the leading cause of both fatal and nonfatal injuries among adults over the age of 65, contributing significantly to long-term disability and mortality in older populations (Kakara et al., 2023). Among these injuries, hip fractures are particularly devastating. After the age of 80, a person is nearly three times more likely to die within a year following a hip fracture—a stark reminder of how a single fall can initiate a rapid and often irreversible decline in health (Katsoulis et al., 2017).

One of the most effective ways to lower the risk of falling is by maintaining lower body power. Lower body power, specifically of the lower limb extensors such as the calf muscles, as well as quadriceps and hips, are the most valuable predictors in forecasting the likelihood of an accidental fall (Simpkins and Yang, 2022).

Slow, shuffling gait and difficulty coordinating foot contact significantly contribute to accidental falls among older individuals. The ability to powerfully toe off during walking and to react quickly plays a crucial role not only in preventing falls but also in preserving overall independence. However, walking speed and lower body power are not just predictors of fall risk; they also serve as broad indicators of overall health. Assessments as simple as a 10-meter walking speed test have been shown to predict functional capacity and general health status, while also being directly associated with cognitive disease, accidental falls, and even all-cause mortality (Middleton et al., 2015). In this way, walking speed offers a simple yet powerful snapshot of an individual's vitality.

A powerful and reactive nervous system plays a key role in the ability to move with intent, react quickly, and stabilize oneself during unexpected movements. Whether it is catching one's balance after tripping or simply participating in one's favorite recreational activity, the ability to generate force rapidly can mean the difference between moving with ease or recovering quickly and a serious fall. From a training perspective, this means consistently training both bilateral and unilateral lower body exercises, skips, hops, jumps, and bounds to maintain the power and coordination of the nervous system.

PROGRAMMING POWER TRAINING: NOT JUST FOR COMPETITIVE ATHLETES

Both coaches and clients often view power training as a form of exercise that should be reserved only for the young and competitive athlete, and while power training is popular among competitive athletes, it should be viewed as a required form of exercise for the aging general-population client as well.

Due to the speed and dynamic nature of power training, it undoubtedly comes with increased risk, especially for the sedentary and untrained client. However, the benefits of progressively exposing our clients to power exercises greatly outweigh the potential risks if we program and coach them intelligently.

The key to programming power exercises such as plyometrics, medicine ball throwing, and heavy-implement power drills for the aging client is to prioritize safety and intelligent progressions that match the client's functional abilities.

CLIENT ASSESSMENT: 30-SECOND SIT-TO-STAND TEST

Benefits

The 30-second sit-to-stand test is a widely used functional capacity test to measure lower body power and functional ability. The sit-to-stand test is low impact and easy to apply, making it a useful assessment for older clients to track progress and ensure they are not losing functional abilities as they age. Research has demonstrated it to be a valid and reliable measure to predict physical independence and fall risk in aging populations (Dos Santos et al., 2017; Hetherington-Rauth et al., 2022).

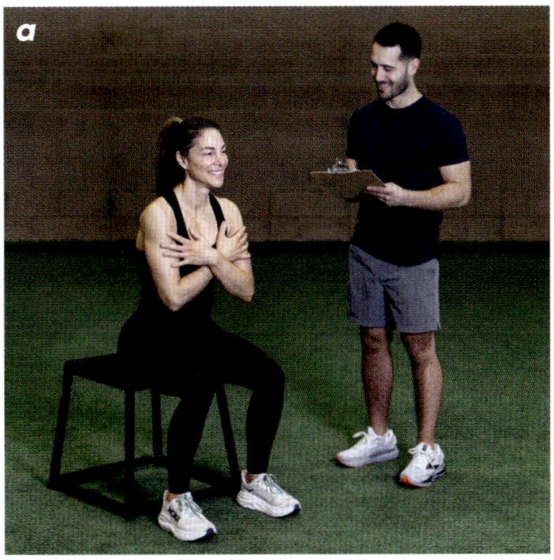
a

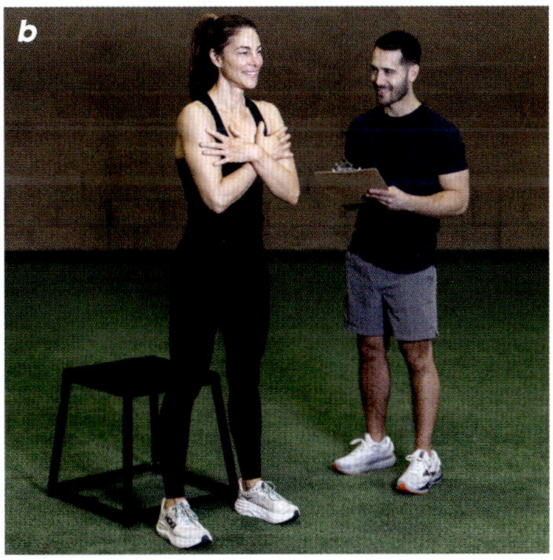
b

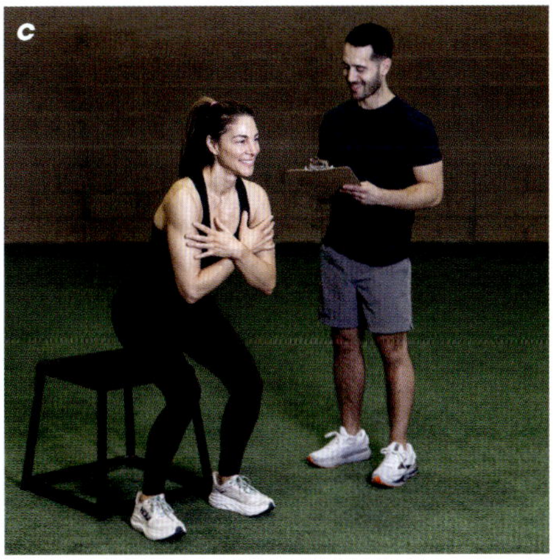
c

Instructions for the Client

1. Start by sitting on an 18-inch (46 cm) plyometric box, bench, or chair with your knees bent to 90 degrees and your feet flat on the floor, shoulder-width apart.
2. Cross your arms over your chest.
3. Once ready to begin the test, start the clock and rapidly sit and stand, touching the box or bench with the glutes without bouncing at the bottom of each repetition.
4. Count the total number of repetitions, and terminate the test after 30 seconds.
5. Table 6.1 displays the minimum recommended scores by age and sex. Scores below the listed cutoff indicate an increased risk for accidental falls and future loss of physical independence.

CLIENT ASSESSMENT: 30-SECOND SIT-TO-STAND TEST *(continued)*

Table 6.1 Minimum Recommended Scores to Avoid Accidental Falls and Future Disability in 30-Second Sit-To-Stand Test

Age range	Men	Women
60-64	Less than 14	Less than 12
65-69	Less than 12	Less than 11
70-74	Less than 12	Less than 10
75-79	Less than 11	Less than 10
80-84	Less than 10	Less than 9
85-89	Less than 8	Less than 8
90-94	Less than 7	Less than 4

Reprinted from National Center for Injury Prevention and Control (U.S.), "Assessment: 30-Second Chair Stand," *STEADI: Stopping Elderly Accidents, Deaths & Injuries* (2017).

LIGHT-IMPLEMENT POWER VERSUS HEAVY-IMPLEMENT POWER

When it comes to training for muscular power, power exercises can be organized into two distinct categories: light-implement power and heavy-implement power. This distinction is centered around the speed and weight of the implements used during the exercises.

- Light-implement power exercises such as plyometrics and medicine ball throws emphasize velocity and speed of movement. These movements improve rate of force development, reactive neuromuscular strength, and the ability to decelerate and stabilize under dynamic conditions. They are especially valuable for enhancing neuromuscular coordination, elasticity, and the ability to manage impulse forces during rapid changes in direction.
- Heavy-implement exercises such as kettlebell swings or dumbbell snatches focus more on the load end of the spectrum. These exercises challenge the body to produce maximal force in a short amount of time against resistance, improving the ability to generate high levels of force under load.

Together, light and heavy power exercises build a more complete and adaptable system, enhancing both the capacity to generate force and the speed at which that force can be applied—two qualities that are critical for fall prevention, athletic performance, and everyday functional movement. Both variations of power exercises are necessary and useful in a functional training program and should be programmed concurrently. Figure 6.2 demonstrates the speed–load continuum of light- and heavy-implement power exercises.

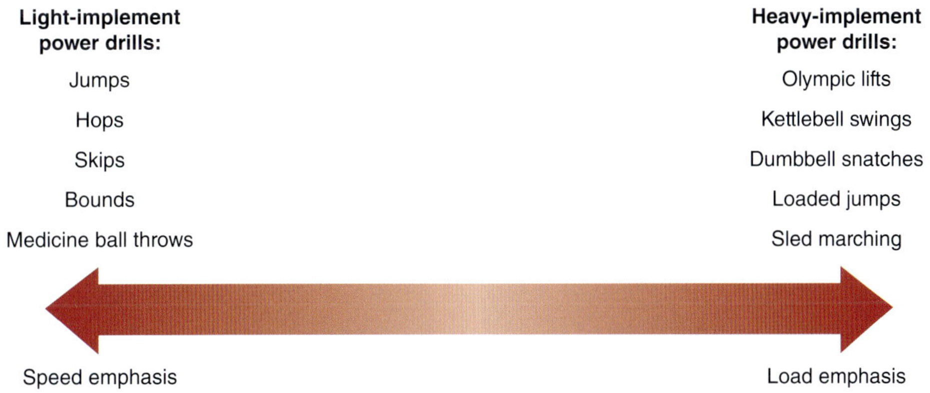

Figure 6.2 Speed–load continuum of light- and heavy-implement power exercises.

PROGRAMMING FOR POWER

When programming heavy- and light-implement power exercises, the primary goal is to enhance neurological output, thereby increasing the speed and force of muscular contractions. Explosive power training specifically targets type II muscle fibers, the motor pathways of the central nervous system, and the phosphagen energy system. While these components of the body can produce high levels of force, they are also highly susceptible to fatigue. Therefore, they should be trained in a way that prioritizes maximal force output and avoids excessive fatigue.

To prioritize speed of movement and maximize force output during training, power exercises should be prescribed before heavy strength training or conditioning work. This approach helps prevent excessive fatigue, which can limit force production capacity. Additionally, power exercises should consist of a low number of repetitions per set, typically ranging from three to five repetitions. It is also important to allow adequate rest between sets to ensure full recovery of the nervous system and the phosphagen energy system.

Plyometrics Progressions: Jump, Hop, Skip, and Bound

Plyometrics are bodyweight exercises that involve rapid contractions of the muscles aimed at improving neuromuscular power and elasticity. Plyometrics have long been programmed for competitive athletes to improve rapid force production and deceleration as a means to improve performance and reduce sport injuries; however they should also be viewed as a vital tool for the general-population client to maintain power and functionality with age.

Jumping, hopping, bounding, and skipping are the primary plyometric exercises that we will use to develop power and elasticity in this program.

Plyometric Terminology

Jump: Taking off on two legs and landing on two legs

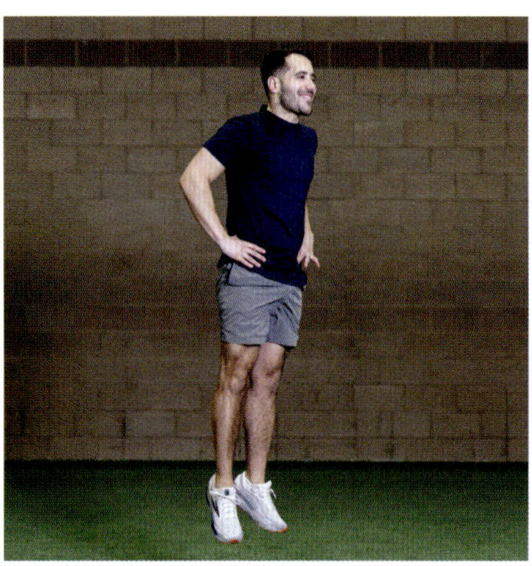

Hop: Taking off on one leg and landing on the same leg

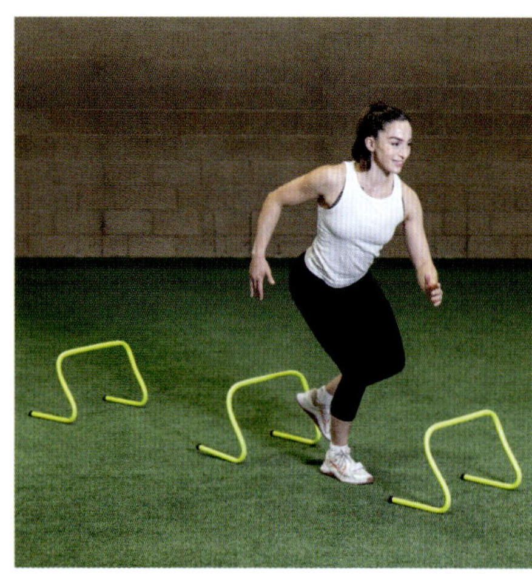

Bound: Taking off on one leg and landing on the opposite leg

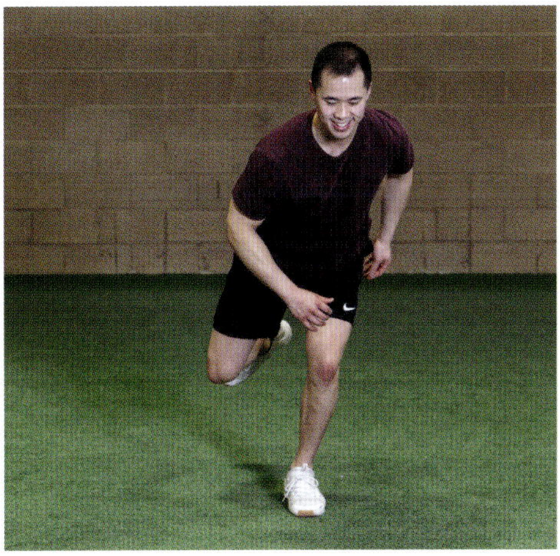

Skip: A light bouncing step from one foot to the other

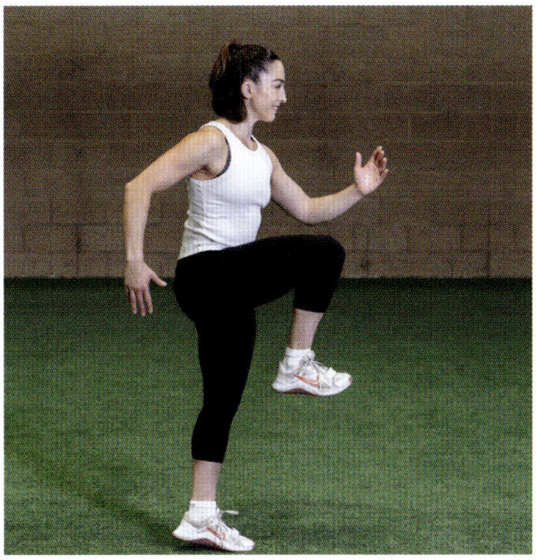

Although power development programs are often viewed as valuable tools to develop concentric force, their most valuable and often overlooked component related to injury reduction is their ability to develop eccentric deceleration and landing skills. The ability to control rapid, eccentric loading is vital to reduce accidental falls and non-contact-related lower body injuries that can occur with recreational sports or activities of daily living.

The musculoskeletal braking system can be developed effectively by programming stability focused plyometrics that emphasize quality, controlled landings to develop the muscles and the nervous system's ability to decelerate the body's forward momentum.

When programing plyometrics it is vital to first focus on developing deceleration skills before progressing to more advanced rapid and elastic focused plyometric drills. First introduce clients to low-speed and low-force plyometrics that cause minimal stress to the tendons and joint and then progressively move toward variations that introduce greater speed and force into the movement. It is recommended to start beginner clients with jumping and bounding variations that require less force and complexity before introducing hopping variations that will be more challenging. Following this progression will ensure safety and reduce the chances of injury during training. Progress all plyometric exercise variations in the following order to progressively increase force, tendon stress, and neuromuscular demand.

Regressions: Box jumping and hopping

Progression 1: Stick landings

Progression 2: Mini bounce

Progression 3: Continuous

Box Jumping and Hopping

Box jumping and hopping are useful plyometric variations that can be used to regress from hurdle hopping and jumping or to introduce plyometric exercises for clients who require less impact force. Jumping or hopping onto an elevated surface, as in a box jump, reduces the overall distance the client's body falls before landing. Less downward acceleration occurs, resulting in a decrease in the velocity at the point of impact. This results in a lower ground reaction force on landing, which means less stress on the joints and connective tissues compared to landing on the ground from the same height.

Stick Landings

Stick-focused landings are slower-speed plyometrics that focus on the deceleration and landing component of the exercise. On each repetition we should cue the client to "stick" and hold the landing position for one to two seconds. Starting with slower-speed, deceleration-focused plyometrics allow us to introduce dynamic jumping, hopping, and bounding drills with low-impact forces and less tendon stress, making them safer and more accessible to the beginner client. It is recommended to stay with these basic plyometrics for an extended period of time to ensure the client can fully adapt before advancing to higher-speed progressions.

Mini-Bounce Plyometrics

Following stick-focused landings, we should move to mini-bounce variations as a means to begin introducing more elasticity and rhythm to the plyometric progressions. On mini-bounce progressions we will add a small pogo-style hop in between each repetition of jump hop or bound. This variation will progressively increase the tendon stress and speed, helping the client to develop more elasticity and springiness in the feet, calves, and Achilles tendons. A risk-versus-reward calculation should be made as it relates to fitness for longevity, and as such, many older clients may not need to progress beyond this variation.

Continuous Plyometrics

Continuous plyometrics are an advanced form of plyometric training where we instruct the client to minimize ground contact time as much as possible between every repetition of jump, hop, and bound. This progression will introduce the highest levels of force, speed, and tendon stress, making it an effective tool for improving power and elasticity while carrying the highest risk for injury. This progression should be reserved for advanced trainees who have mastered all three previous variations.

HURDLE JUMP AND STICK

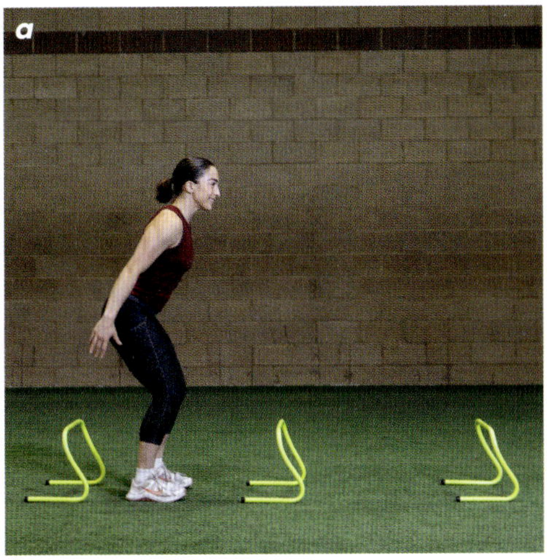

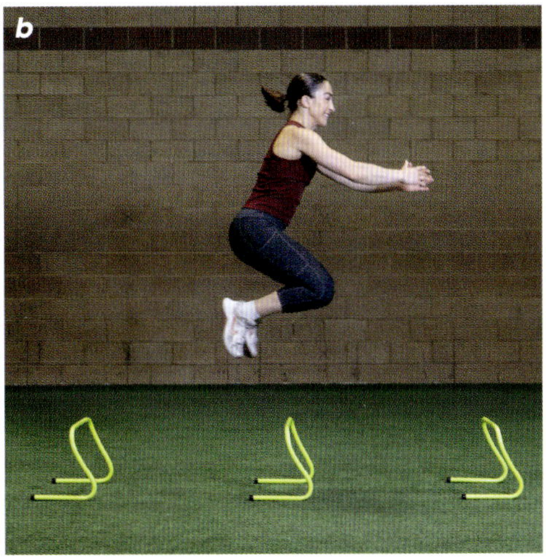

Benefits

The hurdle jump and stick develops bilateral force production and eccentric landing skills in the feet, calves, quads, and hips.

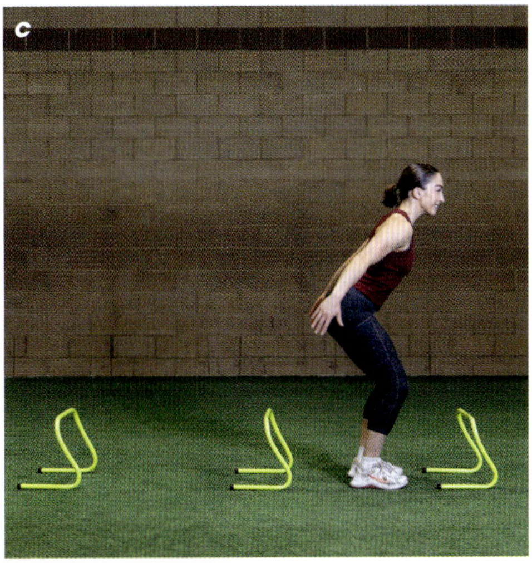

Instructions for the Client

1. Organize a set of hurdles that you feel comfortable jumping over in a straight line, placing them roughly 3 feet (0.9 m) apart.
2. Stand in an athletic position with your feet shoulder-width apart, knees bent, and toes facing straight ahead.
3. Jump over the first hurdle by driving your arms upward, pushing forcefully into the ground, and extending your hips, knees, and ankles.
4. Land softly on the other side of the hurdle, sinking into your hips, knees, and ankles to absorb the landing.
5. Complete the prescribed number of repetitions over the remaining hurdles.

HURDLE JUMP AND STICK *(continued)*

Variations

Regression: Box Jump

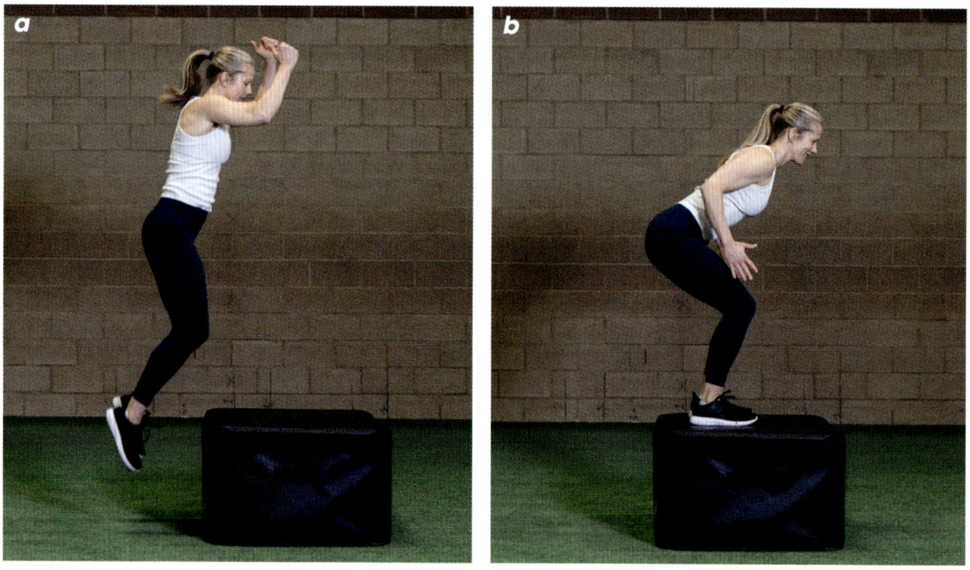

The box jump regression allows clients to learn proper takeoff and landing mechanics while reducing impact forces on the joints and connective tissues. The client jumps onto a box of appropriate height and is cued to land softly and "stick" the landing, holding a stable athletic position for one to two seconds before stepping down.

Progression 1: Hurdle Jump With Mini Bounce

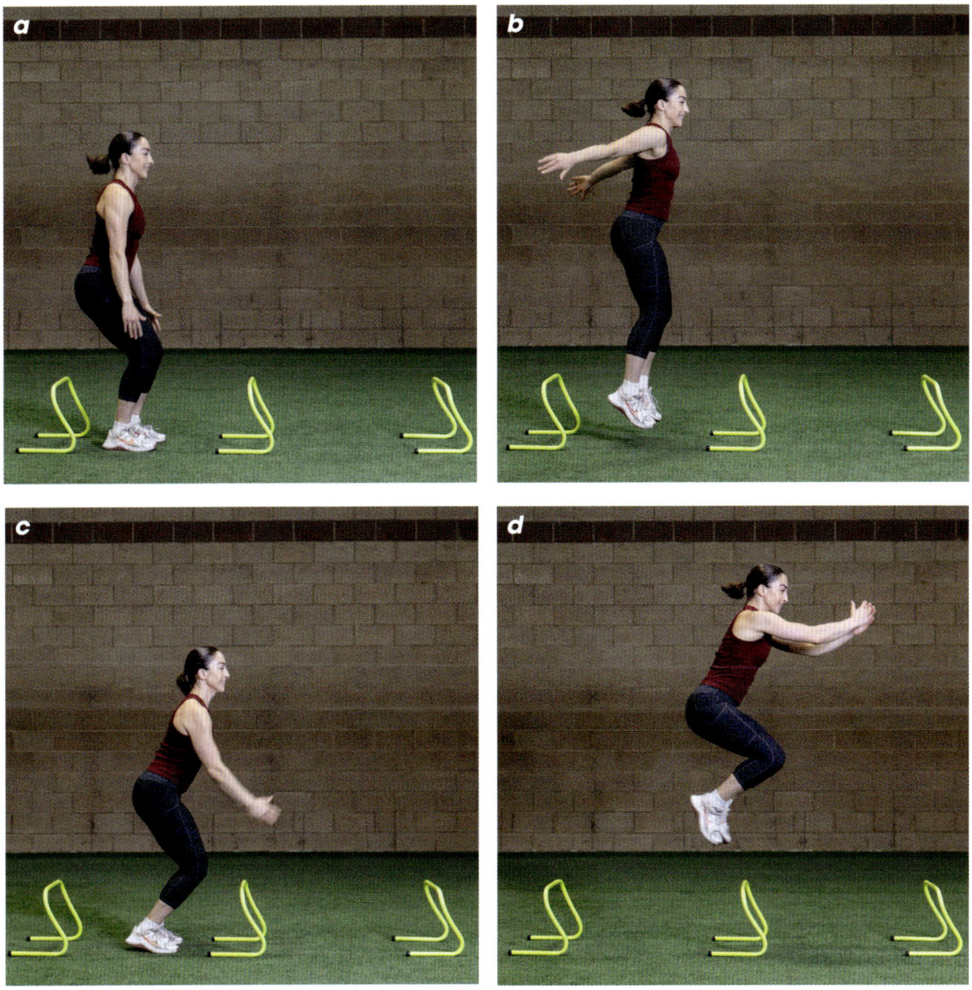

This mini-bounce progression will introduce higher levels of force and speed into the movement to develop elasticity in the foot and lower leg. In this variation, the client performs a hurdle jump and immediately performs a small, controlled, pogo-style bounce before the next repetition. The mini bounce introduces greater speed and elastic demand while still allowing the client to maintain rhythm and control between jumps.

PLYOMETRICS

HURDLE JUMP AND STICK *(continued)*

Progression 2: Continuous Hurdle Jumps

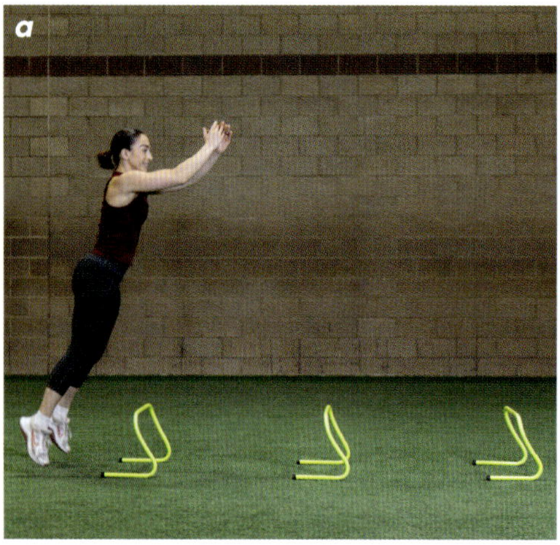

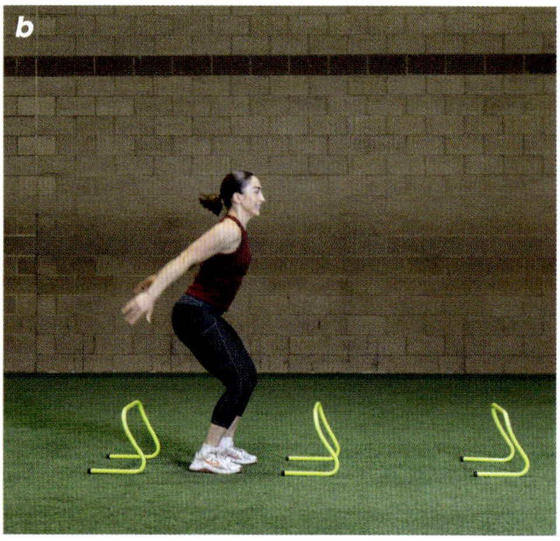

Continuous hurdle jumps are performed by repeatedly jumping over the hurdles with minimal ground contact time between repetitions. The client is cued to stay tall, land softly, and transition quickly from landing to takeoff, emphasizing reactive strength and elastic efficiency. This variation places the highest demands on the neuromuscular and tendon systems and should be reserved for advanced trainees.

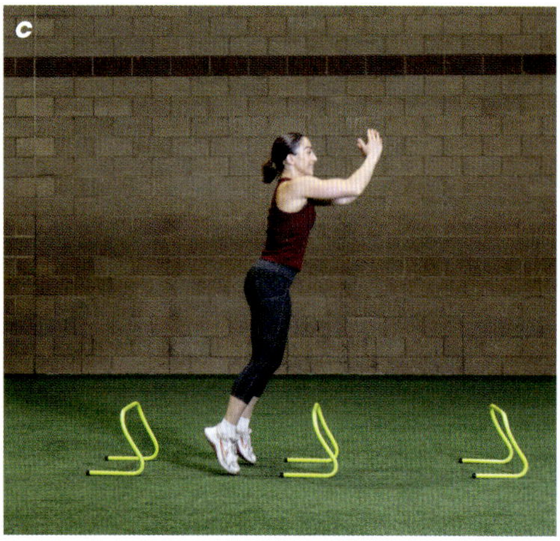

45-DEGREE BOUND AND STICK

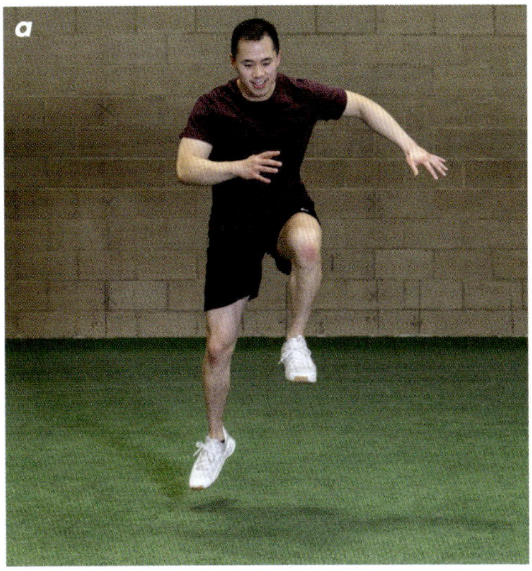

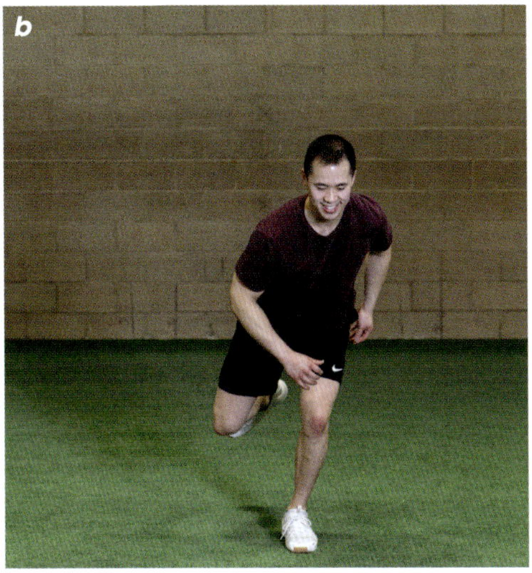

Benefits

Bounding is a valuable exercise to develop unilateral power in the hips, quadriceps, and lower legs. It is recommended to use bounding as an introductory unilateral plyometric exercise, because it requires less coordination and impact force than hopping.

Instructions for the Client

1. Begin in a single-leg athletic position with a slight bend in the knee, ankle, and hip.
2. Bound forward at a 45-degree angle toward the midline by pushing forcefully into the ground.
3. Land softly on the opposite leg in a single-leg athletic position by sinking down into the ankle, knee, and hip and centering yourself over your foot.
4. Hold the position for 2 seconds before repeating on the opposite side.
5. Repeat for the prescribed number of repetitions.

45-DEGREE BOUND AND STICK *(continued)*

Variations

Regression: Lateral Bound and Stick

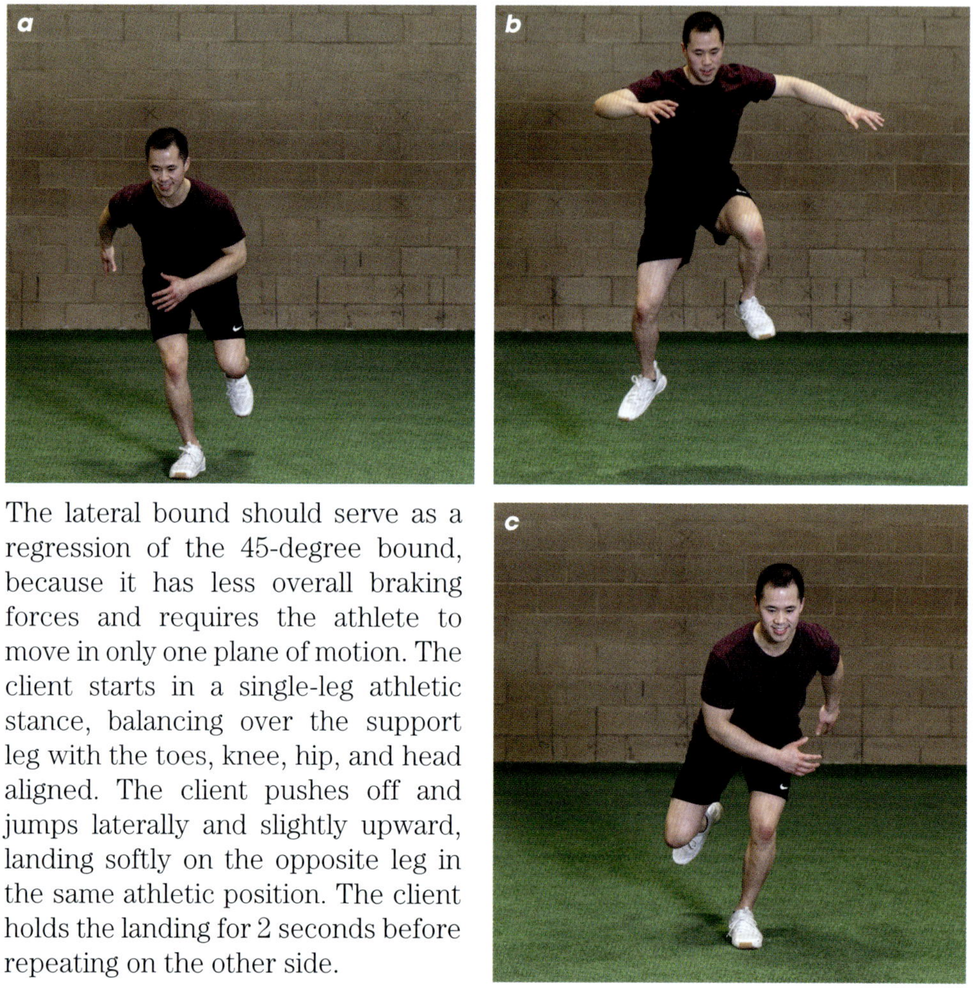

The lateral bound should serve as a regression of the 45-degree bound, because it has less overall braking forces and requires the athlete to move in only one plane of motion. The client starts in a single-leg athletic stance, balancing over the support leg with the toes, knee, hip, and head aligned. The client pushes off and jumps laterally and slightly upward, landing softly on the opposite leg in the same athletic position. The client holds the landing for 2 seconds before repeating on the other side.

Progression 1: 45-Degree Bound With a Mini Bounce

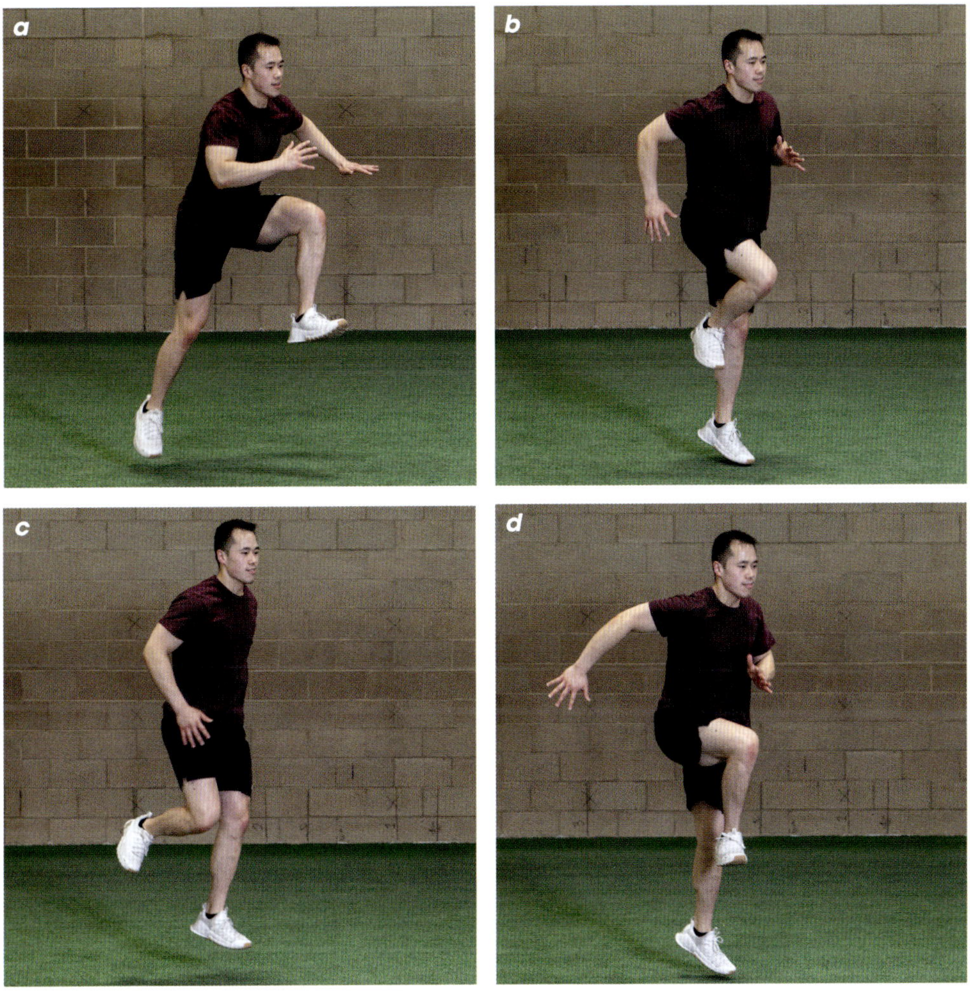

This mini-bounce progression introduces higher levels of force and speed into the movement to develop elasticity in the foot and lower leg. From an athletic stance, the client bounds forward and laterally at roughly a 45-degree angle, landing on the opposite leg. On landing, the client immediately performs a small pogo-style mini bounce before the next repetition.

45-DEGREE BOUND AND STICK *(continued)*

Progression 2: Continuous 45-Degree Bounds

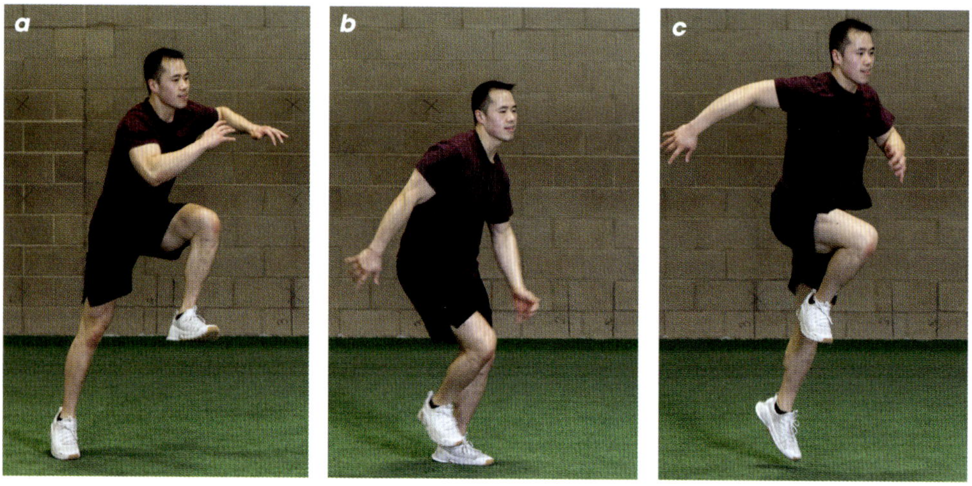

Continuous 45-degree bounds introduce the highest levels of force into the movement and should be reserved for more advanced trainees. The client performs repeated bounds forward and laterally at roughly a 45-degree angle, minimizing ground contact time between landings. Emphasize smooth, rhythmic transitions from landing to takeoff.

LINEAR HURDLE HOP AND STICK

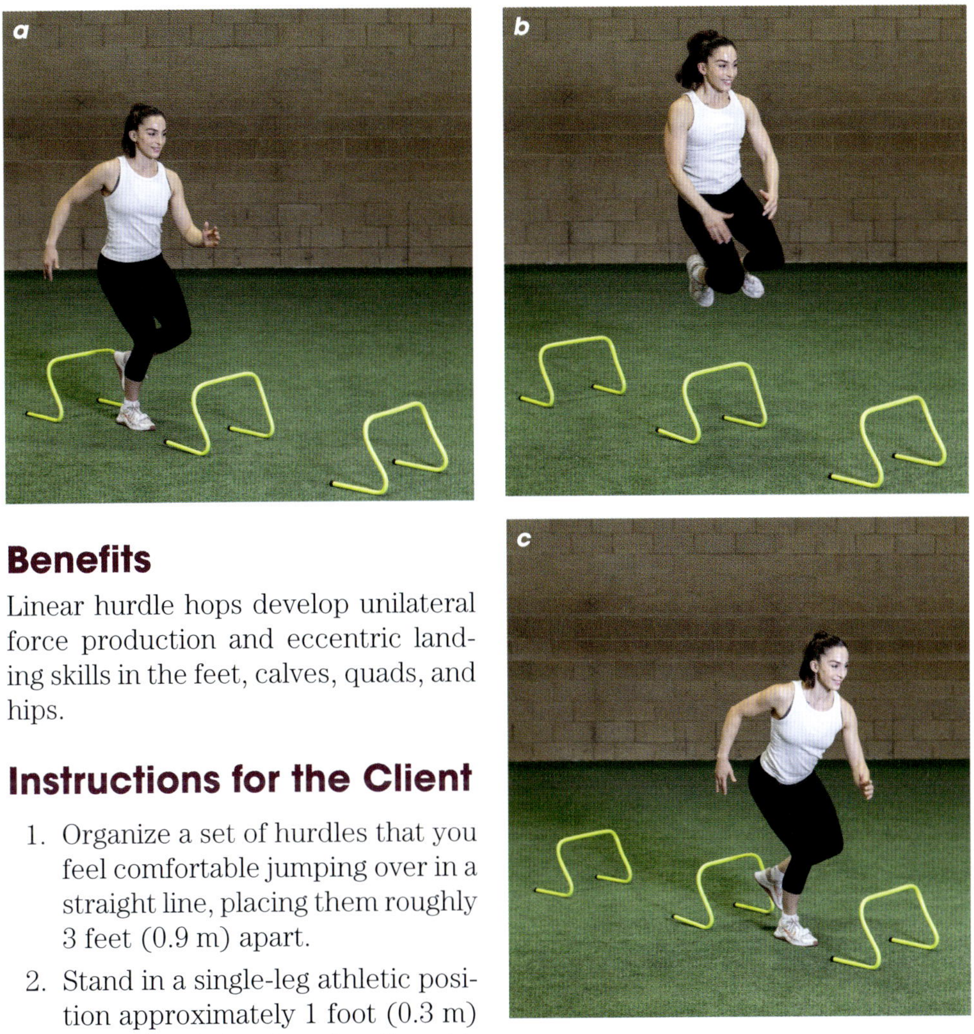

Benefits

Linear hurdle hops develop unilateral force production and eccentric landing skills in the feet, calves, quads, and hips.

Instructions for the Client

1. Organize a set of hurdles that you feel comfortable jumping over in a straight line, placing them roughly 3 feet (0.9 m) apart.
2. Stand in a single-leg athletic position approximately 1 foot (0.3 m) in front of the first hurdle with your knee and hip slightly flexed.
3. Hop over the first hurdle by forcefully pushing into the ground and extending your hips, knees, and ankles.
4. Land softly on the other side of the hurdle on the same leg, sinking into your hips, knees, and ankles to absorb the landing.
5. Complete the prescribed number of repetitions over the remaining hurdles. Repeat on the opposite leg.

LINEAR HURDLE HOP AND STICK *(continued)*

Variations

Regression: Single-Leg Box Hop

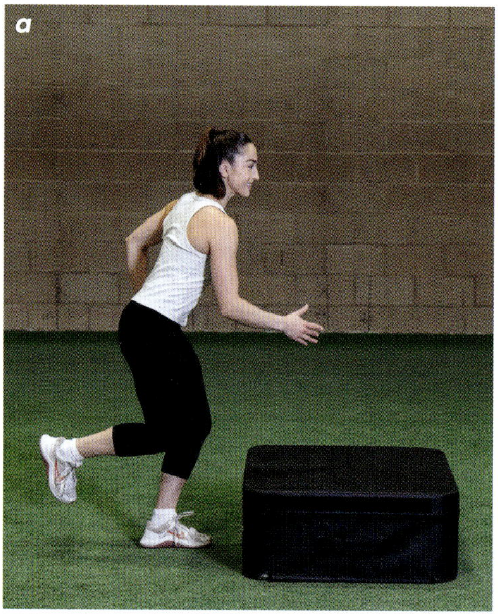

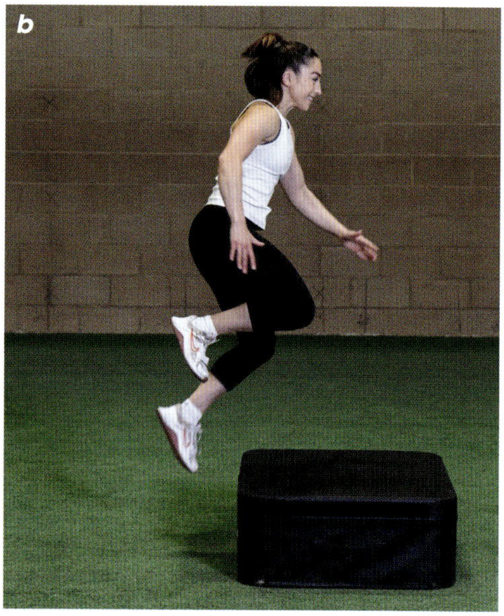

The box-hop regressions help clients learn proper landing mechanics with less impact force and stress on the tendons and joints.

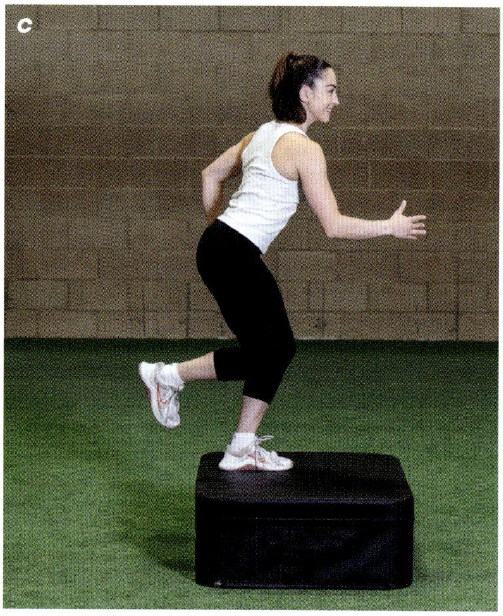

Progression 1: Hurdle Hop With Mini Bounce

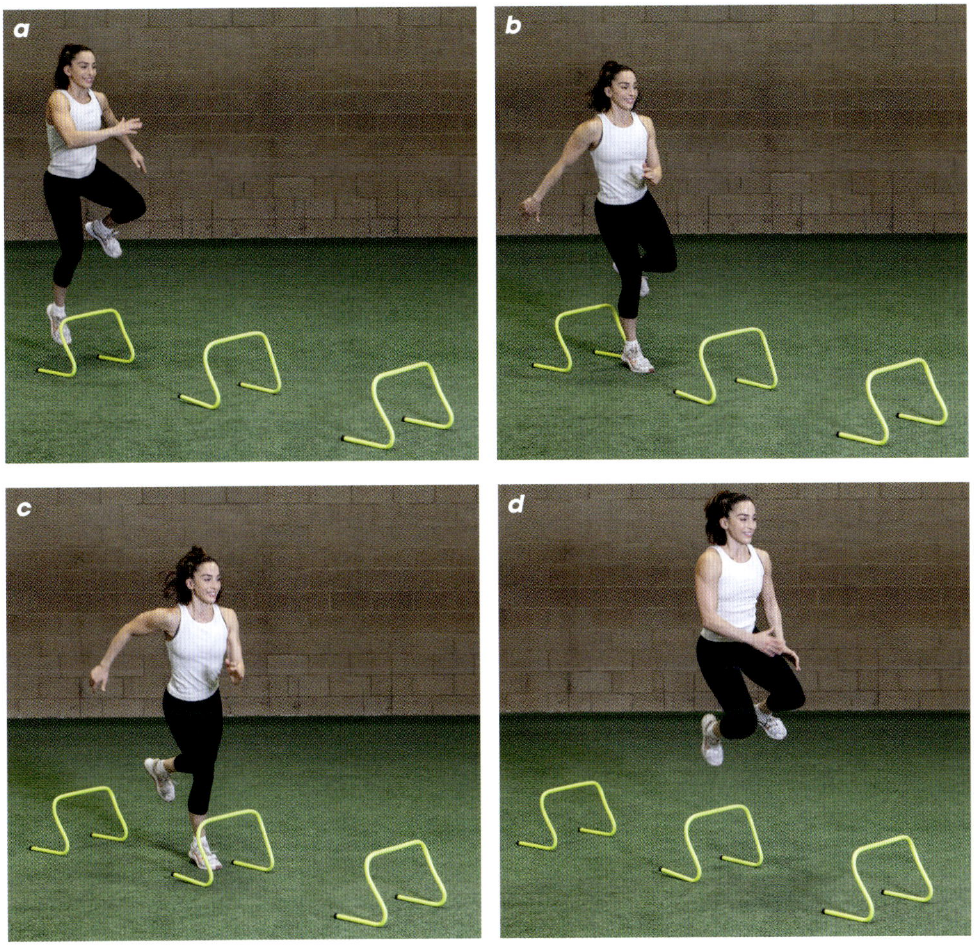

This mini-bounce progression introduce higher levels of force and speed into the movement to develop elasticity in the foot and lower leg.

LINEAR HURDLE HOP AND STICK *(continued)*

Progression 2: Continuous Hurdle Hops

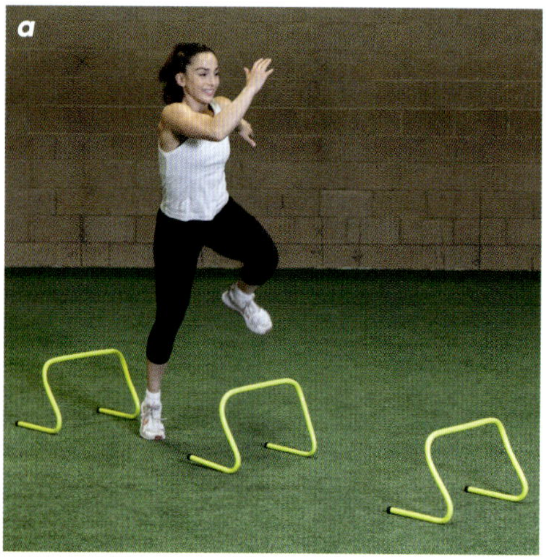

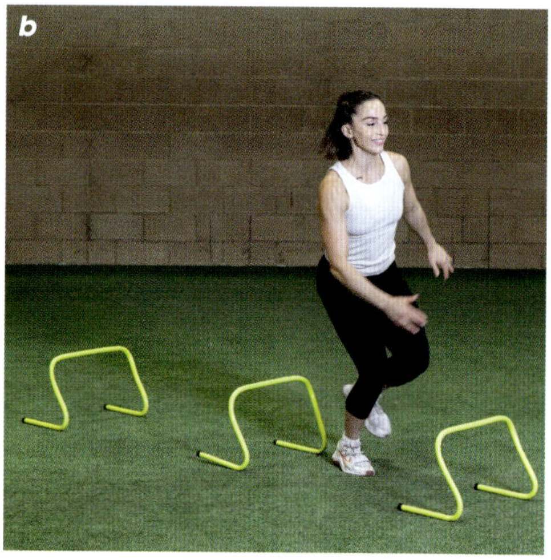

Continuous hop progressions introduce the highest levels of force into the movement and should be reserved for more advanced trainees.

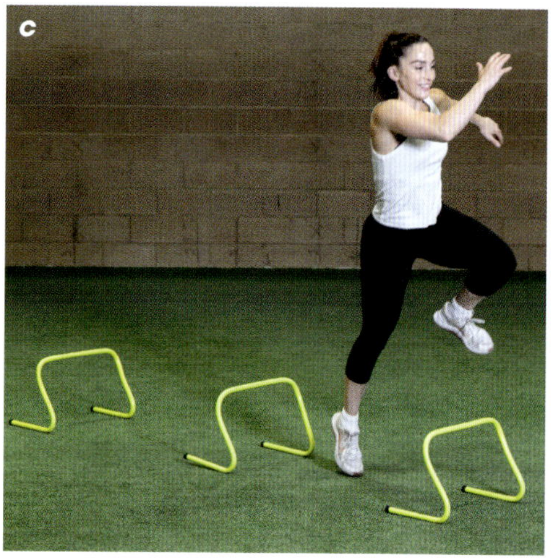

MEDIAL AND LATERAL HURDLE HOP AND STICK

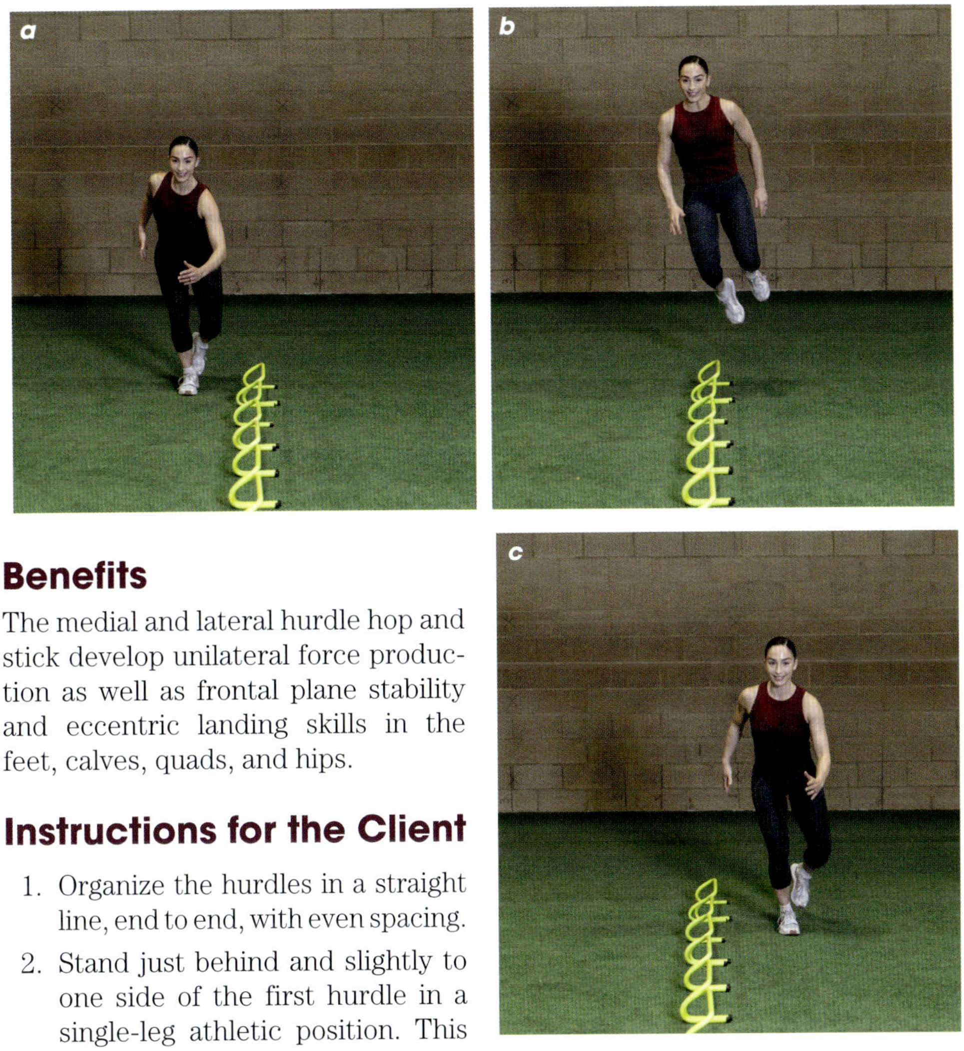

Benefits

The medial and lateral hurdle hop and stick develop unilateral force production as well as frontal plane stability and eccentric landing skills in the feet, calves, quads, and hips.

Instructions for the Client

1. Organize the hurdles in a straight line, end to end, with even spacing.
2. Stand just behind and slightly to one side of the first hurdle in a single-leg athletic position. This will be your working leg.
3. Hop forward and diagonally over the first hurdle on the same leg, pushing forcefully through the foot by extending the hip, knee, and ankle.
4. Land softly on the same leg on the opposite side of the hurdle, sinking into the hip, knee, and ankle to absorb the landing and briefly "stick" the position.
5. Continue hopping forward down the line on the same leg, alternating sides of the hurdles in a zig-zag pattern (medial to lateral, then lateral to medial) with each repetition.
6. Complete the prescribed number of hops, then repeat the drill using the opposite leg.

MEDIAL AND LATERAL HURDLE HOP AND STICK *(continued)*

Variations

Regression: Single-Leg Medial and Lateral Line Hop

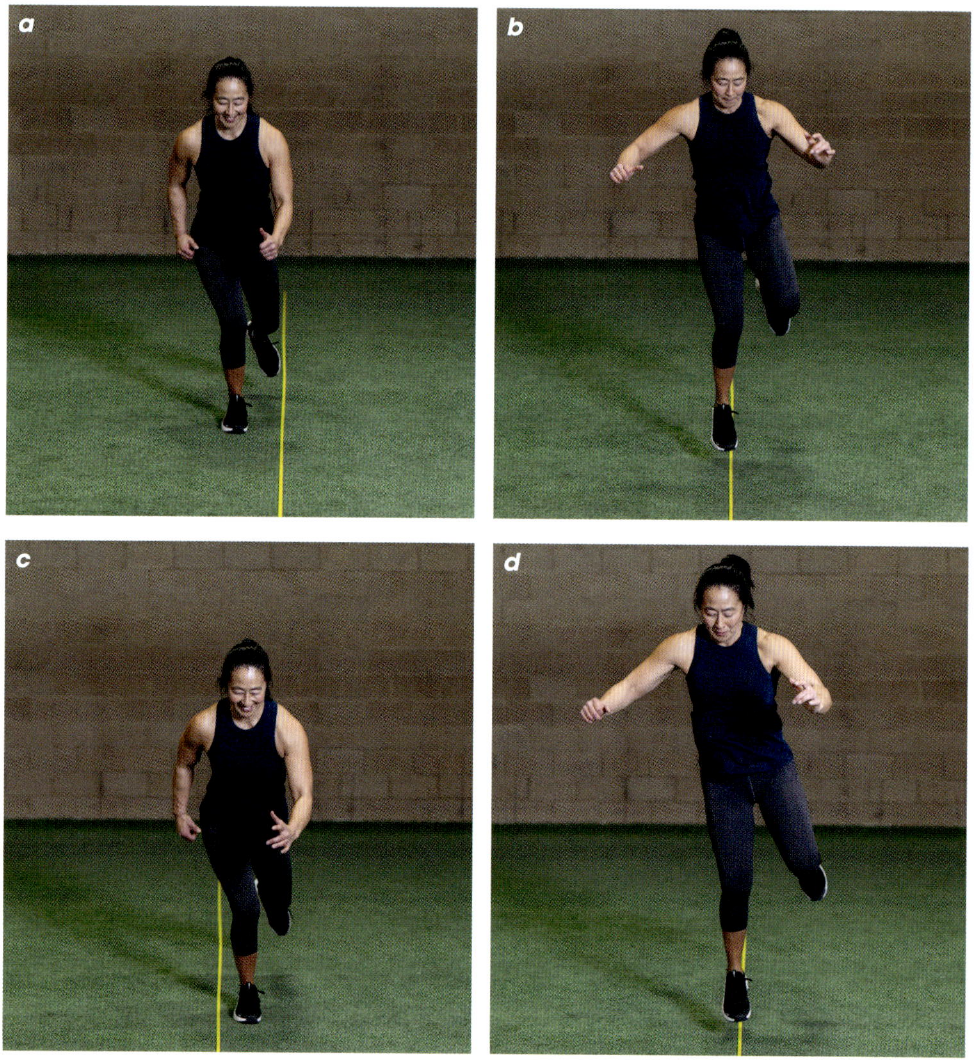

This regression introduces single-leg hopping mechanics with reduced impact by using a line or strip of tape on the ground instead of hurdles. The client hops side to side over the line on the same leg, landing softly and briefly "sticking" each landing to reinforce balance, alignment, and controlled deceleration with minimal stress on the joints and tendons.

Progression 1: Hurdle Medial and Lateral Hop With Mini Bounce

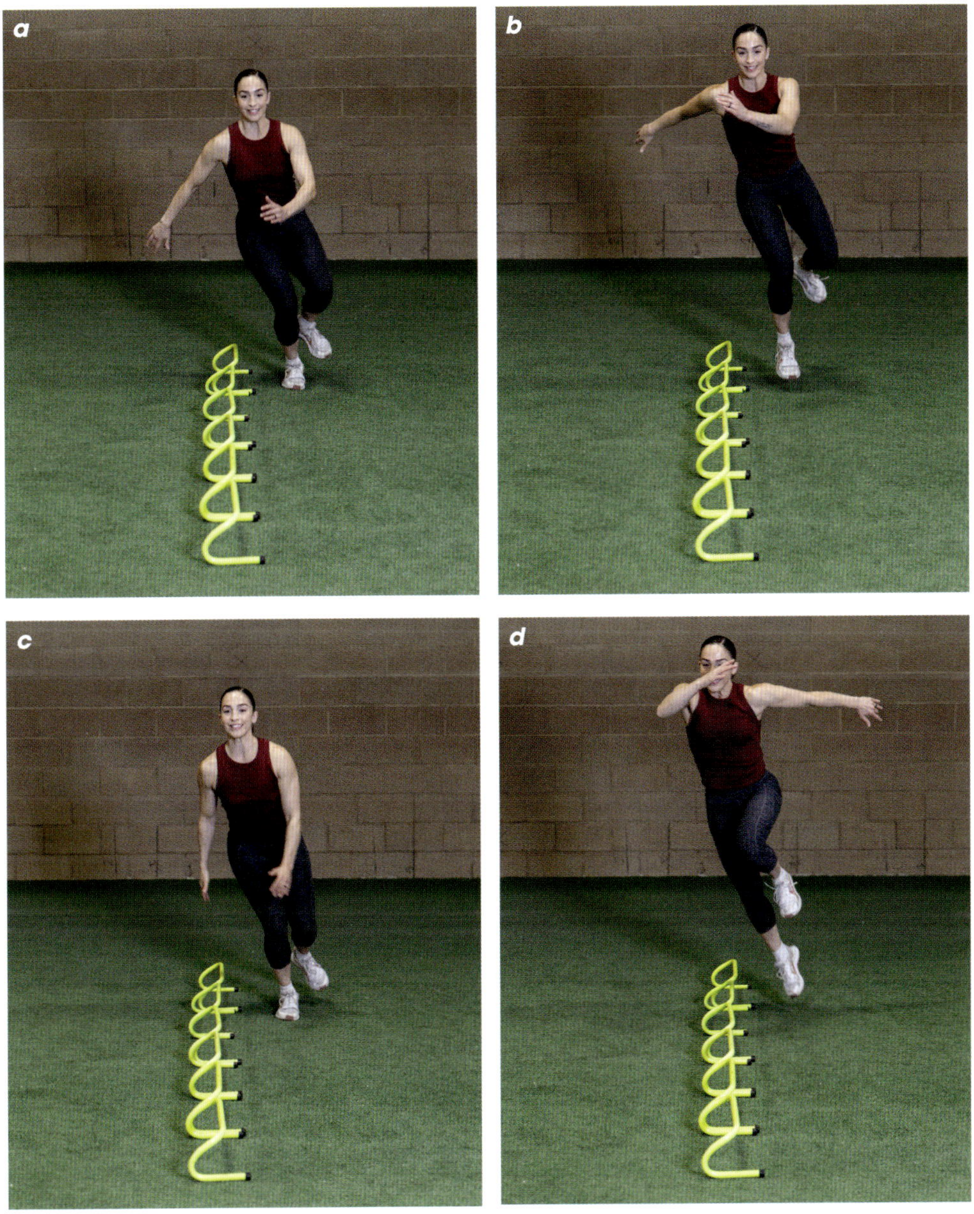

In this variation, the client hops medially and laterally over a low hurdle on the same leg. On landing, immediately perform a small pogo-style mini bounce before the next repetition. The mini bounce increases speed and elastic demand in the foot, calf, and Achilles while still allowing the client to maintain rhythm and control.

MEDIAL AND LATERAL HURDLE HOP AND STICK *(continued)*

Progression 2: Continuous Medial and Lateral Hurdle Hops

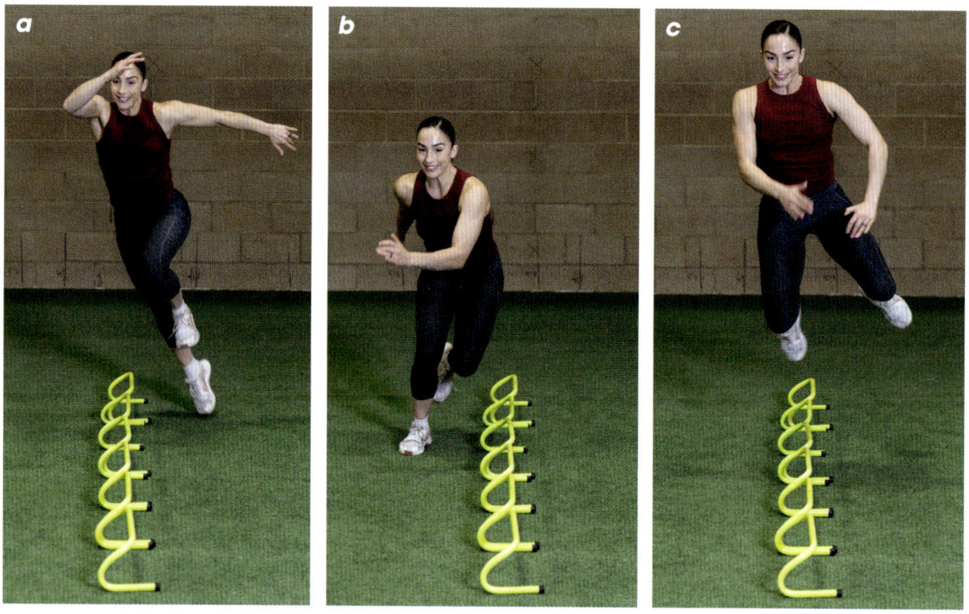

Continuous hurdle hops are performed by repeatedly hopping back and forth over the hurdle on the same leg with minimal ground contact time between repetitions. This progression places the greatest demands on reactive strength, elastic efficiency, and frontal-plane stability and should be reserved for advanced trainees.

POWER SKIP

Benefits

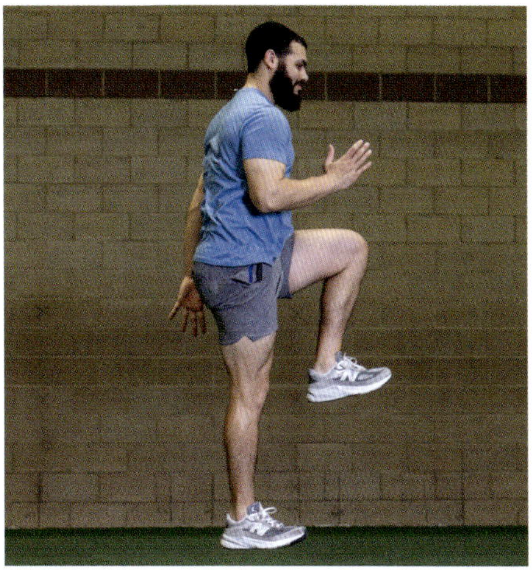

Power skipping is a useful exercise to develop forceful hip extension and plantar flexion as well as contralateral arm and leg coordination. Skipping is particularly valuable for untrained clients because it exposes the body to less total force and requires less coordination than hopping while still developing the powerful lower body extension that translates directly to gait patterning.

Instructions for the Client

1. Stand tall with your arms by your side and your feet hip-width apart.
2. Begin the movement by explosively pushing off of your left foot while simultaneously driving your right knee upward as you move forward. At the same time, drive your left arm up and forward so your arms and legs move reciprocally.
3. Land softly on your left foot and repeat on the opposite side by forcefully pushing downward with your right foot and driving your left knee upward.
4. Focus on producing as much height and propulsion as possible with each skip while maintaining proper posture and coordination.
5. Repeat for the prescribed distance or repetitions.

Variation

Regression: A-Skip

A-skips work on the skipping pattern with less impact on the muscles, joints, and tendons than power skips. The emphasis is on rhythm, coordination, posture, and proper knee drive rather than generating maximal force and height with each skip.

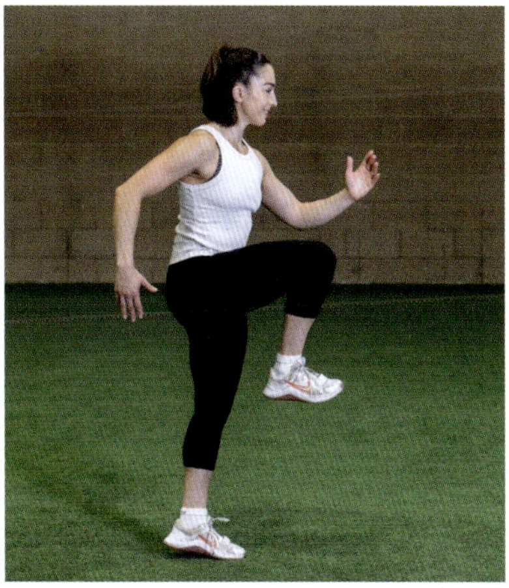

Medicine Ball Throws

Just as plyometric drills can be used for lower body power development, medicine ball drills are safe and effective tools to develop power in trunk and upper body musculature. Medicine ball drills should be performed with light- to moderate-load (2-10 lb [0.9-4.5 kg]) soft, nonbouncing medicine balls to avoid potential injury (see figure 6.3). High-velocity throwing with light medicine balls will help to develop the nervous system and promote high-threshold motor unit recruitment to develop type II muscle fibers. It is recommended to use a variety of throwing variations such as side tosses, overhead throws, chest passes, slams, and shot put throws to develop power in multiple planes of motion and muscles groups.

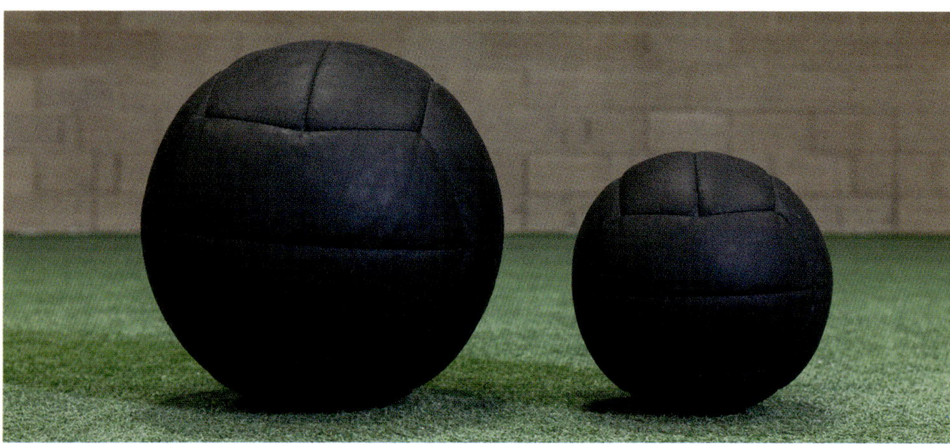

Figure 6.3 Soft, nonbouncing medicine balls designed to minimize rebound and impact forces during training.

STANDING MEDICINE BALL CHEST PASS

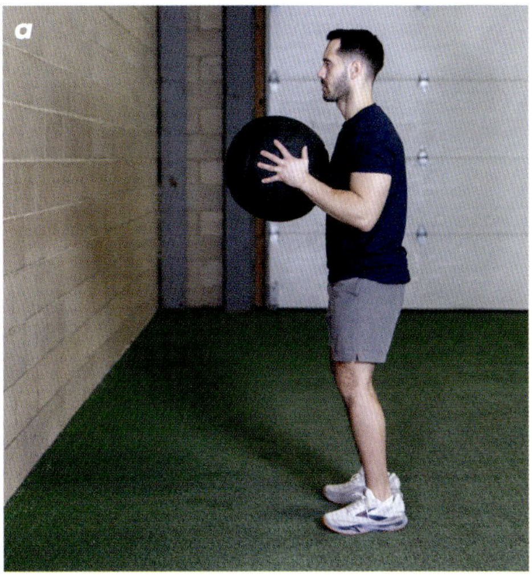

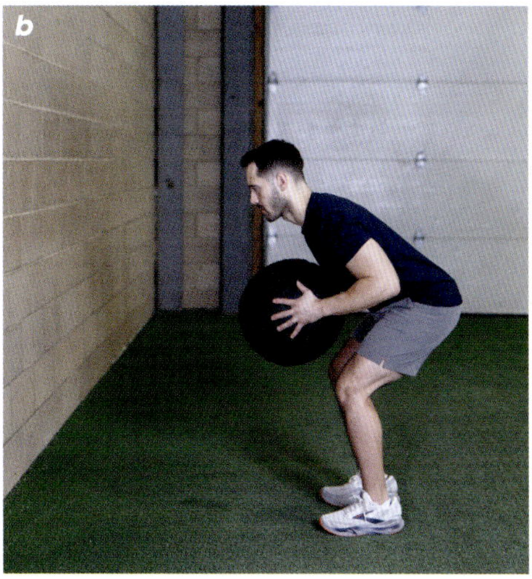

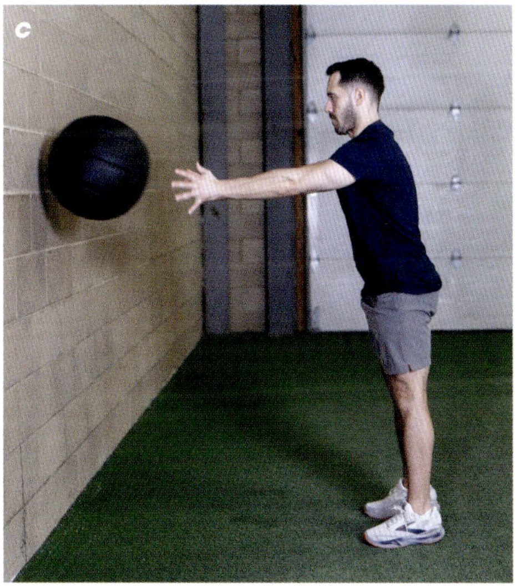

Benefits

The medicine ball chest pass can be used to develop explosive power in the chest and arm musculature.

Instructions for the Client

1. Begin by standing tall with your feet shoulder-width apart roughly 4 feet (1.2 m) from a wall.
2. Holding a 4- to 8-pound (1.8-3.6 kg) medicine ball at your chest, hinge backward into your hips to generate momentum.
3. Forcefully reverse the direction, standing up tall and extending your hips and knees while pushing the ball forward as fast as possible toward the wall.
4. Catch the ball as it bounces off the wall and repeat the exercise for the prescribed number of repetitions.

STANDING MEDICINE BALL CHEST PASS *(continued)*

Variations

Regression: Tall-Kneeling Medicine Ball Chest Pass

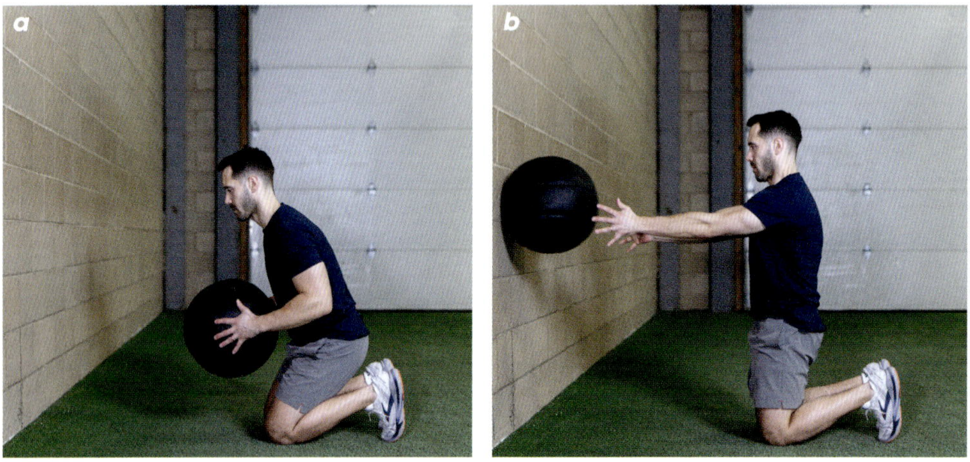

Performing the medicine ball chest pass from a tall kneeling position is an easier variation that produces less force and requires less full body coordination.

Progression: Two-Point Sprint Start Chest Pass

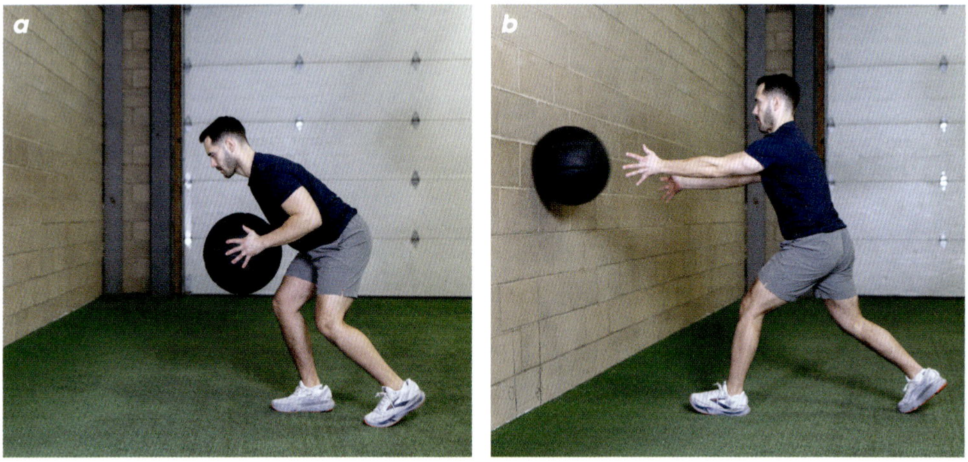

The two-point sprint start chest pass is a progression that performs the chest pass from a sprint start position, turning it into a full-body exercise that develops lower-body power in the hips, quadriceps, and calves.

STANDING MEDICINE BALL SIDE TOSS

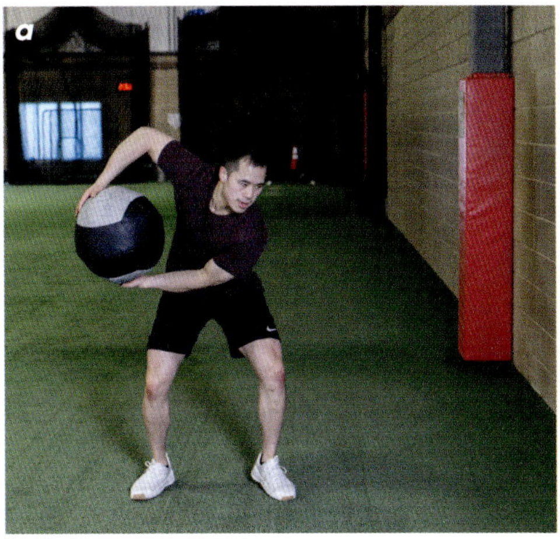

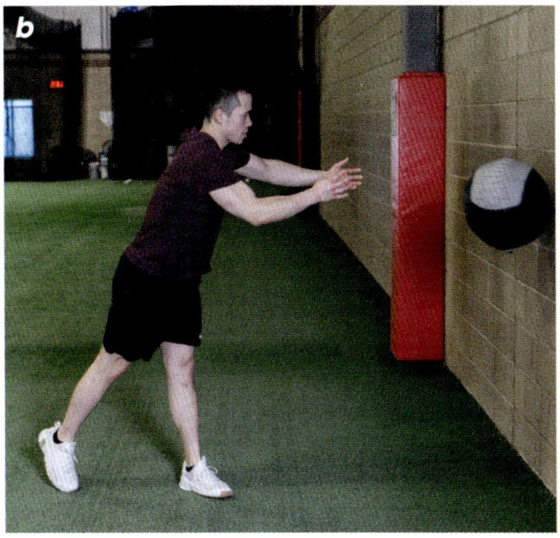

Benefits

The standing medicine ball side toss can be used to develop rotational power in the trunk musculature for both recreational activities as well as activities of daily living.

Instructions for the Client

1. Begin standing in an athletic position approximately 3 feet (0.9 m) from a wall, with the wall positioned directly to your side.
2. Hold a 4- to 8-pound (1.8-3.6 kg) medicine ball at your side in front of the outside hip.
3. Initiate the movement by rotating the hips and torso toward the wall, allowing the ball to travel across the body.
4. Release the ball with a scooping motion, throwing it into the wall at approximately waist height. The outside hand stays on top of the ball with the elbow high, while the inside hand supports the bottom of the ball to guide the upward path of the throw.
5. Catch the ball off the wall, reset to the starting position, and repeat for the prescribed number of repetitions.
6. Repeat on the opposite side.

STANDING MEDICINE BALL SIDE TOSS *(continued)*

Variations

Regression: Half-Kneeling Medicine Ball Side Toss

The half-kneeling medicine ball side toss is a regression from the standing variation that helps to develop trunk and hip stability in the half-kneeling position.

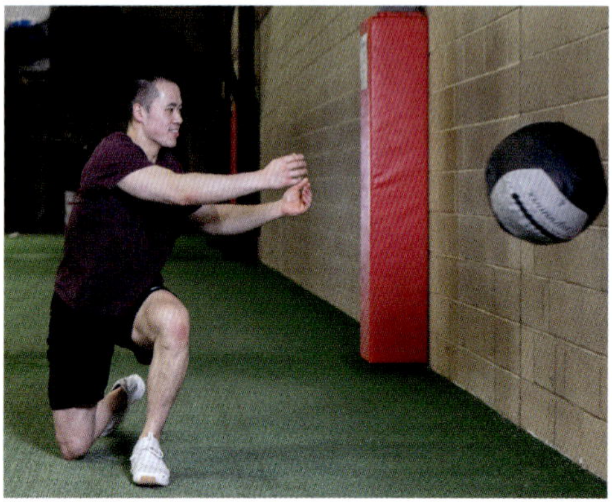

Progression: Medicine Ball Shuffle Side Toss

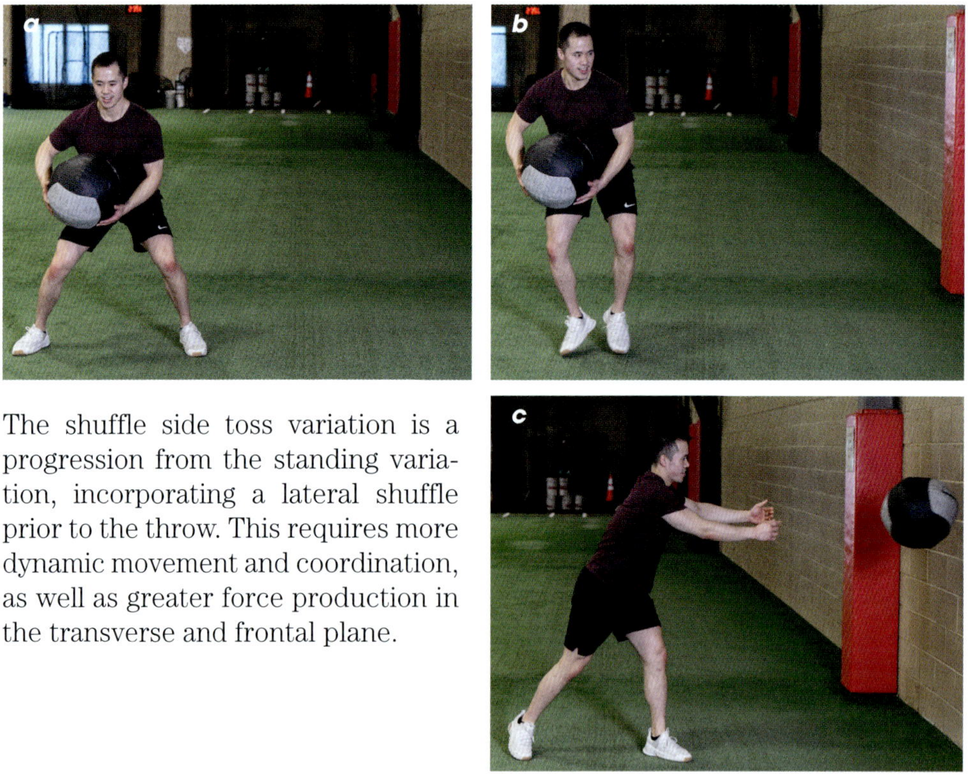

The shuffle side toss variation is a progression from the standing variation, incorporating a lateral shuffle prior to the throw. This requires more dynamic movement and coordination, as well as greater force production in the transverse and frontal plane.

STANDING MEDICINE BALL OVERHEAD THROW

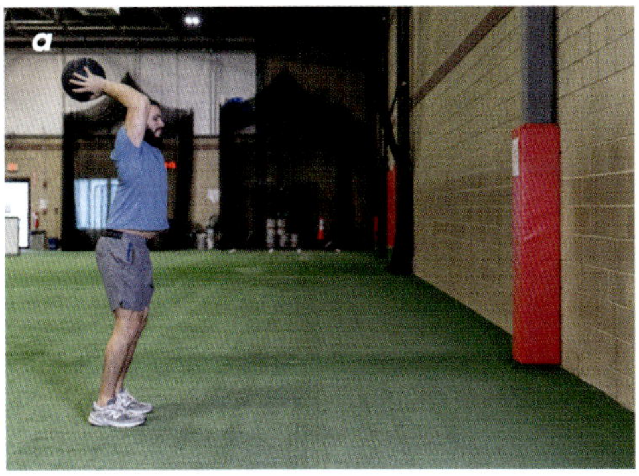

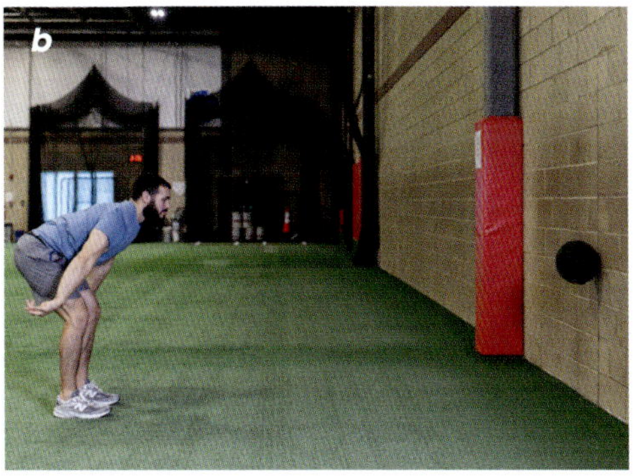

Benefits

The standing medicine ball overhead throw is an effective drill for developing upper body and shoulder power, with a strong emphasis on the anterior core and lat musculature. The movement reinforces coordinated force transfer from the trunk to the arms while teaching athletes to use the lats and core to support powerful overhead activities.

Instructions for the Client

1. Begin standing in an athletic position, facing a wall, with feet shoulder-width apart.
2. Hold a 2- to 4-pound (0.9-1.8 kg) medicine ball at chest height with both hands, elbows slightly bent.
3. Smoothly raise the ball overhead by extending the arms upward, maintaining a braced core and neutral spine.
4. From the fully extended overhead position, forcefully throw the ball forward into the wall.
5. Aim to strike the wall at approximately chest height.
6. Catch or retrieve the ball, reset to the starting position, and repeat for the prescribed number of repetitions.

STANDING MEDICINE BALL OVERHEAD THROW *(continued)*

Variations

Regression: Kneeling Medicine Ball Overhead Throw

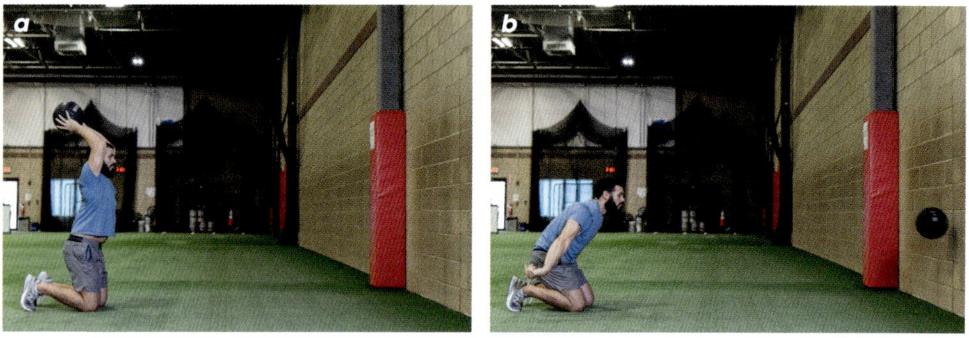

The kneeling overhead throw reduces lower body involvement and helps isolate upper body power while reinforcing anterior core and lat engagement. This variation is appropriate for beginners or for athletes who need to improve trunk control during overhead movements.

Progression: Medicine Ball Overhead Throw With Step

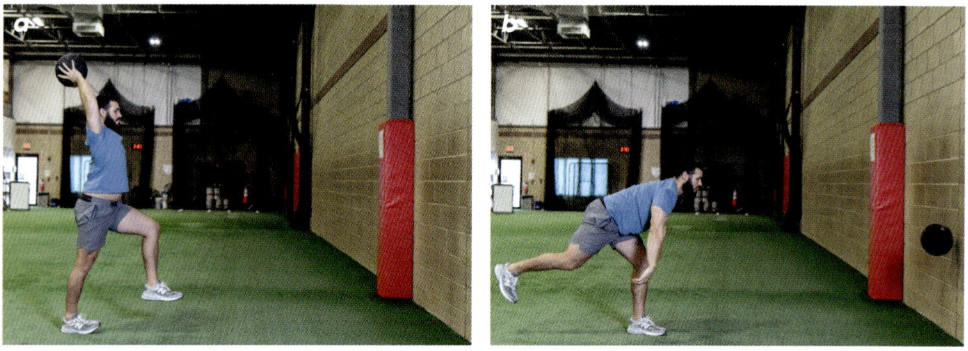

The overhead throw with a step increases the demands on coordination and force transfer by adding a dynamic lower body component. This progression challenges the athlete to maintain core stability and effective lat engagement while producing greater total body power.

STANDING MEDICINE BALL SLAM

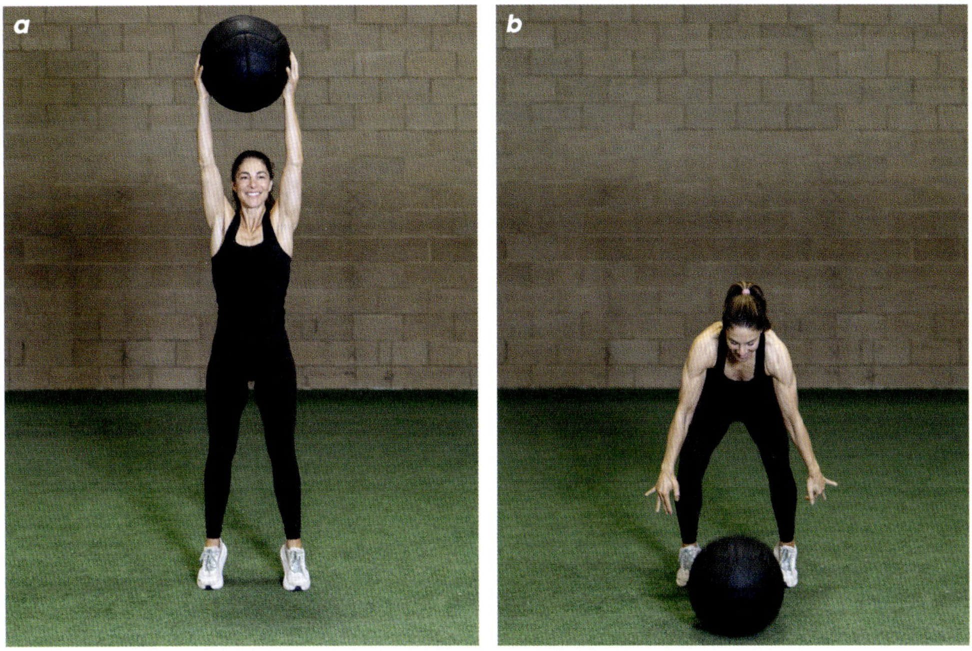

Benefits

The medicine ball slam exercise can be used to develop power in the anterior trunk and latissimus muscles.

Instructions for the Client

1. Begin by standing in an athletic position with your feet shoulder-width apart.
2. Hold a 4- to 8-pound (1.8-3.6 kg) medicine ball in front of you with both hands.
3. Reach the ball up above your head with both hands while simultaneously extending your hips, knees, and ankles.
4. Slam the ball down forcefully in front of you and catch the ball as it bounces.
5. Repeat for the prescribed number of repetitions.

STANDING MEDICINE BALL SLAM *(continued)*

Variation

Progression: Side-to-Side Medicine Ball Slam

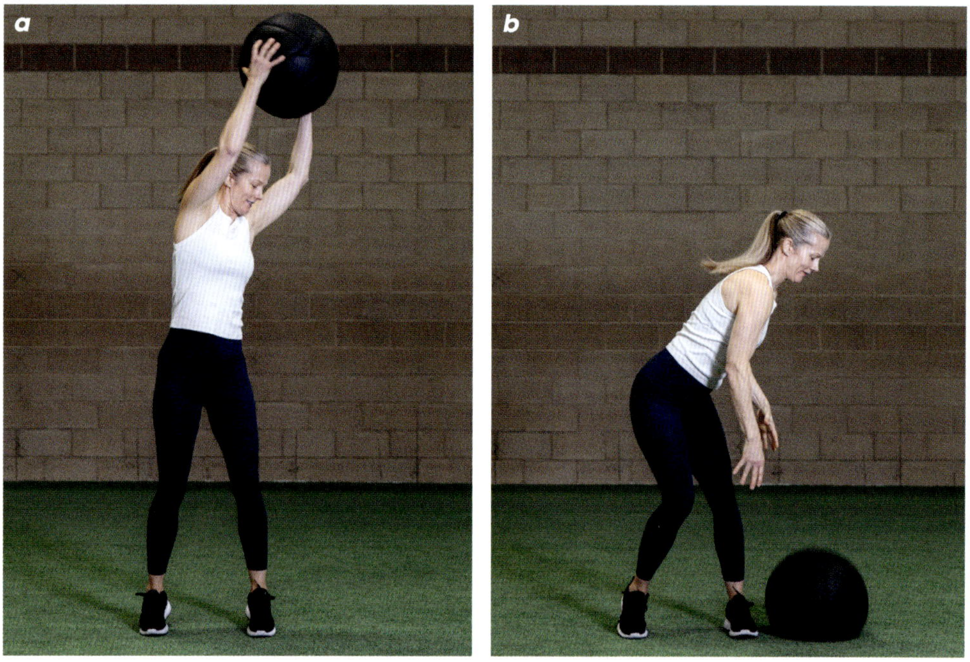

The side-to-side medicine ball slam is a progression that adds a transverse plane component by rotating side to side between slams to develop rotational power in the oblique muscles.

Heavy-Implement Power Exercises

In contrast to light-implement power exercises, heavy-implement power drills emphasize force production against greater external load. Exercises such as kettlebell swings, dumbbell snatches, and loaded jumping variations train the ability to rapidly generate high levels against an external load. Although these movements are performed at lower velocities than plyometrics or medicine ball throws, they remain explosive in intent and are highly effective for developing total body power, particularly through the hips and posterior chain. When properly coached and loaded, heavy-implement power exercises provide a safe and accessible means of improving force-production capacity, making them valuable for both athletic performance and long-term functional resilience.

KETTLEBELL SWING

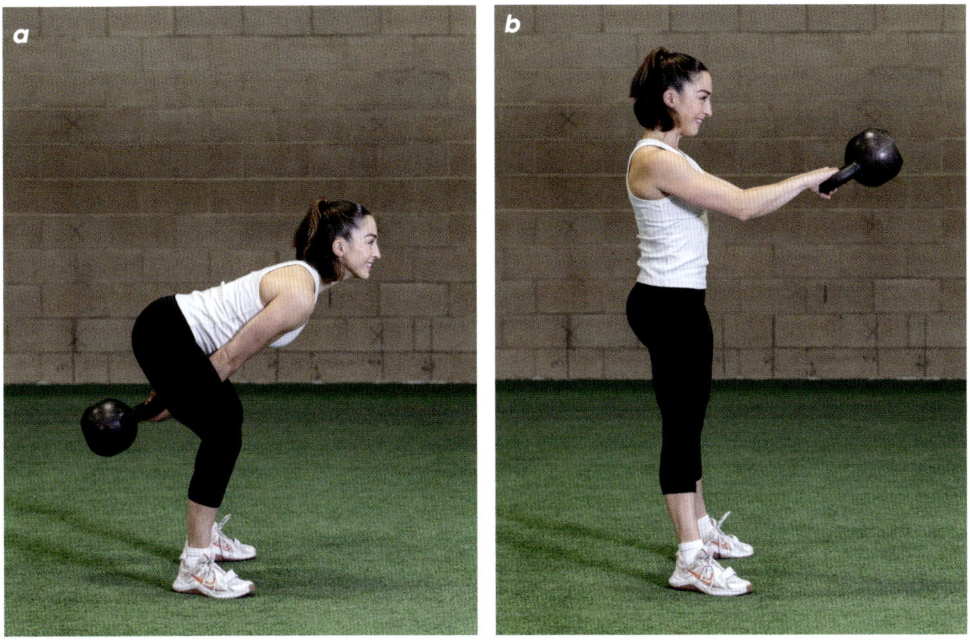

Benefits

The kettlebell swing is a non-impact, hip-dominant exercise that develops power in the hips and hamstrings. The versatility, loading potential, and non-impact nature of the kettlebell swing makes it an especially valuable tool to develop power for the general-population client.

Instructions for the Client

1. Start by standing tall, about 3 feet (0.9 m) behind a kettlebell. Hinge at your hips, bending your knees and pushing your hips back. Your shoulders should be positioned slightly above your hips.
2. Reach forward, fully extending your arms, and grasp the kettlebell with both hands. Hike the kettlebell backward under your hips toward your glutes while maintaining a strong, neutral spine.
3. Reverse the momentum of the kettlebell by forcefully extending your hips, straightening your knees, and lifting your shoulders upward.
4. Stop the motion when your arms reach chest height and are parallel to the ground. Reverse the motion to begin the cycle again, performing the exercise for the programmed number of repetitions.
5. Finally, return the kettlebell safely to the ground in front of you.

KETTLEBELL SWING *(continued)*

Variations

Regression: Kettlebell Deadlift

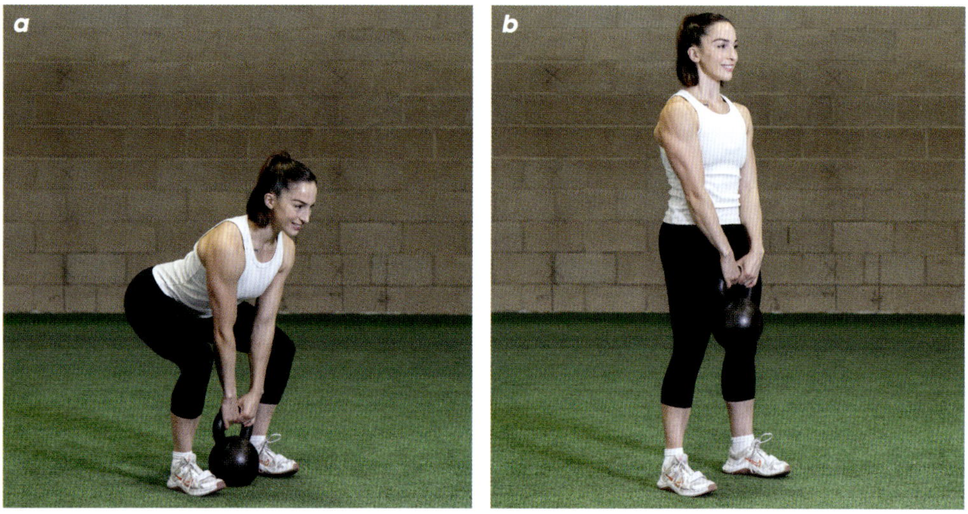

For inexperienced clients or those who struggle with coordination, the kettlebell deadlift should serve as a regression that will help to develop strength in a hinging pattern before progressing to the kettlebell swing.

Progression: Single-Arm Kettlebell Swing

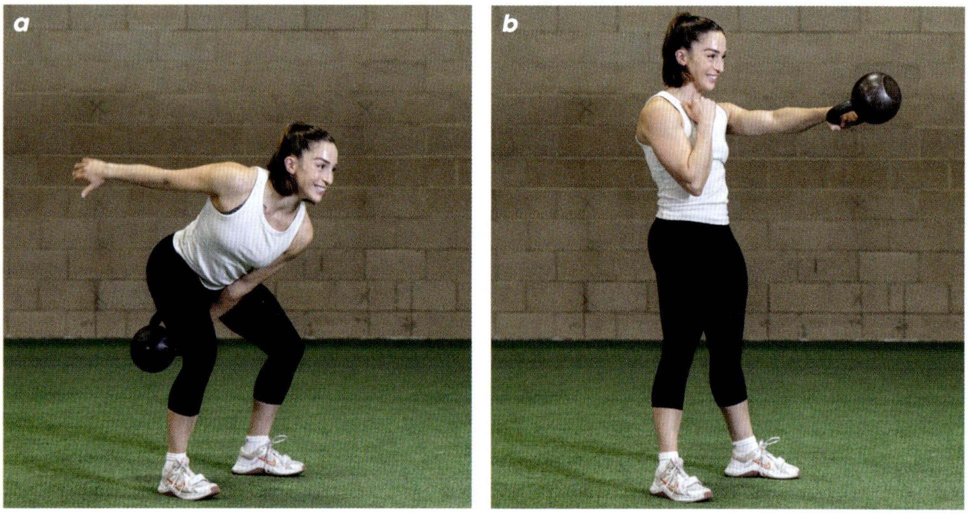

The single-arm kettlebell swing is a progression from the traditional kettlebell swing that will challenge the client's transverse plane trunk stability.

DUMBBELL JUMP SQUAT AND STICK

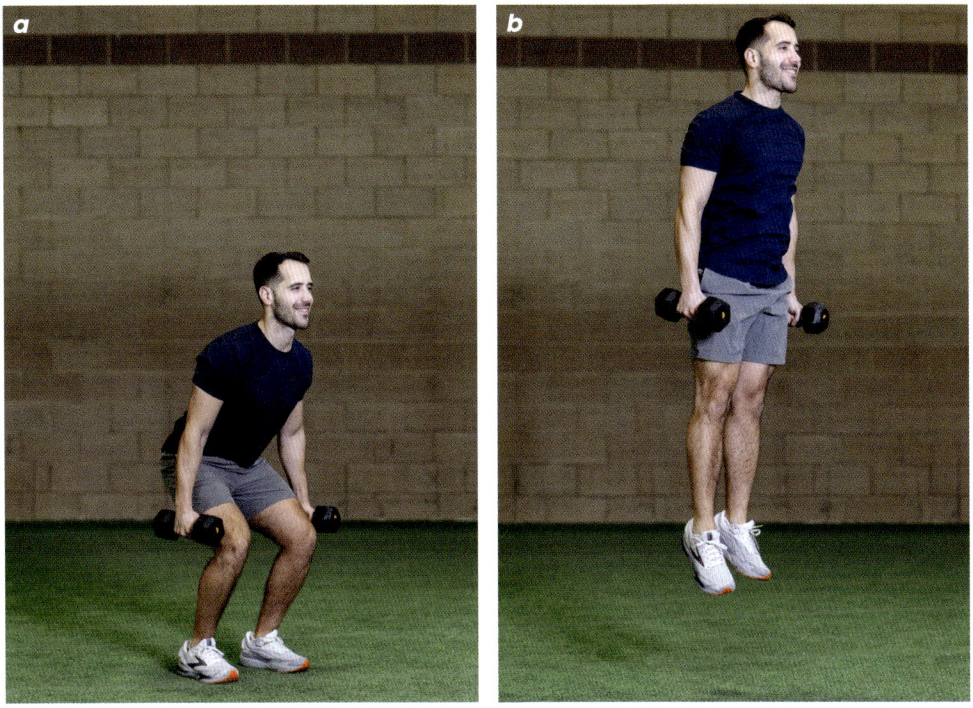

Benefits

The dumbbell jump squat is an impact-based, knee-dominant power exercise that develops the quadriceps, hips, and calves and should be reserved for clients who can tolerate repeated ground contact.

Instructions for the Client

1. Stand in an athletic position with your feet shoulder-width apart and your hips and knees slightly bent.
2. Hold a dumbbell in each hand by your side. If it is your first time doing this exercise, start with a light load of 5 to 10 pounds (2.3-4.5 kg) in each hand and progress as you feel comfortable.
3. Keeping your arms straight and by your side, jump upward forcefully as high as you can.
4. Land softly and hold the landing position for 2 seconds before repeating for the prescribed number of repetitions.

DUMBBELL JUMP SQUAT AND STICK *(continued)*

Variations

Regression: Bodyweight Jump Squat

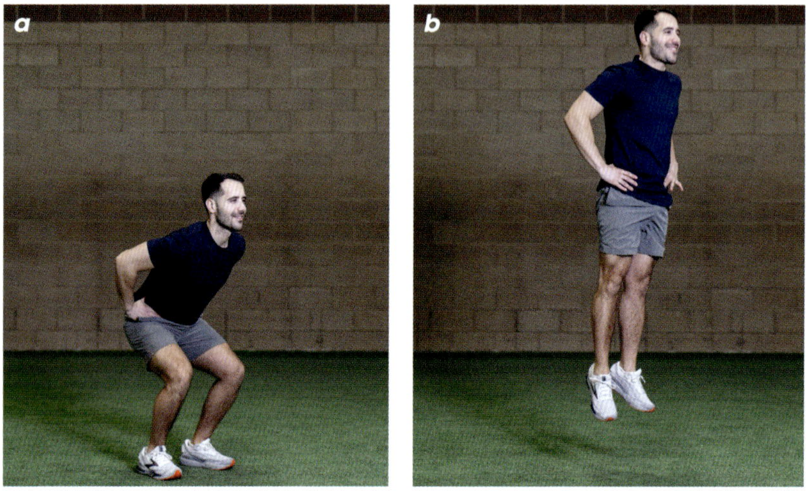

Clients who are inexperienced or may have a history of lower body injuries should start with a simple jump squat and stick without load to allow them to acclimate to impact forces.

Progression: Continuous Dumbbell Jump Squats

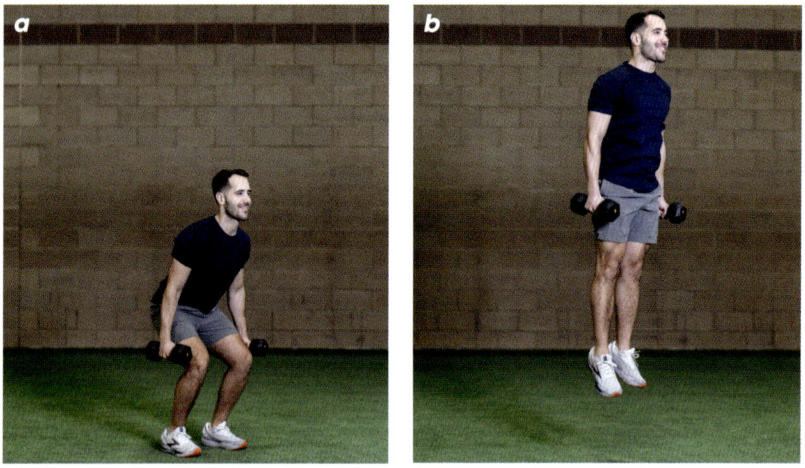

In this progression, the client performs repeated dumbbell jump squats with minimal pause between repetitions. Rather than sticking the landing, the client transitions quickly from landing into the next jump, increasing speed, elastic demand, and overall impact exposure. This variation should be reserved for clients who demonstrate excellent landing mechanics and tolerance to repeated ground contact.

DUMBBELL SNATCH

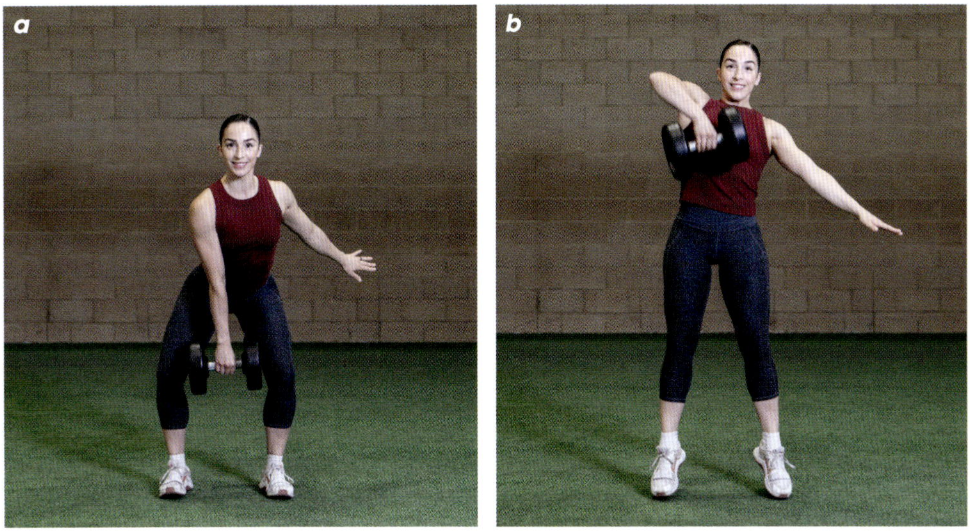

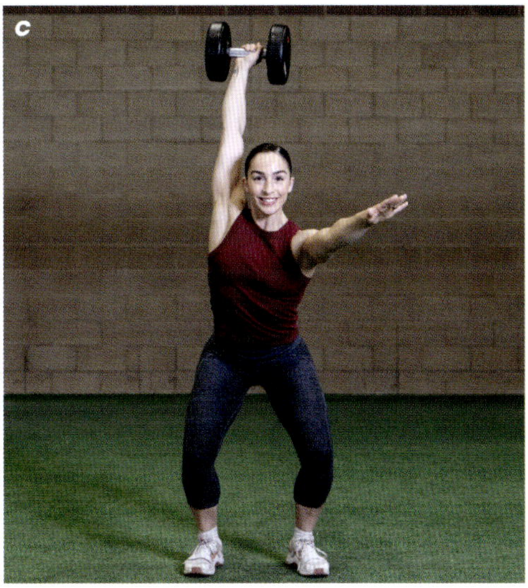

Benefits

The dumbbell snatch is a valuable exercise to develop full body power, targeting the calves, glutes, quadriceps, shoulders, and upper back musculature.

Instructions for the Client

1. Stand in an athletic position with your feet shoulder-width apart and your hips and knees slightly bent.
2. Hold a dumbbell in one hand directly in front of you so that it is positioned between the knees with your palm facing toward you.
3. Keeping the dumbbell close to your body, jump upward while simultaneously pulling the dumbbell upward to propel it overhead.
4. Finish the movement with the dumbbell overhead with your shoulder and elbow locked straight and your hips and knees bent.
5. Return the dumbbell back to starting position safely and repeat for the prescribed repetitions.
6. Repeat on the other side.

SLED MARCH

Benefits

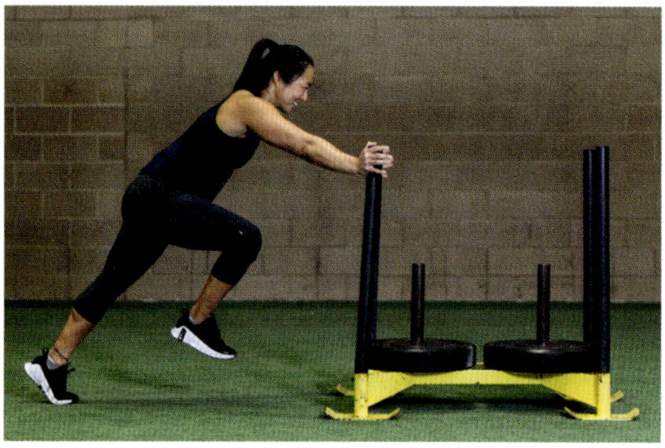

The sled march is a lower-body strength and power exercise that develops hip extension and lower-limb power through a gait-specific movement pattern.

Instructions for the Client

1. Load a sled with weight that you can comfortably push with good form in a continuous marching pattern.
2. Lean against the sled at a 45-degree angle with your hands on top of the handles and your elbows locked straight.
3. Begin marching, driving your knees upward and striking the ground down and back behind you.
4. Maintain an upright torso posture, ankle dorsiflexion, and a steady marching pattern for the prescribed distance.

Variation

Progression: Fast Sled Push

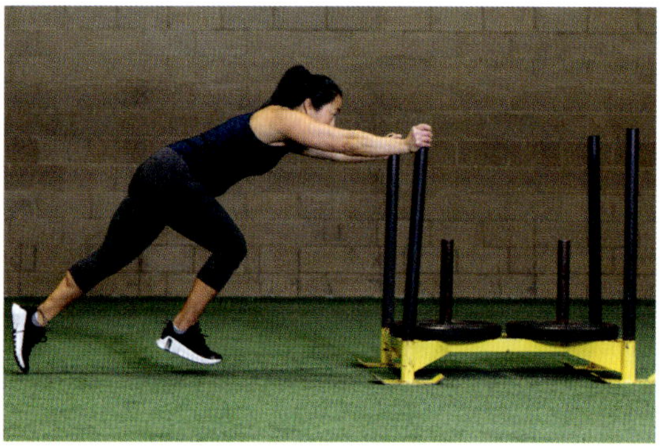

In this progression, the client performs the sled push at a higher rate of speed. Rather than using a slow, steady marching pattern, the client drives the sled forward as quickly as possible. This progression places greater demand on the lower body musculature, including the glutes, hamstrings, calves, and feet and helps develop lower body extension power.

Case Study: Maria

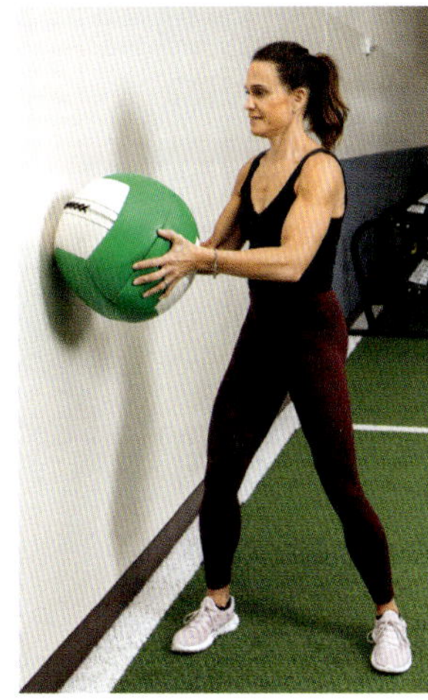

Maria is a 41-year-old sedentary woman who began an exercise program to improve her metabolic health and physical capacity. Although she has no diagnosed chronic illnesses, she had recently noticed increasing difficulty with everyday tasks like housework, walking her dogs, and climbing stairs—activities that previously felt effortless.

When we began designing her program, Maria was initially hesitant to include power training. She associated power-based movements with a high risk of injury and felt they were unnecessary for someone who was not actively participating in sport. We discussed the role of power as a key determinant of functional independence, particularly its importance in tasks such as rising from a chair, climbing stairs, reacting to loss of balance, and reducing fall risk with age. We agreed to implement a gradual and well-structured approach that would safely introduce power-based activities using dynamic warm-up drills and both light- and heavier-implement power exercises.

Maria participated in a twice-per-week functional training program that included mobility, strength training, and cardiovascular conditioning in addition to the dynamic warm-up and dedicated power circuits, outlined here. Her program included supersets, which is the performance of multiple exercises together in a pairing.

DAY 1

Dynamic Warm-Up

- A-skips: 20 yards
- High-knee run: 20 yards
- Lateral skip: 10 yards each direction
- Lateral shuffle: 10 yards each direction
- Carioca: 10 yards
- Backpedal: 10 yards

Light-Implement Power

- A1—Box jump: 3 × 5 reps
- A2—Tall-kneeling medicine ball chest pass: 3 × 10 reps

(continued)

Case Study: Maria *(continued)*

Heavy-Implement Power

- B1—Loaded jump squat: 3 × 5 reps
- B2—Front plank: 3 × 30 seconds

DAY 2

Footwork and Coordination: Ladder Drills

- 1-2 stick (forward and backward)
- In-in-out-out (sideways, both directions)
- In-in-out-out (forward and backward)
- Cross in front (forward and backward)
- Cross behind (forward and backward)

Light-Implement Power

- A1—Lateral bound and stick: 3 × 5 reps per side
- A2—Half-kneeling medicine ball side toss: 3 × 5 reps per side

Heavy-Implement Power

- B1—Kettlebell swing: 3 × 10 reps
- B2—Side plank: 3 × 30 seconds per side

After the first two training sessions, Maria's initial apprehension surrounding dynamic movement and power training began to fade. She recognized that power could be developed in a safe, controlled, and accessible manner. As the program progressed, we gradually increased the complexity and intensity of the movements to continue developing her power and coordination.

Over time, Maria reported improved confidence, quicker movement, and greater ease performing activities of daily living. By reframing power training as a tool for function rather than athletic performance, we were able to enhance her physical capacity while building confidence and long-term adherence.

Following the completion of power exercises such as plyometrics, medicine ball throws, and loaded power drills, the next priority is building strength. Power training helps to keep the nervous system fast and reactive, but power can only be expressed when the client has a foundation from which to produce force. Strength training builds the capacity to tolerate load, protect joints, and create the reserve that makes everything else in training and life safer and easier. In the next chapter, we will break down how to develop strength in a way that supports performance, injury resistance, and long-term independence.

Chapter 7

Strength Training

When it comes to the recipe for improving longevity, the main ingredient is strength training. If I were forced to choose a single mode of exercise for the rest of my life to ensure that I stay fit, vibrant, and independent, it would be lifting weights. Although a well-rounded program should include more than just resistance training, the quest for improved health and longevity should be focused heavily on the development of muscular strength.

Strength training provides people with a foundation of structural integrity, allowing them to be active, independent, and resilient to physical stressors in daily life. As I once heard strength coach Brett Jones say succinctly, "Absolute strength is the glass. Everything else is the liquid inside the glass. The bigger the glass, the more of 'everything else' you can do."

If living longer relies on staying physically active, then staying physically active relies on maintaining musculoskeletal integrity. If unchecked, the progressive loss of muscular strength that comes with aging will make it much harder to complete tasks of daily living and to participate in voluntary physical activity. The result is a downward spiral of increasing sedentary behavior, declining metabolic health, and a loss of physical independence. Alternatively, if people are able to build and maintain a large reserve of muscular strength over their lifetimes, it will allow them to access a wide array of physical activities into their later years.

REDUCING DISEASE RISK

Strength training serves as a form of preventive medicine that can break the cycle of physical decline associated with aging. The regular stress placed on muscle and bone slows the natural losses that drive sarcopenia and osteoporosis while also reducing risk of other conditions related to inactivity. In the section ahead, we will look more closely at these conditions and highlight how regular resistance training serves as a vital tool to preserving health and function with age.

Sarcopenia

Sarcopenia is a syndrome that is characterized by the progressive loss of muscle mass and function with age, which often leads to physical frailty, loss of independence, and metabolic dysfunction. Sarcopenia affects between 10 and 16 percent of older adults worldwide and has a significant impact on quality of life (Yuan and Larsson, 2023). The stark reality is that as people age, if they are not actively working to develop strength and muscle mass, they are losing it. After the age of 50, if people do not strength train, the average person can expect to lose 1 to 2 percent of muscle mass and 3 percent of muscle strength per year (Haehling et al., 2010). Extreme cases of sarcopenia can account for a loss of 50 percent of muscle mass by the eighth decade of life (Wilkinson et al., 2018).

The impact of the loss of muscle that comes with sarcopenia extends beyond physical appearance. Losing muscle mass and strength has serious consequences on health and longevity. Preserving muscular strength throughout aging is vital to maintaining physical independence; in fact, having low muscle mass and function makes people over 12 times more likely to lose their physical independence as they age (Dos Santos et al., 2017). Moreover, sarcopenia is an independent predictor of all-cause mortality in adults aged 65 years or older (Liu et al., 2017).

We often accept physical frailty as a simple fact of the aging process. Although progressive loss of muscle mass and strength with age can be partly explained by natural changes in endocrine functions and neuromuscular signaling, many age-related declines in strength can be mediated by participating in a basic strength training program.

The progressive frailty that happens as we age is more often a result of disuse than natural biological decline. The side effect of sedentary behavior and physical inactivity is an inadequate physical strain required to stimulate protein synthesis and muscular development. Over time physical frailty becomes a self-fulfilling prophecy as we enter a cycle of sedentary-driven weakness that is tough to escape.

Although sarcopenia doesn't appear until later in life, preventing it starts much earlier. The muscle mass we develop and maintain in our 20s, 30s, and 40s is the same muscle mass that will support us into our golden years. With this in mind, we should be focused on developing as much muscular strength as possible to give ourselves a head start later on in life.

Osteopenia and Osteoporosis

Muscles aren't the only tissues in the body that dissipate with age; bones do as well. As we age, the trabecular structure that gives bones their strength and stiffness begins to break down due largely to changes in the balance of activity in bone remodeling. *Osteoclasts*, the cells that are responsible for breaking down bone, progressively begin to outpace the activity of *osteoblasts,* which are the cells that rebuild bone. This process results in a slow chipping away of bone density.

The average person can expect to experience a decline in bone mineral density of 0.2 to 0.5 percent per year after the age of 30 (Dobbs et al., 1999).

For women, this decline accelerates significantly after menopause—up to 50 percent faster than in men (Heaney et al., 2000). Globally, approximately one in three women over the age of 50 will develop osteoporosis, and women account for nearly 80 percent of all cases (Melton et al, 1992; Benjamin, 2010). Women are disproportionately affected by osteoporosis because on average they accumulate less bone mineral density at a young age and lose it much faster due to sharp reductions in estrogen levels following menopause. Estrogen plays a vital role in bone health by supporting the function of osteocytes, promoting bone remodeling and limiting bone reabsorption (Khosla et al., 2012).

As estrogen levels fall during menopause, the body's ability to stimulate bone formation diminishes. This hormonal shift marks a transition from a state of bone building to one of bone breakdown. With bone formation slowing and bone resorption by osteoclasts continuing or even accelerating, women experience a progressive loss of bone density over time.

Fortunately, strength training is the most powerful tool for building and maintaining bone density with age. Mechanical loading on bones via compression and mechanical tension from muscular contractions stimulates osteoblasts to create and maintain collagen bone matrix. Strength training is not just a defense against age-related decline; it is an investment in long-term skeletal health, starting from a young age.

While osteoporosis is a condition that emerges in the second half of life, the roots of the disease begin much earlier. The bone mass accumulated in youth serves as a critical reserve that sustains adults in the second half of life. After the third decade of life, building new bone mass becomes more challenging, but consistent strength training and proper nutrition can help maintain and, in many cases, improve bone density while slowing its progressive decline. This makes weightlifting especially important for children, particularly females, to maximize bone density while it is still possible. The bone gained in adolescence and early adulthood provides crucial support later in life. Figure 7.1 illustrates the typical progression of female bone density over a lifetime and the impact of regular mechanical loading and menopause.

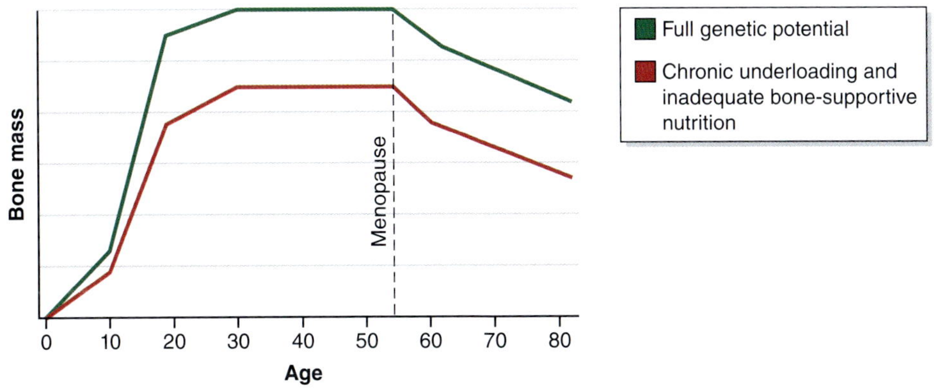

Figure 7.1 Bone density progression over a lifetime (Heaney et al., 2000).

Why Is It So Essential to Maintain Bone Density Throughout Aging?

Accidental falls are a massive driver of mortality as people reach age 60 and beyond because of the impact that broken bones can have on overall health, independence, and physical activity. In fact, an estimated one in two women over the age of 50 will experience a fragility fracture in their lifetime, highlighting how common and clinically significant these events are (Crandall et al, 2014). Mortality risk increases by a startling 178 percent following a hip fracture that occurs after 60 years old. Stated another way, the hazard ratio of breaking a hip after 60 years old is 2.78, meaning someone is 2.78 times more likely to die in the year following a hip fracture than someone who did not break their hip (Katsoulis et al., 2017).

While the movement and power training drills discussed in chapters 5 and 6 can help prevent falls, strength training plays a crucial role in ensuring the body is resilient enough to withstand a fall if it occurs. The exercises presented in this chapter form the foundation of a comprehensive training program, providing the mechanical loading necessary to build and maintain strength, preserve bone mass, and support long-term structural integrity.

Following a progressive weightlifting program at a young age and continuing it throughout life is the most effective way to preserve bone density. A well-rounded functional training program that uses free weights in various movement patterns ensures the entire body experiences the necessary stress to stimulate bone strengthening.

MUSCLE AS AN ORGAN

Losing muscle mass does more than just put people at risk for physical frailty; it can also wreak havoc on numerous physiological processes throughout the body. Most people think of muscles as nothing more than mechanical pulleys that help them to move throughout the day. However, the function of muscles has an extensive impact on the metabolic health and function of the entire body.

Having more skeletal muscle has a significant impact on metabolism, increasing resting metabolic rate, increasing fat oxidation, and, probably most significantly, affecting blood glucose levels and insulin sensitivity.

Maintaining skeletal muscle mass throughout aging is essential to managing glucose metabolism. Muscles are the largest organ in the body and are responsible for up to 80 percent of glucose uptake following a meal (Merz and Thurmond, 2020). Essentially, muscles serve as a reservoir for glucose uptake and storage; the more muscle one has, the more glucose one can take up from the blood stream and use in muscles for energy. The research is clear that the increased muscle mass and regular participation in strength training, independent of aerobic activity, is directly correlated with reduced rates of developing dysregulated glucose metabolism and diabetes (Merz and Thurmond, 2020; Grøntved et al., 2012).

Additionally, emerging research has shown that muscles function as endocrine organs that release signaling molecules called *myokines*, which are proteins that are released from contracting skeletal muscles in the body that have hormone-like effects on virtually every system in the body. Over 650 different myokines have been identified that serve purposes such as regulating metabolism, reducing inflammation, improving glucose metabolism and insulin sensitivity, and improving cognitive function (Severinsen and Pedersen, 2020).

Interleukin 6 (IL-6) is the most widely studied and systemically significant myokine in the human body. IL-6 is released from satellite cells in the muscles following contraction. It can improve insulin sensitivity and glucose uptake, increase lipolysis and fat-burning, reduce systemic inflammation, and even suppress tumor growth (Severinsen and Pedersen, 2020).

Losing muscle mass has a wider systemic impact on the body than just affecting how well people move. Muscles function as the body's own internal pharmacy, releasing chemicals in response to physical activity that help the body to fine-tune its vital functions in an effort to maintain homeostasis.

STRENGTH TRAINING AND MENTAL HEALTH

The impact of strength training even appears to extend beyond muscles to brains, affecting mental health and well-being. Research has begun to demonstrate the wide-ranging impact that regular participation in resistance training can have on conditions such as anxiety and depression.

A meta-analysis of 33 clinical trials involving over 1,800 participants found that participation in strength training significantly reduced depressive symptoms, regardless of a person's health status, the total prescribed training volume, or even measurable improvements in strength (Gordon et al., 2018). A similar meta-analysis examining the impact of resistance training on anxiety symptoms found that resistance training significantly reduced anxiety symptoms in both healthy and clinically diagnosed patients regardless of varieties in program design or significant improvements in strength (Gordon et al., 2017).

Simply participating in a strength training program can help alleviate anxiety and depressive symptoms, even without significant strength gains. This suggests that the psychological benefits of resistance training may stem from physiological responses to exercise, such as the release of myokines and hormones, rather than improvements in muscle strength and hypertrophy itself. While strength training should not replace clinical or pharmacological treatment for mental health conditions, it should be recognized as a valuable tool in promoting long-term psychological well-being and healthy aging.

INCREASING STRENGTH SPAN

The concept of strength span developed by Faigenbaum (2024) refers to a continuous measure of physical strength over a life span that contributes to improved health outcomes and longevity. Extending strength span preserves the capacity to live independently, function safely, and participate in a wider range of physical activities well into older adulthood.

Building a reserve of physical strength early in life and consistently working to preserve it extends strength span across the lifespan. Rather than simply slowing decline, this approach raises the baseline from which age-related losses occur, allowing individuals to maintain functional capacity, independence, and resilience well into older adulthood. In this way, strength span is not just about how strong someone is at a given moment, but how long they can maintain meaningful levels of strength across their life.

Data summarized in *Physiology of Sport and Exercise* (Kenney et al., 2025) illustrate how dramatically strength span can diverge depending on training habits across a lifetime. Muscular strength begins to decline as early as the third decade of life in untrained individuals. However, individuals who consistently participate in strength training can maintain substantially higher levels of strength into older age and in some cases demonstrate levels of strength comparable to untrained individuals 40 years younger than them. These age-related declines in strength closely mirror reductions in muscle cross-sectional area, underscoring the central role of preservation of muscle mass in sustaining functional capacity over time (Kenney et al., 2025).

Figure 7.2 demonstrates the typical deterioration of strength span over the course of a lifetime and that of an individual who actively works to maintain muscular strength.

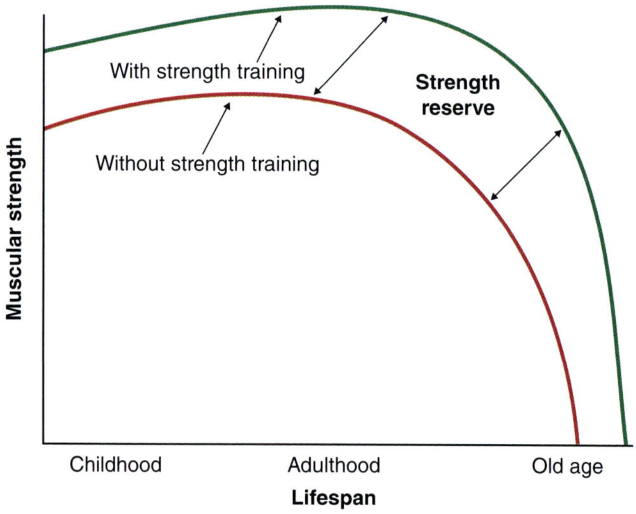

Figure 7.2 Strength span over a lifetime.

Reprinted by permission from A.D. Faigenbaum, A. Garcia-Hermoso, J.P. MacDonald, et al., "Bridging the Gap Between Strengthspan and Lifespan," *British Journal of Sports Medicine* 58, no. 14 (2024): 758-60, with permission from BMJ Publishing Group Ltd.

The earlier someone begins weight training, the better. Research shows that those who engage in strength training during youth not only build immediate strength and fitness but are also more likely to remain physically active and healthy later in life. Developing healthy exercise habits and positive experiences with weight training at a young age helps people build greater reserve of muscle and bone mass while fostering long-term fitness behaviors that last a lifetime (Fraser et al., 2017).

While starting weight training at a young age is ideal, it is never too late to start benefiting from resistance training. As the old saying goes, "The best time to plant a tree was 30 years ago; the second best time is now." Untrained older clients can see significant improvements in strength, muscle mass, and functional abilities, such as stair climbing, walking, and the ability to stand up from a chair, with as little as three 45-minute strength training sessions per week (Meigh et al., 2021). Clients who are 80 years old can expect to see changes in strength and muscle mass similar to people who are decades younger than them when they commit to resistance training (Hikida et al., 2000). Additionally, research shows that resistance training can significantly reduce markers of systemic inflammation, a major driver behind chronic disease.

At our training facility, we regularly work with clients in their 70s and 80s who are starting weight training for the first time. Many experience life-changing results, gaining the strength and confidence to live more active, independent lives with less fear of falls.

MUSCULAR STRENGTH AS THE FIFTH VITAL SIGN

There are four basic vital signs: body temperature, heart rate, blood pressure, and respiratory rate. Anyone who has been to the hospital or had a basic yearly physical exam has had these measures checked. While these measures are unquestionably valuable and predictive of overall health and chronic disease, they are inadequate to assess a person's muscular strength. Thankfully, research has begun to show that measures of muscular strength, such as grip strength and quadriceps strength, can serve as useful proxy measures that are predictive of overall health and longevity.

Simple measures of grip strength and quadriceps strength have both been found to be independent predictors of all-cause mortality, meaning that these measures of strength could be used to predict longevity independent of the presence of other disease such as diabetes or heart disease (Newman et al., 2006). Grip strength alone has been shown to be predictive of numerous health outcomes including cardiovascular risk (Rein et al., 2016), length of hospital stays (Kerr et al., 2006), likelihood of surgical complications (Chen et al., 2011), and all-cause mortality for patients as young as 35 years old (Sasaki et al., 2007).

Recent research has even demonstrated a direct association between grip strength and cognitive health. In a study of over 450,000 participants, having low grip strength was associated with a 72 percent increased risk of developing dementia and a 87 percent risk of dying from dementia over a 10-year follow-up independent of lifestyle factors and other diseases such as heart disease and diabetes (Esteban-Cornejo et al., 2022). Figure 7.3 demonstrates the association of grip strength and relative risk for all-cause mortality in men and women.

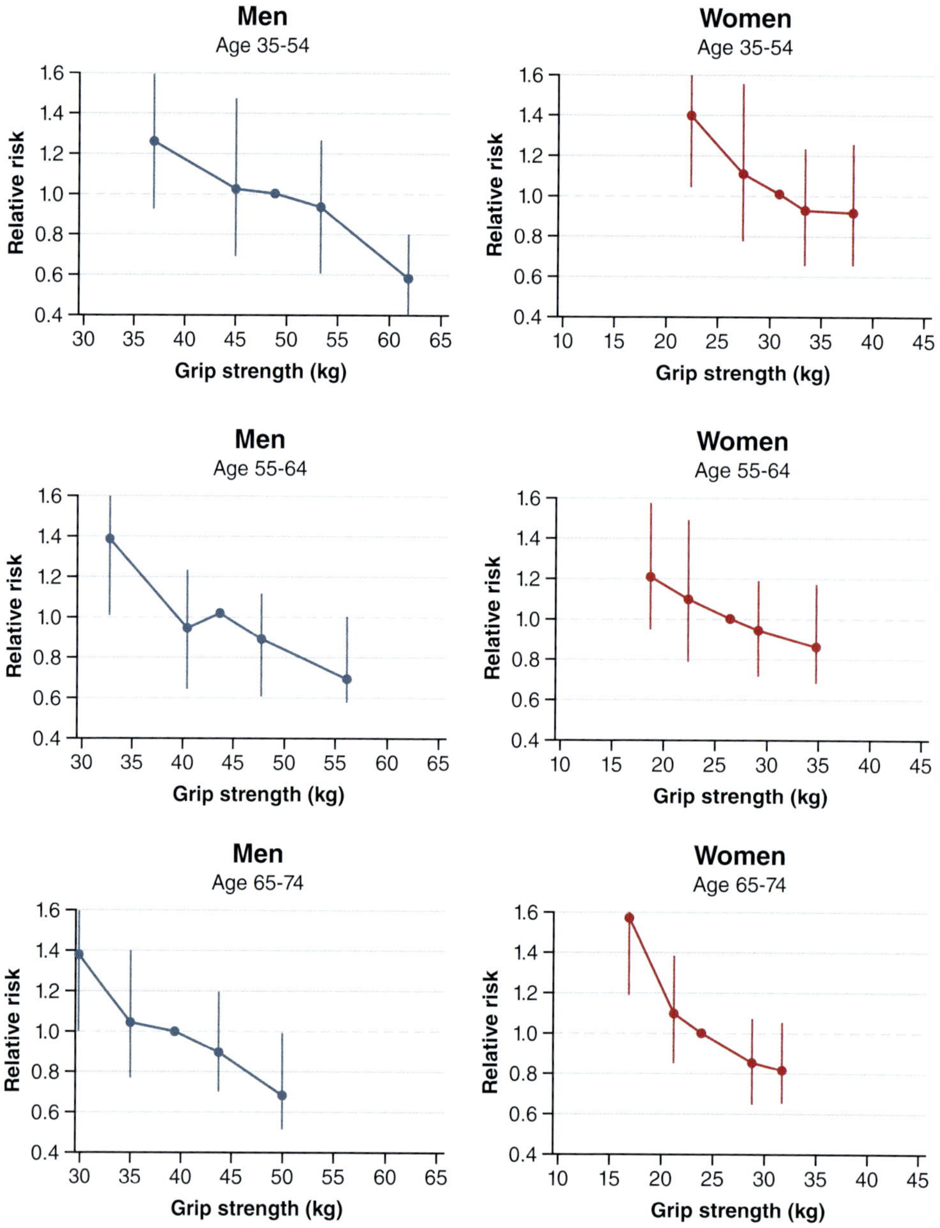

Figure 7.3 Grip strength and relative mortality risk by age and gender.

Adapted by permission from H. Sasaki, F. Kasagi, M. Yamada, and S. Fujita, "Grip Strength Predicts Cause-Specific Mortality in Middle-Aged and Elderly Persons," *The American Journal of Medicine* 120, no. 4 (2007): 337-42, with permission from Elsevier.

The value of these measures comes from the fact that they are representative of full body strength, vitality, and physical robustness. Someone with a strong grip likely has the upper body strength to lift, carry, and easily complete physical tasks of daily living. Someone with adequate quadriceps strength can walk, climb stairs, and move throughout their day without physical limitations. Grip strength is an especially valuable measure due to its simplicity and practicality. With minimal barriers to assessment, it can be performed in a gym by a coach, in a clinical setting, or at home by a client.

Measures of upper body strength such as push-up capacity also have been shown to be useful predictors of longevity. In a study of over 1,000 participants, push-up capacity was inversely associated with 10-year risk of heart attack among men aged 21 to 66 years. Participants able to perform as little as 11 or more push-ups at baseline had significantly reduced risk of a subsequent cardiovascular event. Men able to do more than 40 push-ups had a 96 percent reduced risk of cardiovascular events compared with those who were able to do less than 10 push-ups (Yang et al., 2019). When looking at this data it is reasonable to say that push-up capacity is a simple, no-cost measure that can provide an estimate of functional status and cardiovascular risk among middle-aged men.

As a coach, regularly measuring improvements in upper and lower body strength can be a simple and effective way to track progress and stratify relative risk in our training clients.

CLIENT ASSESSMENT

CLIENT ASSESSMENT: GRIP STRENGTH TEST

1. Stand tall with a grip dynamometer in one hand with that arm flexed to 90 degrees at the elbow and your upper arm by your side.
2. Squeeze the grip dynamometer with maximum force, taking care not to move your upper arm away from your body or contort your torso.
3. Repeat the test on the opposite side and average the two scores together.
4. Use figure 7.4 to compare yourself to the average grip strength relative to your age and sex.

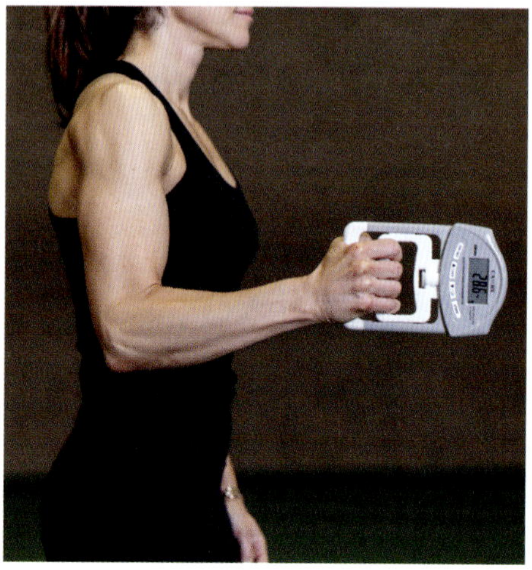

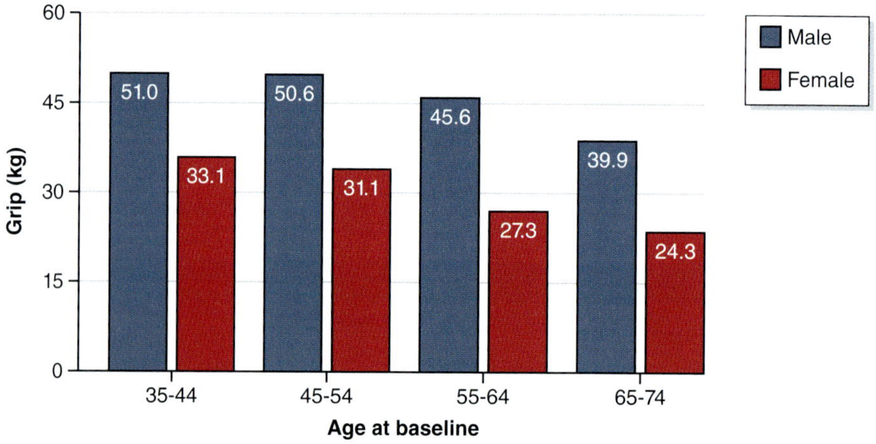

Figure 7.4 Grip strength average by age and sex.

Adapted by permission from H. Sasaki, F. Kasagi, M. Yamada, and S. Fujita, "Grip Strength Predicts Cause-Specific Mortality in Middle-Aged and Elderly Persons," *The American Journal of Medicine* 120, no. 4 (2007): 337-42, with permission from Elsevier.

CLIENT ASSESSMENT: PUSH-UP CAPACITY TEST

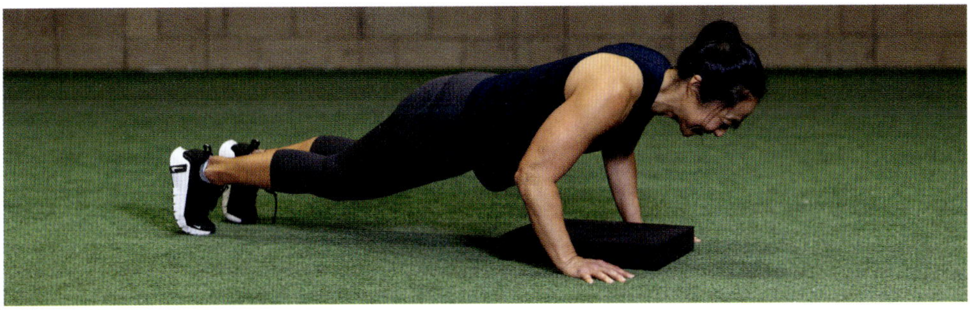

1. Get into a push-up position on the ground with your legs and feet together and your arms slightly outside of shoulder-width apart.
2. Place an Airex pad or other object about 3 to 4 inches (8-10 cm) high between your hands to serve as a depth marker.
3. Complete as many consecutive push-ups as possible until failure. Be sure to touch your chest to the pad on every repetition while maintaining a straight torso.
4. Use figure 7.5 to categorize your push-up total by age and sex.

Fitness categories for the push-up – men

Age	20-29	30-39	40-49	50-59	60+
Excellent	>35	>29	>24	>20	>17
Very good	29-35	22-29	17-24	13-20	11-17
Good	22-28	17-21	13-16	10-12	8-10
Fair	17-21	12-16	10-12	7-9	5-7
Poor	<17	<12	<10	<7	<5

Fitness categories for the push-up – women

Age	20-29	30-39	40-49	50-59	60+
Excellent	>29	>26	>23	>20	>16
Very good	21-29	20-26	15-23	11-20	12-16
Good	15-20	13-19	11-14	7-10	5-11
Fair	10-14	8-12	5-10	2-6	2-4
Poor	<10	<8	<5	<2	<2

Figure 7.5 Fitness categories for the push-up by age and sex.

Adapted by permission from American College of Sports Medicine, *ACSM's Guidelines for Exercise Testing and Prescription*, 12th ed., edited by C. Ozemek, A.R. Bonikowske, J.W. Christle, and P.M. Gallo (Wolters Kluwer, 2026), 103, permission conveyed through Copyright Clearance Center, Inc.

CLIENT ASSESSMENT: SINGLE-LEG SQUAT TEST

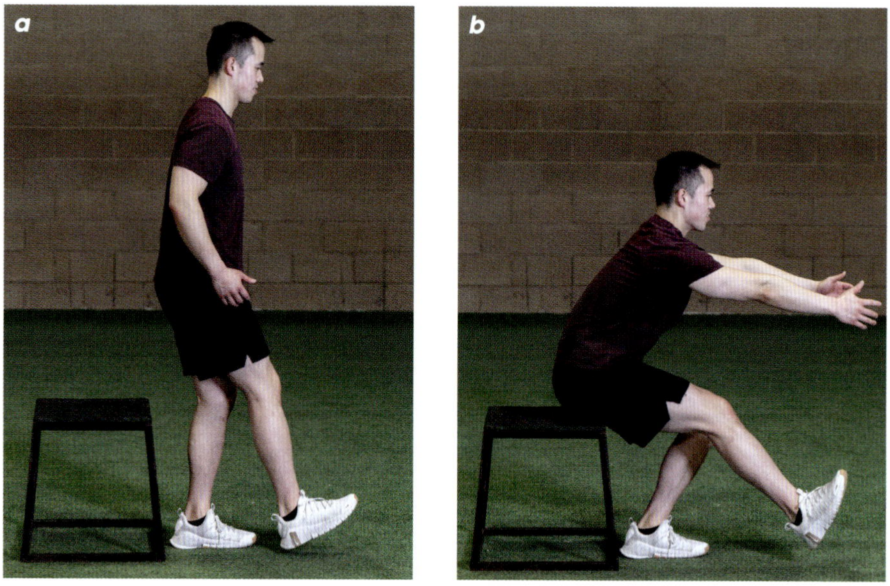

1. Stand tall in front of an 18-inch (46 cm) plyometric box or exercise bench. Pick up one leg off the floor so you are standing in a single-leg stance position.
2. Squat down on one leg, lightly tapping the box with your bottom, and return to the standing position. Repeat as many times as possible until failure.
3. Be sure not to bounce off the box or push off the ground with your inactive leg.
4. To ensure optimal independent function with age, the goal should be to complete 10 unassisted repetitions on each side successfully.

FUNCTIONAL STRENGTH TRAINING PROGRAMMING

When building strength training programs with the goal of improving health and longevity, we should focus on three key variables: safety, efficiency, and functionality.

First and foremost, design strength training programs that are safe and minimize injury risk for clients. If clients are injured during the training process, it directly contradicts the goal of the program to enhance their function and quality of life. With this in mind, we should be cautious with our exercise selection and load management to not put clients at risk for musculoskeletal injury.

Second, build strength training programs that maximize the client's time and efficiency in the gym. With most clients having limited time to devote to organized exercise programs, we should select compound exercises that maximize muscular stimulation. Finally, select exercises that have maximum functional carryover to everyday activities. Resistance training performed with free weights that require multiplanar stability will have a greater carryover to the dynamic nature of everyday activities than isolated machine-based exercises. Although machine-based exercises may be necessary for detrained or injured individuals to begin developing strength, progress toward standing, multiplanar exercises that use free weights to maximally develop joint stability and mobility and therefore carry over to everyday life.

Strength Training Tools

One of the greatest values of a functional strength training program is that it does not require expensive and space-consuming machines to be effective. Most beginners will not need much more than their body weight, dumbbells or kettlebells, and bands or a cable machine to build a complete exercise program. It is important to remember that, for lower body exercises especially, body weight may be sufficient early on to begin providing an adequate stimulus to develop muscle mass and strength.

How Much Strength Training to Do

In addition to recommending 150 to 300 minutes of moderate-intensity or 75 to 150 minutes of vigorous-intensity cardiovascular exercise per week, the U.S. Department of Health and Human Services also advises engaging in muscle-strengthening activities at least two days a week. These activities should target all major muscle groups, including the legs, hips, back, abdomen, chest, shoulders, and arms (Piercy et al., 2018). This stresses the importance of not just completing one or the other but participating in both cardiovascular exercise and strength training as a means to promoting a well-rounded approach to health and fitness.

Strength Training Program Structure

A quality strength training program for health and longevity should consist of two to three full body strength workouts per week. In total strength training should take around 35 minutes and should fit into a complete 60- to 75-minute program in addition to mobility, warm-up, power, and cardiovascular conditioning.

Full body strength training programs provide a well-rounded stimulus and maximize the training effect while allowing time for adequate recovery in between consecutive training sessions.

When building strength training programs, categorize exercise selection via movement patterns rather than individual muscle groups. While traditional bodybuilding-focused programs often are focused on isolated exercises and the development of individual muscles, functional strength training programs should be more concerned with the development of movement patterns to ensure greater carryover to daily functional activities. Table 7.1 outlines the primary strength movement pattern categories used throughout this book, along with representative exercise examples for each.

Table 7.1 Strength Exercise Categories

Strength training categories	Description	Sample exercise image
Knee dominant	Lower body exercises that involve squatting, split squatting, and lunging variations that primarily focus on movement through the knee joint and loading of the surrounding muscles	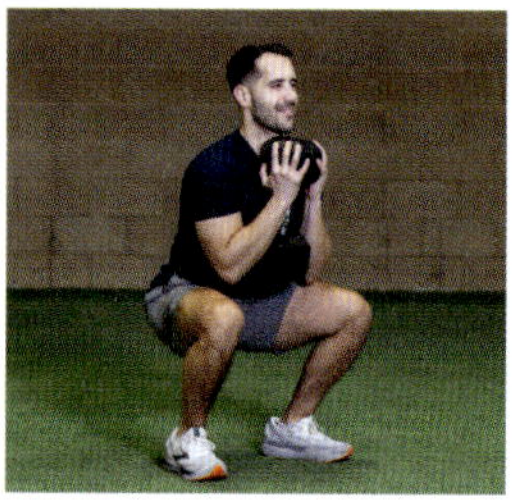
Hip dominant	Lower body exercises such as hinging and bridging variations that primarily focus on movement through the hip joint and loading of the surrounding muscles	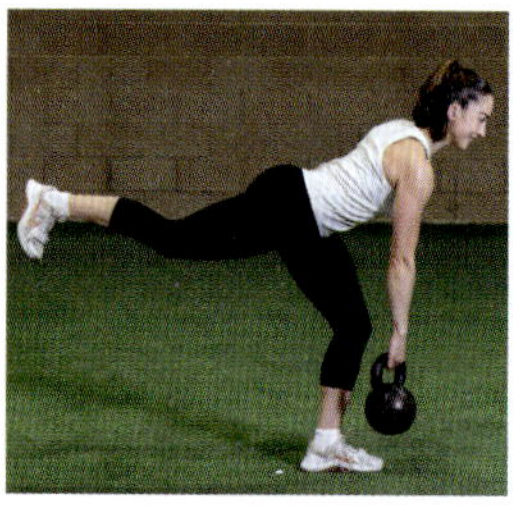
Upper body pushing	Upper body exercises that involve pressing a weight vertically or horizontally and that primarily focus on movement through the shoulders and arms and load the muscles on the anterior side of the body (e.g., pectoralis, triceps, and deltoids)	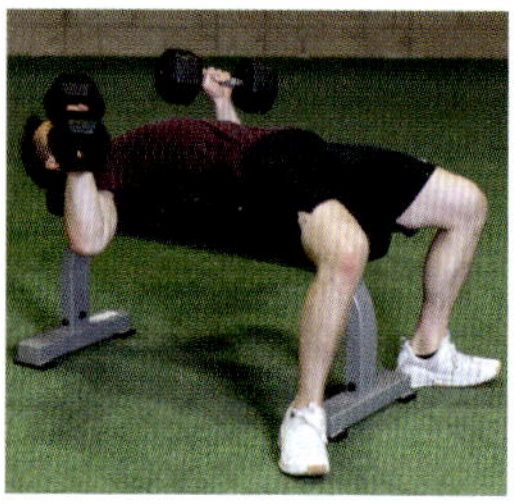

Strength training categories	Description	Sample exercise image
Upper body pulling	Exercises that involve pulling a weight toward the body either horizontally or vertically, that primarily focus on movement through the shoulders and arms, and that load the muscles on the posterior side of the body (e.g., lats, rhomboids, and trapezius)	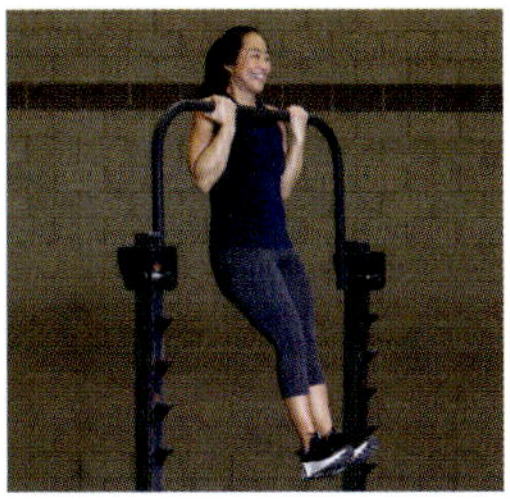
Trunk exercises	Exercises that primarily load the trunk and core muscles (e.g., rectus abdominis, obliques, transverse abdominis and erector spinae)	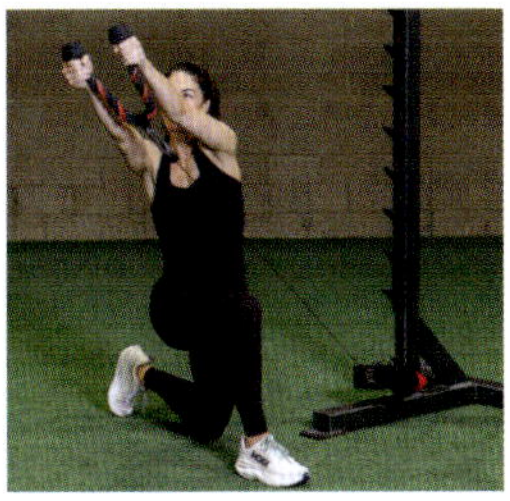

Programming Supersets

Maximizing efficiency is vital to building training programs for clients and providing the most valuable training experience possible. With most gymgoers citing lack of time as the number one reason for not meeting exercise guidelines, we should look to provide as much value as possible in every session (Felicia et al., 2022).

A superset is the performance of multiple exercises together in either a pairing, where the client performs two exercises, or a tri-set, when the client performs three exercises cyclically, as in a circuit. It is recommended to program noncompeting pairings and tri-sets, meaning two or three exercises grouped together that target different areas of the body. This allows one muscle group to rest and recover while a different area of the body is trained at the same time.

An example of a tri-set would be performing a set of bench presses, then a set of split squats, and then a front plank, repeating the cycle multiple times for the prescribed number of sets.

Tri-Set Sample

A1: Bench press (horizontal push)

A2: Split squat (unilateral knee dominant)

A3: Front plank (sagittal plane trunk)

Programming exercise in this way increases the efficiency by creating more workout density. Supersets allow clients to get more work done per unit of time than if they just rested and did nothing between sets.

This approach works well for the general population, whose goals are primarily centered around general health and body composition, because it increases the total amount of work done during the session.

It should be noted that performing supersets does not mean "no rest" or rushing between sets of exercises as quickly as possible; it simply is a programming method that allows us to maximize the allotted exercise time. Intelligently using noncompeting supersets allows us to train a client's strength and power in one body segment while simultaneously resting in another, with minimal interfering fatigue.

Organizing a Strength Training Program

In the interest of developing a balanced full body program, distribute the various strength movement patterns evenly throughout each training session and across the training week, as shown in the following example of a balanced two-day full body strength training program organized using this approach.

SAMPLE STRENGTH TRAINING PROGRAM

DAY 1

- *A1:* Deadlift (bilateral hip dominant)
- *A2:* Front plank (sagittal plane trunk)
- *A3:* Inverted row (horizontal pull)
- *B1:* Split squat (unilateral knee dominant)
- *B2:* Half-kneeling overhead press (vertical push)
- *B3:* Half-kneeling cable chop (transverse plane trunk)

DAY 2

- *A1:* Goblet squat (bilateral knee dominant)
- *A2:* Side plank (frontal plane trunk)
- *A3:* Chin-up (vertical pull)
- *B1:* Single-leg deadlift (unilateral hip dominant)
- *B2:* Push-up (horizontal push)
- *B3:* Half-kneeling cable lift (transverse plane trunk)

By organizing a program in movement patterns as just shown, we can evenly distribute various movement types across each training day and throughout the overall program. This approach ensures a well-rounded strength training program that targets all major muscle groups, movement patterns, and planes of motion.

Programming Load, Sets, and Reps

While many methods for strength programming have been established, one of the simplest and most effective approaches is to use basic linear periodization and progressive resistance to create an overload effect in the muscles to develop strength and hypertrophy. Linear periodization creates an overload effect by either increasing volume weekly (adding more repetitions at the same weight) or increasing intensity weekly (adding more load each week). For novice trainees, consider alternating periods of accumulation (increasing total volume) and intensification (increasing total load) in four-week blocks for a very long period of time and continue to see improvements in strength and hypertrophy. This method provides a varied stimulus, promoting both the neurological adaptations for force production and the physiological adaptations for muscle hypertrophy.

When introducing strength training to a new client, it is best to start with a 4- to 6-week phase focused on anatomical adaptation. During this phase, programming a low total volume with moderate loads allows clients to adjust to strength training, learn fundamental movement patterns, and minimize soreness and injury risk.

Because untrained clients require minimal stimulus to improve strength, high repetition volumes or heavy loads are unnecessary. I recommend starting with two sets of five to eight repetitions in the first week. This provides enough stimulus to initiate adaptation without causing excessive delayed onset muscle soreness (DOMS) and fatigue. From there, we can gradually increase volume throughout the initial phase to develop increased work capacity. Following is an example of a strength training progression over three four-week phases.

Phase 1: Anatomical Adaptation

Week 1: 2 × 6 reps
Week 2: 3 × 6 reps (increase volume)
Week 3: 3 × 8 reps (increase volume)
Week 4: 3 × 10 reps (increase volume)

Phase 2 Progression: Intensification (Increased Load)

Week 1: 3 × 10 reps (increase load)
Week 2: 3 × 8 reps (increase load)
Week 3: 4 × 6 reps (increase load)
Week 4: 4 × 5 reps (increase load)

Phase 3: Accumulation (Increased Volume)

Week 1: 3 × 10 reps (increase volume)
Week 2: 3 × 12 reps (increase volume)
Week 3: 3 × 14 reps (increase volume)
Week 4: 3 × 16 reps (increase volume)

Exercise Execution

How an exercise is performed is just as important as which exercise is selected or how much load is used. Proper execution ensures that the intended muscles are trained effectively while minimizing unnecessary stress on joints and connective tissues.

Strength training exercises should be performed through a full, controlled range of motion whenever possible. Working through a full range allows for more complete muscular development, improves joint mobility, and ensures that strength is built across the entire movement.

Tempo and control are also critical. Repetitions should be performed with intent, maintaining control throughout both the lifting and lowering phases of the movement. Avoid rushing through repetitions or relying on momentum, as this reduces the effectiveness of the exercise and can increase injury risk.

Coaches should also be conservative when introducing new exercises. Load should be kept light until the client demonstrates control, coordination, and an understanding of the movement pattern. Progressing load too quickly before a movement is mastered increases the risk of compensation patterns and injury.

Effort is another key component of execution. To stimulate strength and hypertrophy, sets should be performed to or near muscular failure. This does not mean training to absolute exhaustion on every set, but rather reaching a level of effort where only a few repetitions remain in reserve while maintaining proper form.

Finally, exercises should be performed without pain. While discomfort and fatigue are expected during challenging training, sharp or persistent pain is a signal that the exercise may need to be modified. Coaches should adjust load, range of motion, or exercise selection to ensure that training remains both effective and safe.

Progressive Overload

The key to an effective strength training program is progressive overload. To build strength and muscle mass, we must consistently challenge the muscles and nervous system with increasing stress, prompting the body to adapt and grow stronger.

This means performing strength exercises with enough intensity or volume that sets are taken close to failure, providing a sufficient stimulus for adaptation. When training is performed to or near muscular failure, improvements in strength and muscle mass can occur across a wide range of loading schemes, from heavier loads lifted for fewer repetitions to lighter loads lifted for higher repetitions. In other words, progressive overload does not require lifting the heaviest loads possible; it requires working near failure regardless of load or repetition range.

From a practical standpoint, progression can take many forms. Adding as little as 1.25 to 2.5 pounds (0.6-1.1 kg) to a lift, completing one additional repetition with the same load, or executing the movement with better control and consistency while maintaining proximity to failure all represent valid and sustainable ways to apply progressive overload. Although these changes may seem small, they are realistic and repeatable and compound over time, leading to meaningful improvements in strength and work capacity over the long haul.

Programming Sets and Repetitions

A well-designed strength program should incorporate a broad repetition range, typically between 5 and 20 repetitions per set. This range allows coaches to develop their clients' strength, hypertrophy, and muscular endurance while accommodating individual tolerance, joint health, and training history. Importantly, recent evidence indicates that when sets are performed to a high level of effort—near failure—muscle hypertrophy is largely independent of whether heavier or lighter loads are used so long as near-maximal effort is used (Lees et al., 2025).

As a result, coaches have considerable flexibility when prescribing sets and repetitions. For most general-population clients, one to two challenging working sets per exercise are sufficient to stimulate adaptation when taken close to failure. A simple three-set structure may include an initial lighter warm-up set, followed by one primary working set performed near volitional fatigue. A third set can then be adjusted based on performance—adding load, reducing load, or maintaining the same resistance depending on readiness and execution quality.

This approach emphasizes consistency, effort, and long-term adherence over rigid loading prescriptions. Rather than fixating on a specific repetition target or percentage of one-repetition maximum, effective programming focuses on selecting loads that allow clients to train hard, recover well, and continue progressing over time.

Shown here is an example of how to effectively progress load over three sets.

Example: Bench Press

- *Set 1—Warm-Up:* 135 lb × 5 reps (easy)
- *Set 2—Working Set:* 155 lb × 5 reps (hard)
  - » If easy, increase weight by 2.5 to 5 pounds.
  - » If moderate, keep the same weight.
  - » If hard, decrease weight by 5 to 10 pounds.
- *Set 3—Adjusted Working Set:* Based on set 2 performance

STRENGTH TRAINING EXERCISES

GOBLET SQUAT

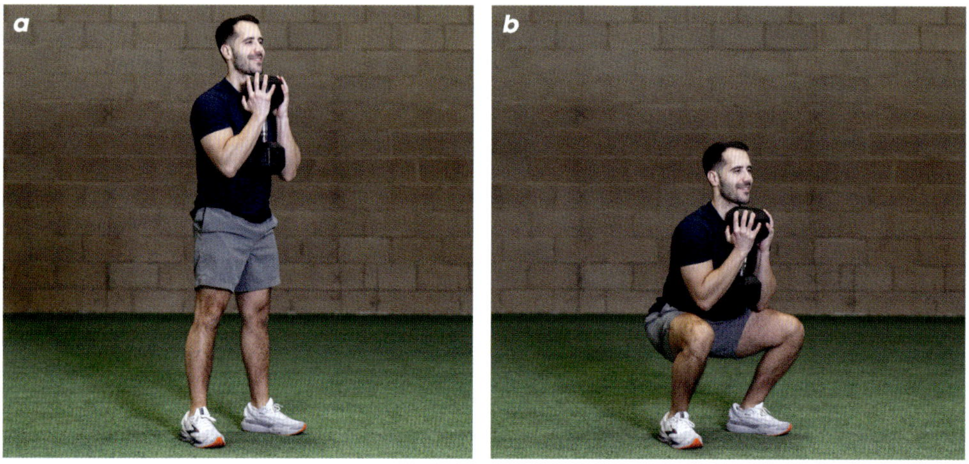

Benefits

The goblet squat strengthens the quadriceps, glutes, and hamstrings while reinforcing trunk strength in a bilateral stance. This foundational movement supports daily physical activities while also building lower body strength that protects joint health and promotes long-term independence.

Instructions for the Client

1. Begin by standing with your feet shoulder-width apart or slightly wider with your toes pointing straight ahead. Hold a dumbbell or kettlebell tightly to your chest with both hands.
2. Brace your abdominals tightly and create tension in your hips by externally rotating and screwing your feet into the floor.
3. Maintain a tall posture with your chest as you lower yourself downward with control until your femurs are parallel to the floor and your elbows come to the inside of your knees.
4. Reverse the motion and drive upward forcefully to the starting position. Repeat for the prescribed number of repetitions.

Variations

Regression: Squat With Medicine Ball Press-Out

In the squat with medicine ball press-out, the client holds a light medicine ball at the chest and reaches it forward while squatting. This variation reduces the external load while encouraging an upright torso, making it an effective regression for those still developing squat mechanics.

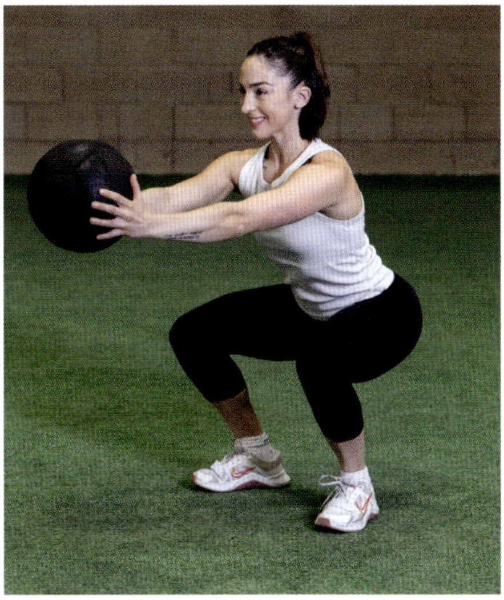

Progression 1: Offset Kettlebell Front Squat

This is a progression from the goblet squat that involves holding a kettlebell on one side of the body, challenging motor control and trunk stability by forcing the client to resist lateral flexion.

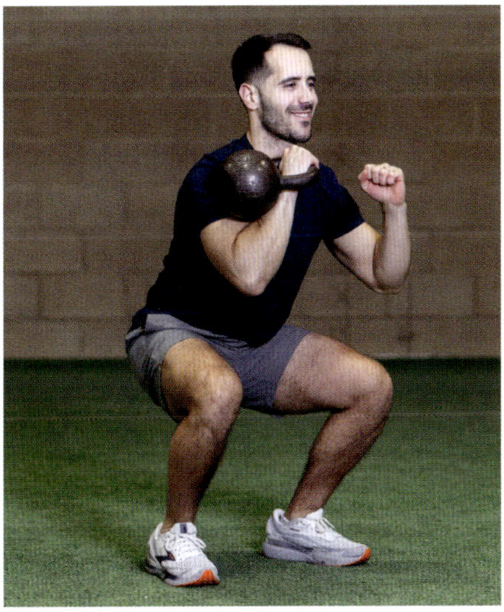

Progression 2: Double Kettlebell Front Squat

This is a progression from the goblet squat or offset squat, holding a kettlebell in each hand in the front rack position to allow for greater external load, challenging both trunk and leg strength.

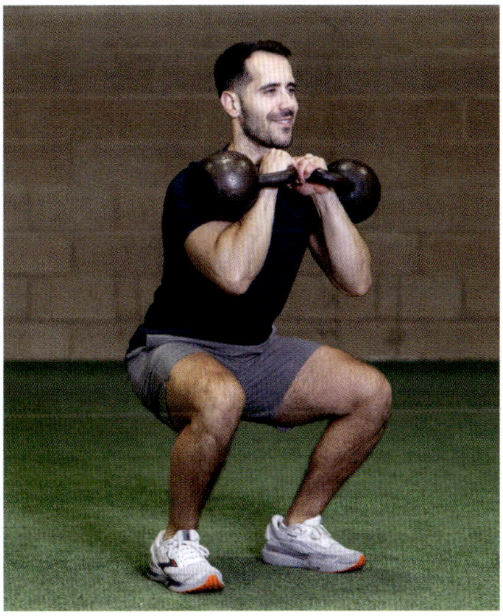

GOBLET SPLIT SQUAT

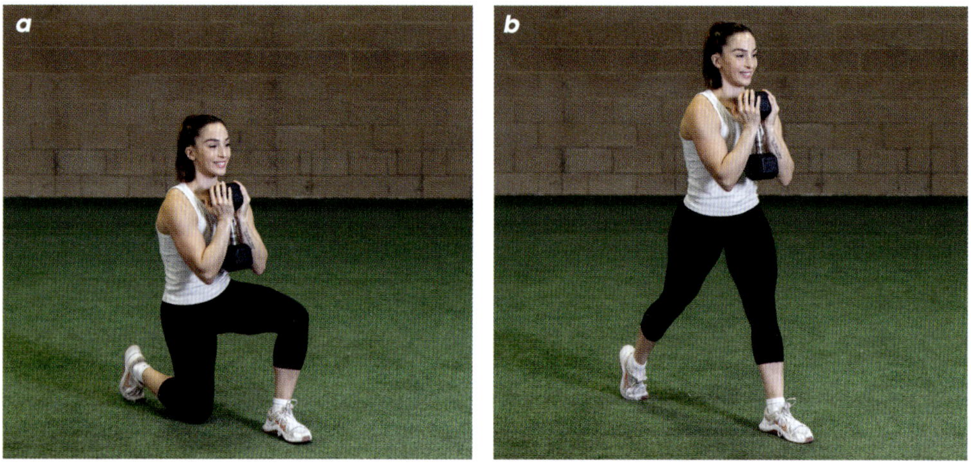

Benefits

The goblet split squat builds lower body strength in a split stance, targeting the quadriceps, glutes, and hamstrings. This movement improves balance, hip stability, and unilateral strength, which are essential to athletic performance, injury reduction, and everyday activities.

Instructions for the Client

1. Begin in a half-kneeling position with your left leg in front and your right leg behind you. Your left knee should be flexed to roughly 90 degrees, with your knee over your midfoot. Your right knee should be resting on the ground under your right hip, with your ankle flexed and toes tucked into the ground.
2. Hold a dumbbell or kettlebell tight to your chest with both hands, with elbows tucked downward by your sides.
3. Maintaining a tall posture with your torso, drive your left foot into the ground, pushing you away from the floor until your left knee is almost fully extended.
4. Lower yourself under control back to the ground, and softly tap your right knee on the floor. Perform for the prescribed number of repetitions and then repeat on the opposite side.

Variations

Regression: Bodyweight Split Squat

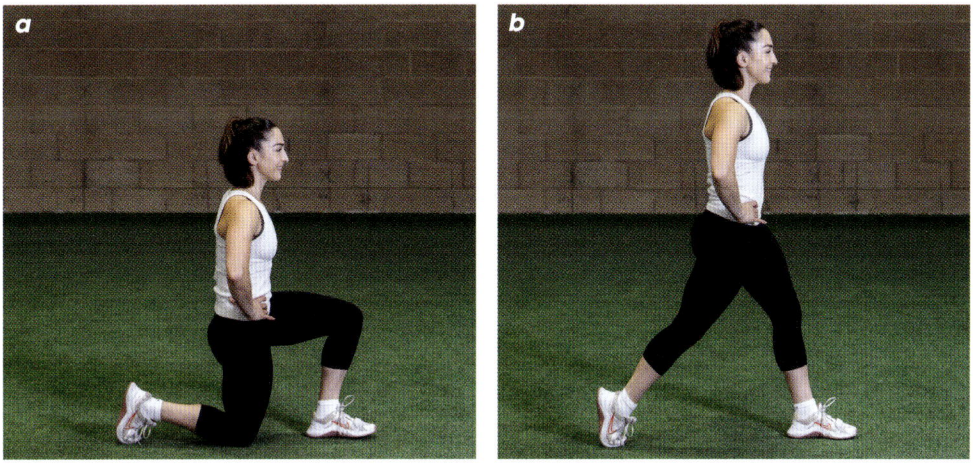

The bodyweight split squat is a regression that removes the external load, allowing the client to develop single-leg strength and focus on proper form and balance.

Progression: Two-Dumbbell Rear-Foot-Elevated Split Squat

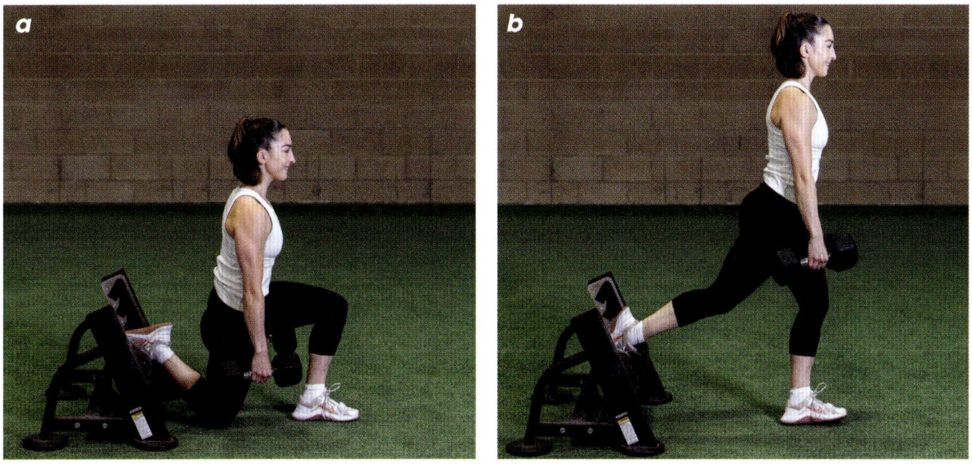

The two-dumbbell rear-foot-elevated split squat increases the challenge on the working leg by holding a dumbbell in each hand while the rear foot is elevated on a bench or split squat stand, increasing the external load and reducing assistance from the rear leg. This variation allows for greater loading to further develop single-leg strength, balance, and hip stability.

SINGLE-LEG SQUAT TO BOX

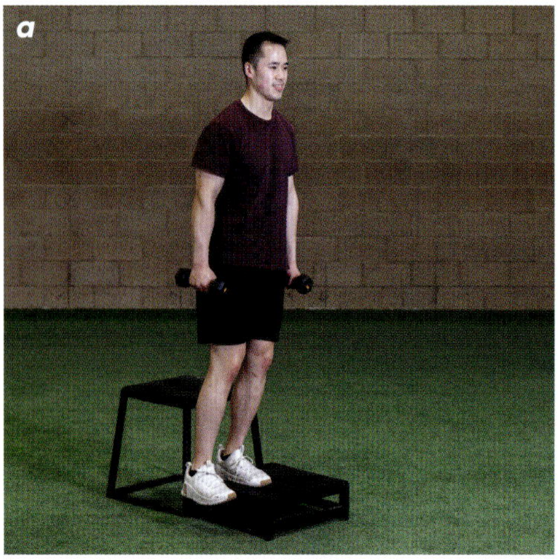
a

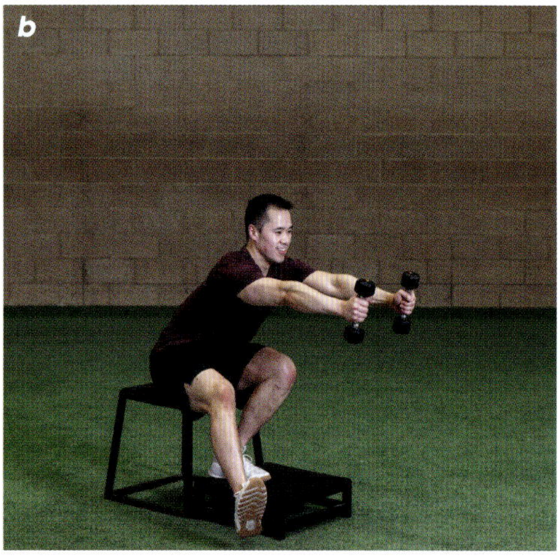
b

Benefits

The single-leg squat emphasizes true unilateral loading, strengthening the quadriceps, glutes, and hamstrings while improving balance and hip stability, which are essential qualities for injury reduction and long-term independence.

Instructions for the Client

1. Stand in front of an 18-inch (46 cm) plyometric box or bench with a 5-pound (2.6 kg) weight in each hand and your arms by your side.
2. Balance on one leg and begin squatting down under control, lowering your hips toward the box. At the same time, raise both arms straight in front of you to shoulder height.
3. Lightly tap the box with your glutes (do not sit or bounce), then push through your standing leg to return to the starting position, lowering your arms back to your side.

Variations

Regression: Goblet Slide Board Reverse Lunge

The goblet slide board reverse lunge serves as a regression from the single-leg squat, holding a dumbbell or a kettlebell in a goblet position while the rear leg slides backward on a slide board, reducing the relative load and balance demands on the working leg while still developing single-leg strength.

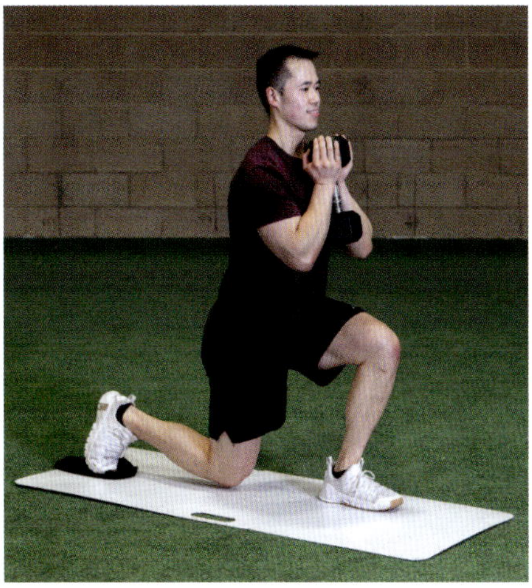

Progression: Zercher Loaded Single-Leg Squat

To progress the single-leg squat, increase squat depth and add a Zercher load with a sandbag. In the Zercher position, the weight is held in the elbow creases in front of the body, which increases trunk demand and allows the client to use greater external load while maintaining an upright posture.

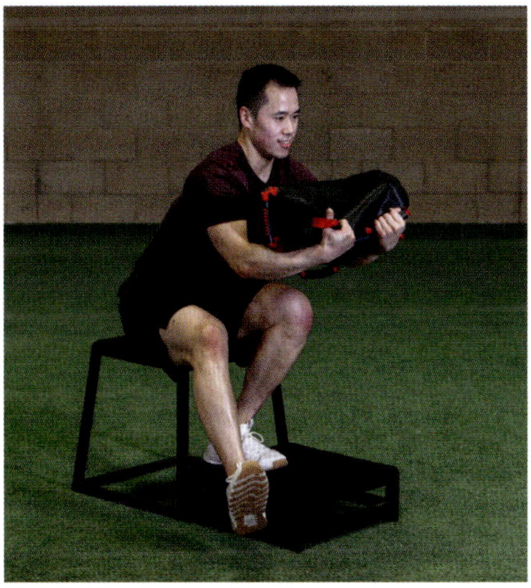

GOBLET LATERAL SQUAT

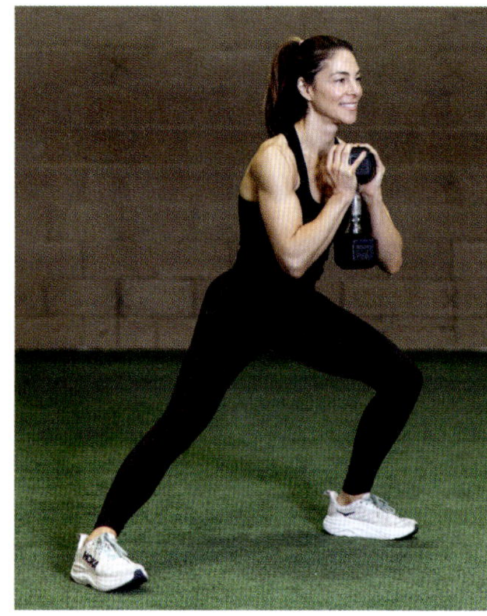

Benefits

The goblet lateral squat helps to strengthen the quadriceps, glutes, and adductors while improving hip mobility in the frontal plane. This variation helps to develop strength with moving laterally, supporting hip and knee health and general movement skills.

Instructions for the Client

1. Begin by standing tall with your feet placed wide apart, approximately 2 times shoulder width, allowing for significant hip abduction with your toes pointing straight ahead. Hold a dumbbell or kettlebell in a goblet position at the chest.
2. Shift your bodyweight to one side, bending the knee and hip while keeping the opposite leg straight and foot flat.
3. Lower under control until the working thigh is parallel to the ground or as deep as your mobility allows while maintaining an upright torso.
4. Push through the working leg to return back to the starting position.
5. Complete the prescribed number of repetitions, alternating sides.

Variations

Regression: Medicine Ball Reaching Lateral Squat

The reaching lateral squat reduces the load and helps teach the movement pattern by holding a medicine ball and reaching it outward during the squat, encouraging the client to shift their weight posteriorly and develop proper control before progressing to the loaded variation.

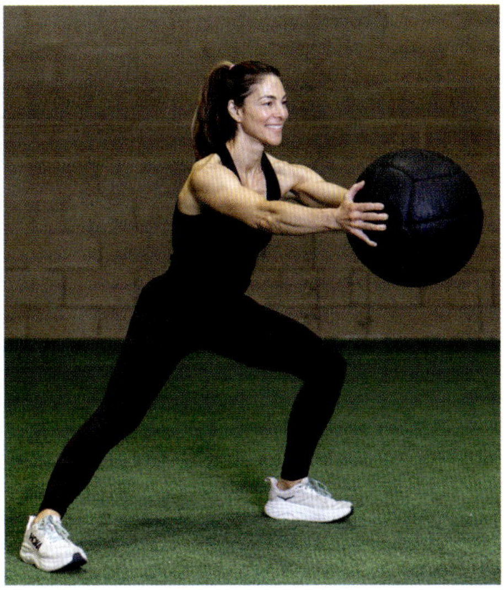

Progression: Goblet Lateral Lunge

The goblet lateral lunge progresses the movement by stepping out to the side into each repetition, introducing a dynamic deceleration component and further challenging coordination and strength of the ankle, knee, and hip.

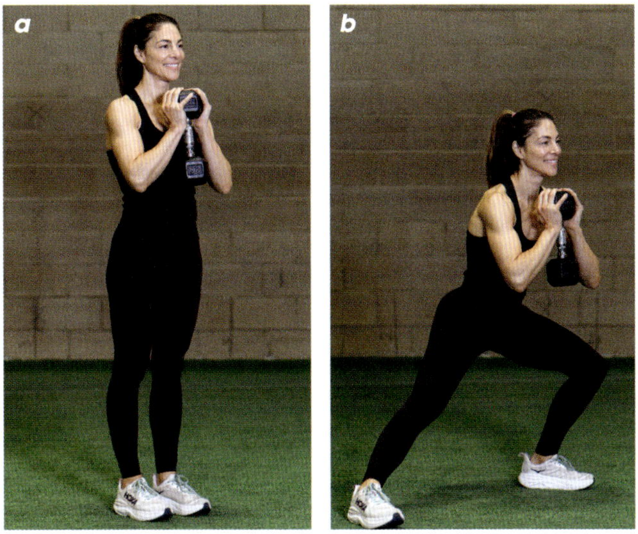

ONE-KETTLEBELL SINGLE-LEG DEADLIFT

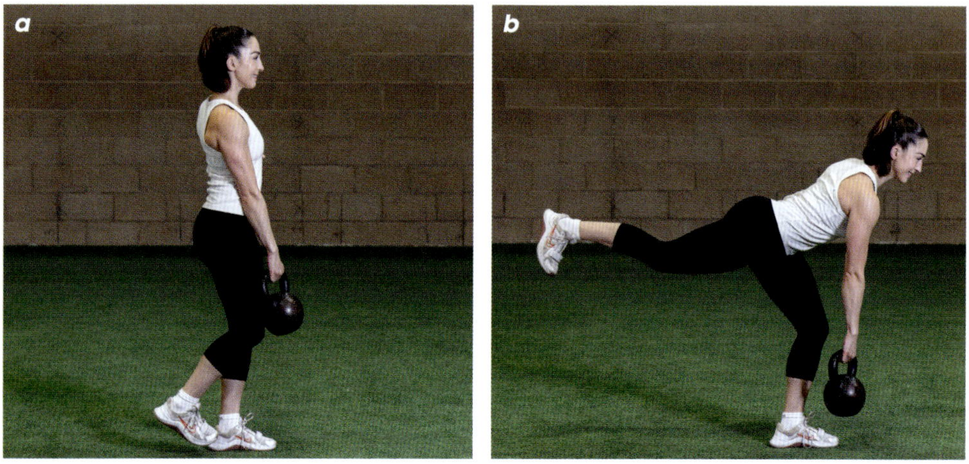

Benefits

The one-kettlebell single-leg deadlift strengthens the hamstrings and glutes while challenging balance and hip stability in a single-leg stance. This variation builds posterior chain strength and supports hip and low back health for performance and longevity.

Instructions for the Client

1. Begin by standing tall with your feet together, with one kettlebell in your right hand in front of your right leg.
2. Lift your right foot off of the floor and extend it behind you.
3. Begin hinging at the hips and slightly bending your left knee.
4. As you lower the kettlebell toward the floor, be sure to maintain a flat back and erect torso.
5. Once your torso is parallel to the floor, reverse the direction by forcefully contracting your glute and hamstring to return yourself to the upright position.
6. Complete the prescribed number of repetitions and repeat on the opposite side.

Variations

Regression: Bodyweight Reaching Single-Leg Deadlift

The bodyweight reaching single-leg deadlift allows the client to learn the movement pattern by reaching the arm opposite the stance leg forward while extending the non-stance leg behind. This reciprocal reaching pattern promotes multiplanar hip stability and balance before progressing to an external load.

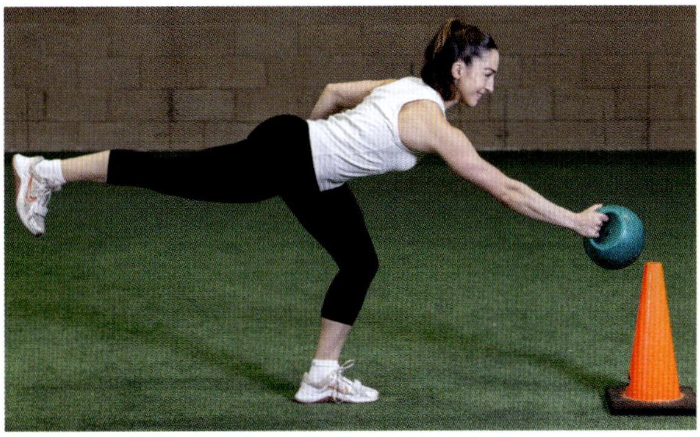

Progression: Two-Kettlebell Single-Leg Deadlift

The two-kettlebell single-leg deadlift increases difficulty by holding a kettlebell in each hand, adding greater external load and further challenging hamstring and glute strength and hip stability.

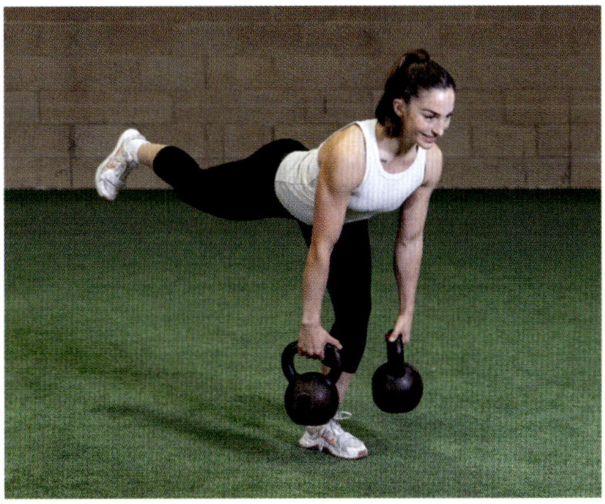

SKATER SQUAT

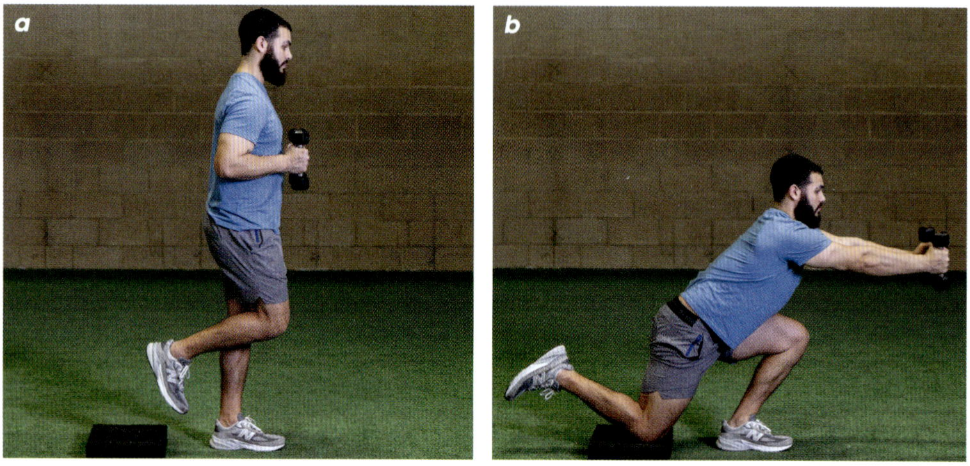

Benefits

The skater squat strengthens the quadriceps, glutes, and hamstrings while challenging balance and stability in a single-leg stance. This exercise variation helps to build hip stability and strength, supporting joint health and functional independence.

Instructions for the Client

1. Begin by standing tall with your feet together, with 5-pound (2.3 kg) dumbbells in each hand and a small Airex pad or other object about 3 to 4 inches (7.6-10.2 cm) high behind you.
2. Lift your right foot off the floor, and try to bring your right heel toward your glute.
3. Lift the weights upward in front of you to shoulder height with the elbows straight while simultaneously lowering yourself down to the pad by hinging at your hips and flexing your left knee.
4. Lightly tap your right knee on the pad while keeping your right foot off the floor and your back flat.
5. Reverse the motion while lowering your arms back down to your sides as you return to the starting position.
6. Complete the prescribed number of repetitions and repeat on the opposite side.

Variations

Regression: Reduced Range of Motion Skater Squat

Performing the skater squat with a reduced range of motion by adding pads under the rear knee to limit depth allows beginners to develop hip stability and balance with greater control before progressing to the full depth variation.

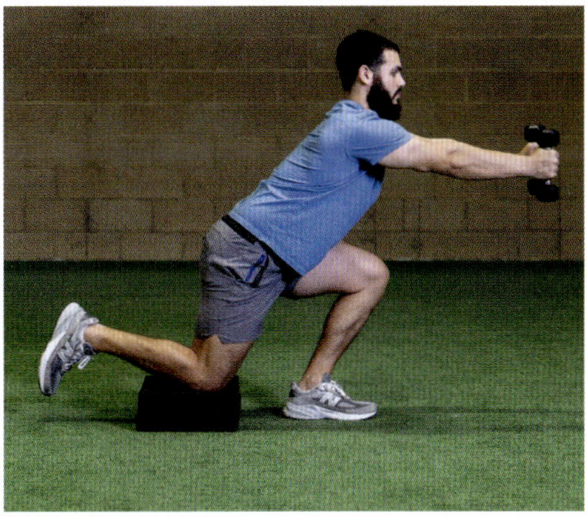

Progression: Sandbag Zercher Loaded Skater Squat

The sandbag Zercher loaded skater squat increases difficulty by adding external load, demanding greater trunk stability and lower body strength.

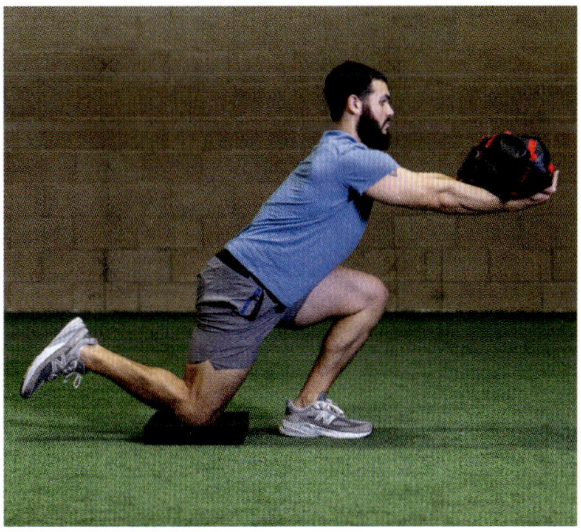

SINGLE-LEG SHOULDER-ELEVATED HIP LIFT

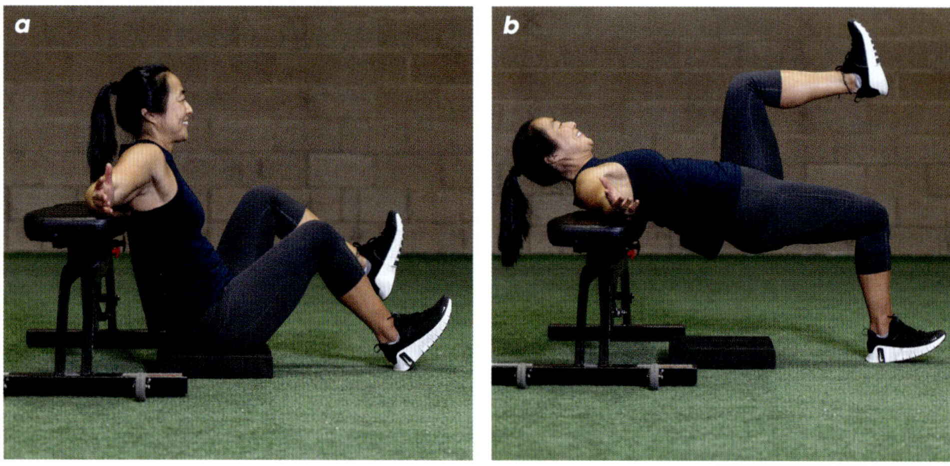

Benefits

The single-leg shoulder-elevated hip lift targets the glutes and hamstrings while challenging trunk stability in the presence of hip extension. This variation builds hip extension strength and improves control of the spine and pelvis to support low back and hip health.

Instructions for the Client

1. Begin by sitting on the ground with your upper back against the side of a weight bench. Your shoulder blades should be positioned above the edge of the bench with your arms stretched out to the sides.
2. Flex both of your knees with your heels pressing into the ground and your ankles dorsiflexed upward.
3. Flex your left hip, bringing your left knee as close as possible to the chest and bringing your left foot off the floor.
4. Drive your right heel into the ground to extend your right hip, lifting your body off the floor until your torso is parallel to the floor, creating a straight line from your knee to your shoulder.
5. Lower yourself back to the floor slowly, lightly tapping the floor with your hip in between repetitions.
6. Complete the prescribed number of repetitions and repeat on the opposite side.

Variations

Regression: Single-Leg Hip Lift on the Floor

This regression of the hip lift exercise is performed while lying on the back on the floor, reducing the overall load and range of motion and making it easier for a beginner to control hip extension and trunk positioning before progressing to the single-leg shoulder-elevated hip lift.

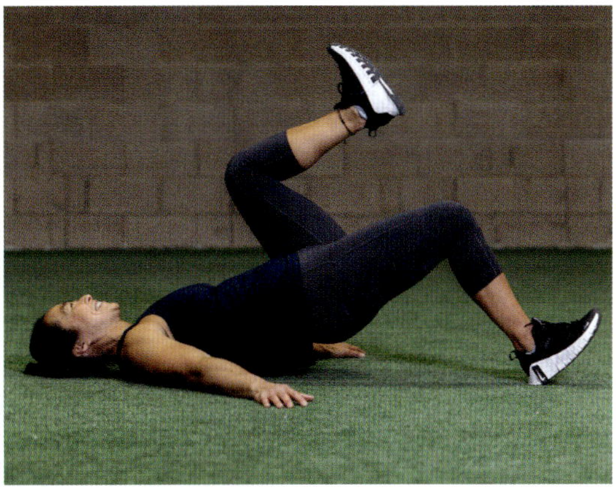

Progression: Loaded Shoulder-Elevated Single-Leg Hip Lift

The loaded shoulder-elevated single-leg hip lift is performed with the shoulders elevated on a bench and a weight held across the hips, increasing difficulty by adding external resistance and further challenging glute and hamstring strength while reinforcing pelvic and core stability.

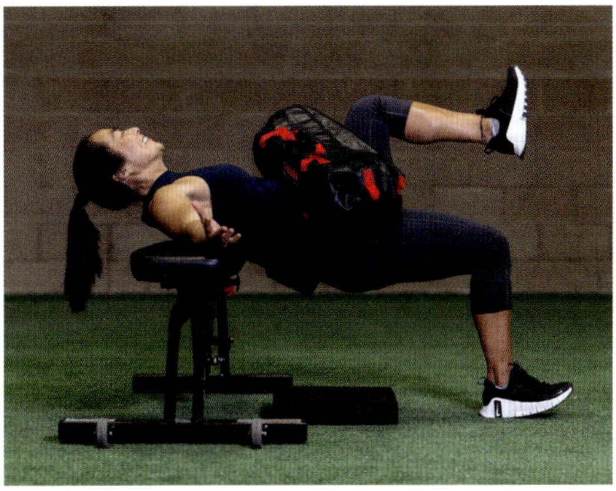

KETTLEBELL DEADLIFT

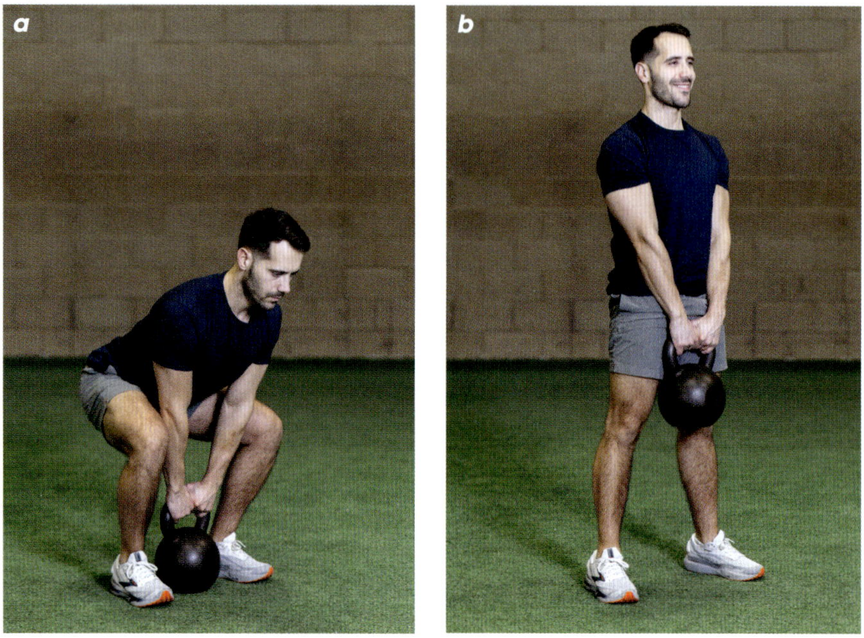

Benefits

The kettlebell deadlift is the most efficient way to teach deadlifting while also strengthening the hamstrings, glutes, and lower back. This is a foundational movement to develop posterior chain strength, support spinal health, and improve functional capacity for daily activities.

Instructions for the Client

1. Stand with your feet shoulder-width apart with a kettlebell placed on the floor directly between your feet. Hinge at your hips and slightly bend your knees as you grab the kettlebell tightly with both hands.
2. Use the glutes and hamstrings to extend the hips forcefully while maintaining a flat back all the way to a tall standing position.
3. Reverse the motion by sitting your hips back and lowering the kettlebell back down to the starting position.
4. Repeat for the prescribed number of repetitions.

Variations

Regression: Chest-Loaded Hip Hinge

The chest-loaded hip hinge serves as a regression from the kettlebell deadlift. Starting in a standing position and holding the weight at the chest allows the client to more easily shift their weight posteriorly and learn the hip hinge pattern before progressing to deadlifting from the ground.

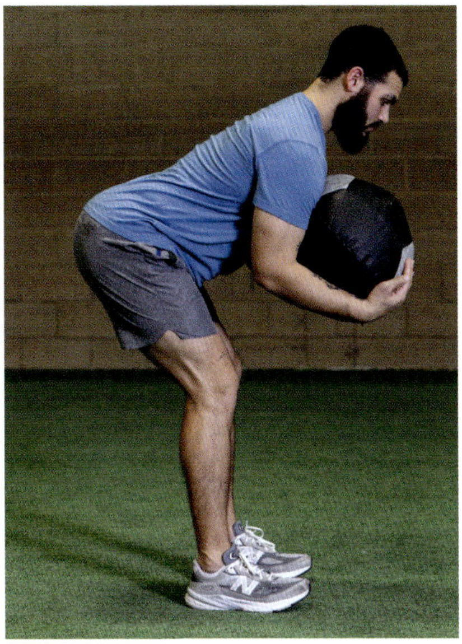

Progression: Trap Bar Deadlift

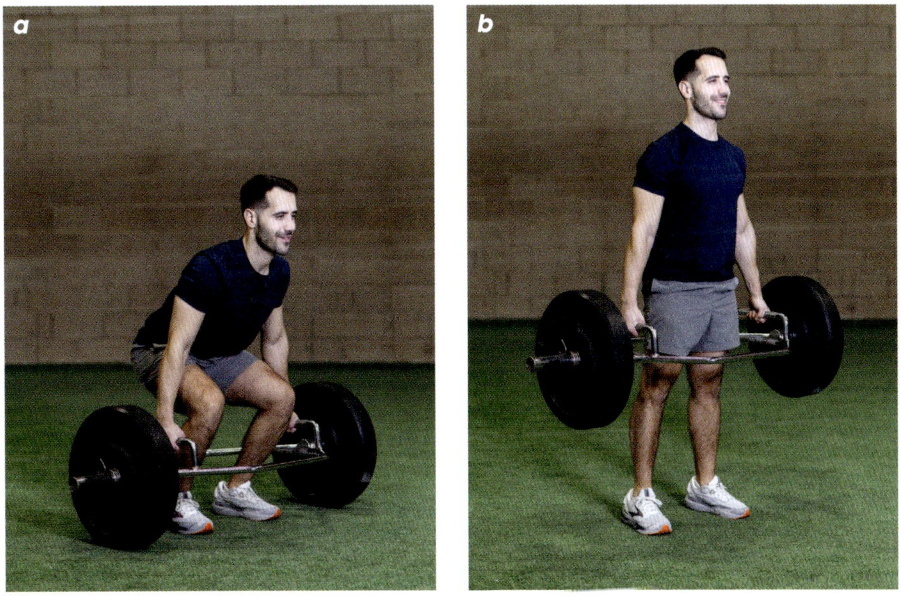

The trap bar deadlift progresses from the kettlebell deadlift by allowing greater external loading to develop strength in the glutes, hamstrings, and lower back.

SLIDING LEG CURL

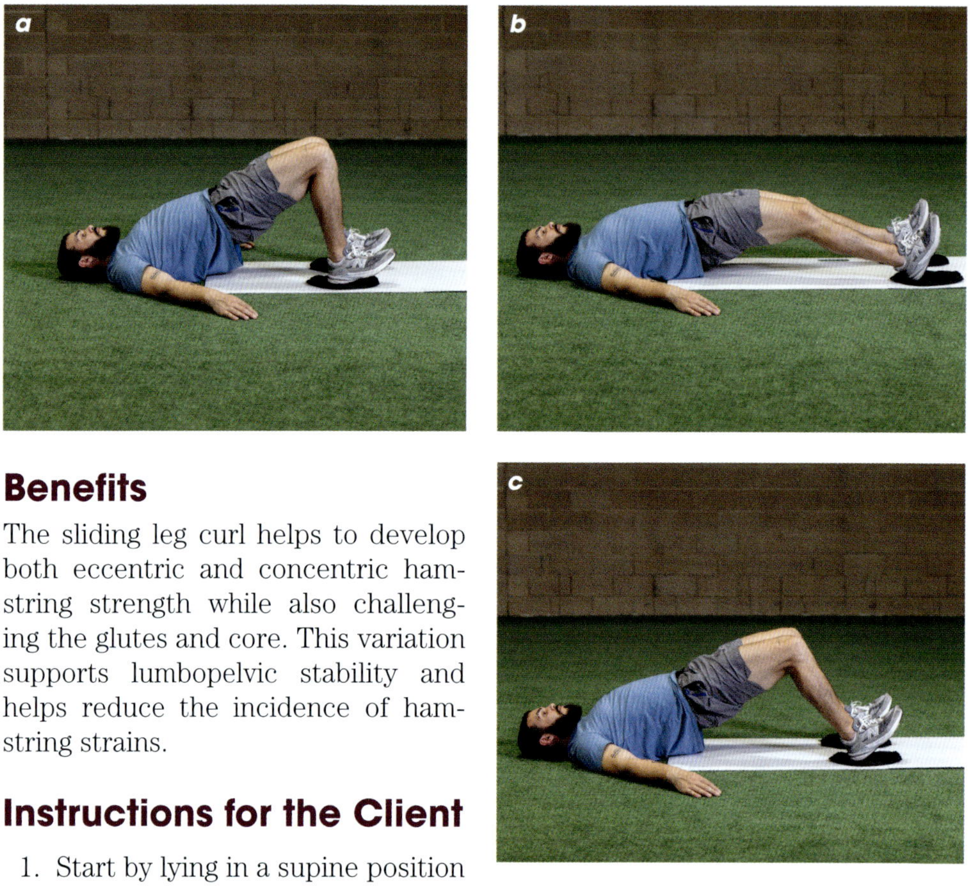

Benefits

The sliding leg curl helps to develop both eccentric and concentric hamstring strength while also challenging the glutes and core. This variation supports lumbopelvic stability and helps reduce the incidence of hamstring strains.

Instructions for the Client

1. Start by lying in a supine position with your knees bent and feet on the floor with your ankles dorsiflexed upward. Place plastic sliders or a towel on a slide board or hardwood floor under your heels so that your feet can slide.
2. Lift your hips up into a bridge position so that you have a straight line from your shoulders to your knees. Slowly extend your knees and begin sliding your heels away from you while maintaining full hip extension.
3. Once your knees are fully extended, reverse the motion by flexing the knees and bringing your heels toward you until you reach the starting position. Be sure to maintain abdominal tension and full hip extension throughout the movement.
4. Repeat for the prescribed number of repetitions, keeping the hips lifted throughout.

Variations

Regression: Eccentric-Only Slide Board Leg Curl

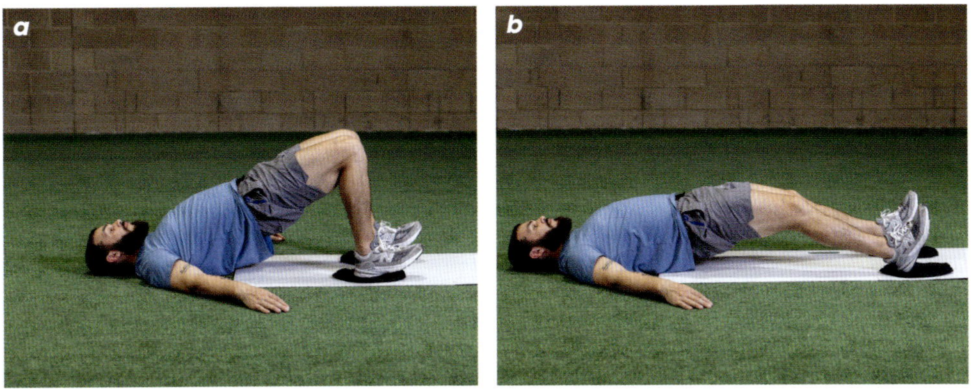

The eccentric-only slide board leg curl reduces difficulty by focusing only on the lowering phase of the movement. This variation helps beginners develop hamstring strength and lumbopelvic control before progressing to the full sliding leg curl.

Progression: Eccentric-Only Single-Leg Slide Board Leg Curl

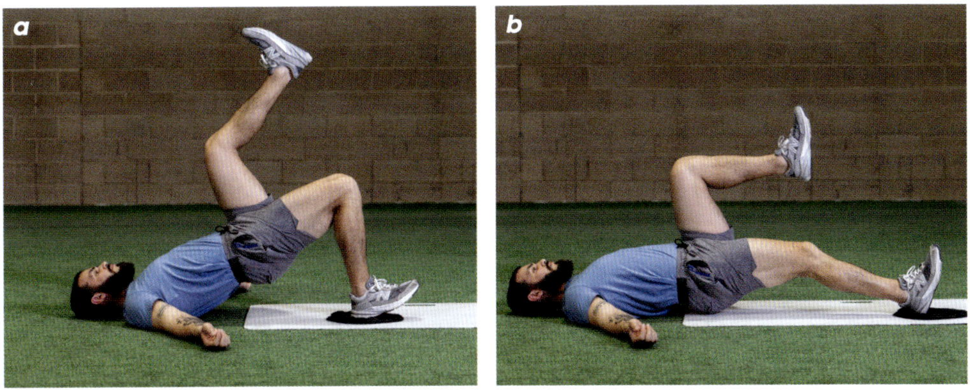

The eccentric-only single-leg slide board leg curl increases difficulty by isolating one leg at a time, demanding greater hamstring strength and core stability.

PUSH-UP

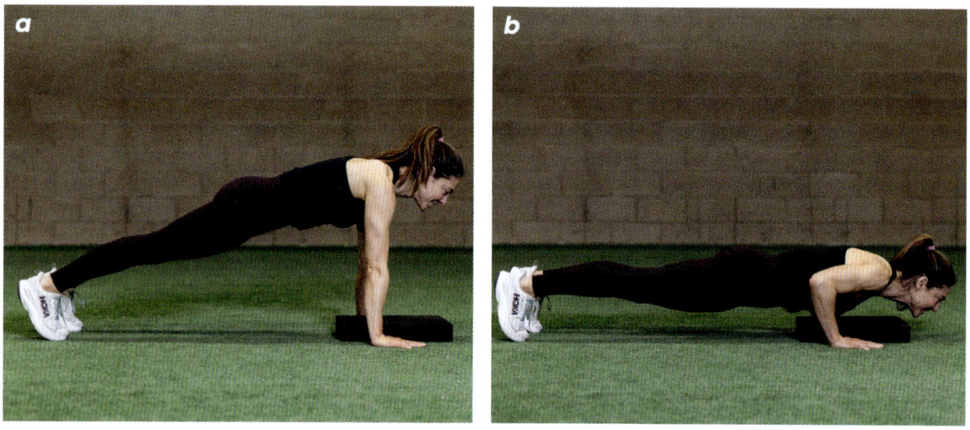

Benefits

The push-up builds upper body strength in the chest, shoulders, and triceps while also developing core strength and stability. This combination of upper body and trunk strength carries over directly to both athletic performance and activities of daily living.

Instructions for the Client

1. Position yourself in a prone plank position with your hands just outside your shoulders, arms locked straight, and feet and legs together. Your abs should be braced tight so that you maintain a straight line from your head to your hips.
2. Slowly lower yourself down toward the floor until you are approximately 3 inches (8 cm) from the floor. In the bottom position, your arms should be abducted roughly 45 degrees from the midline of your body.
3. Drive up from the ground forcefully, maintaining a straight alignment of your body throughout the entire movement and locking out your arms in the top position.
4. Repeat for the prescribed number of repetitions.

Variations

Regression: Incline Push-Up

By elevating the hands on a barbell, box, or bench, this variation allows the client to learn the push-up with reduced load and increase the challenge by lowering closer to the floor until a regular push-up can be completed.

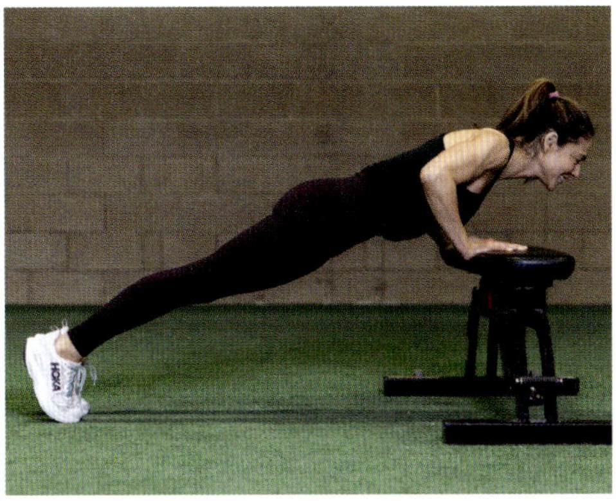

Progression: Weighted Push-Up

The weighted push-up progresses the standard push-up by adding external load, increasing the challenge to the chest, shoulders, triceps, and core muscles.

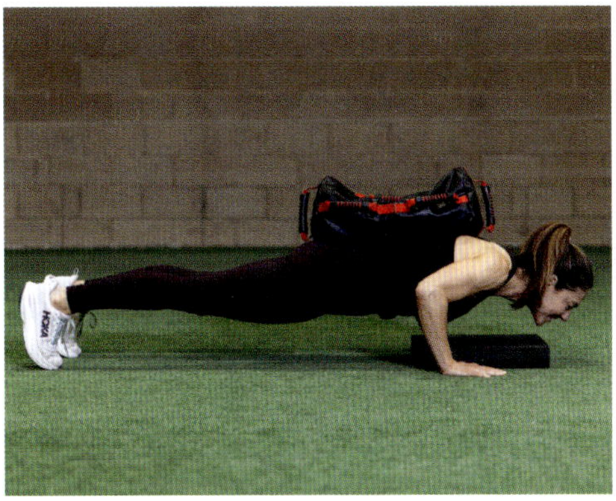

DUMBBELL BENCH PRESS

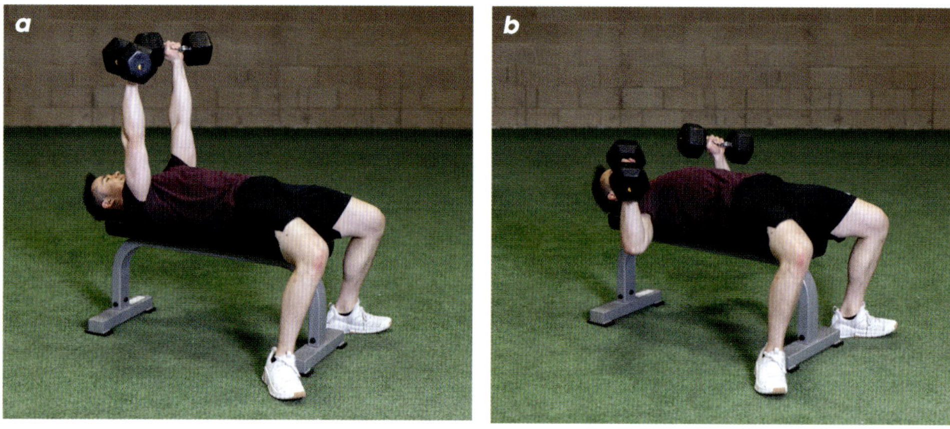

Benefits

The dumbbell bench press strengthens the chest, shoulders, and triceps while allowing for greater variability in movement than barbell pressing, making it a more joint-friendly option for general-population clients with limited shoulder mobility.

Instructions for the Client

1. Begin by lying in a supine position on a flat exercise bench with your feet firmly planted on the floor and a dumbbell in each hand.
2. Create tension in the shoulders by pinning the shoulder blades down and back against the bench. Slowly lower the dumbbells down toward your body so that your arms are at a 45-degree angle from the midline of your body.
3. Once you bring the dumbbells down to the chest, forcefully drive them back up until your arms are locked straight in the starting position. Keep your hips on the bench and your feet on the ground throughout the entire exercise.
4. Repeat for the prescribed number of repetitions.

Variations

Regression: Two-Arm Standing Cable Press

The two-arm standing cable press is a horizontal pressing regression from the dumbbell bench press that allows greater scapular motion, helping to develop greater shoulder stability in clients with a history of pain or limited shoulder mobility.

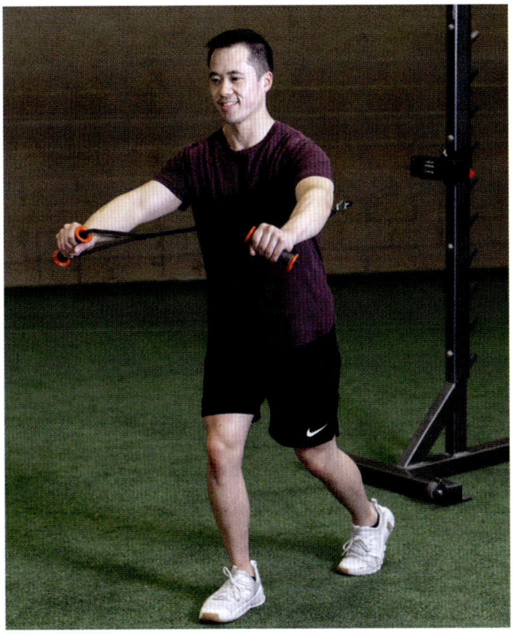

Progression: Single-Arm Dumbbell Bench Press

The single-arm dumbbell bench press progresses the traditional dumbbell bench press by adding an antirotation demand on the trunk. This variation continues to build chest, shoulder, and triceps strength while also developing trunk strength.

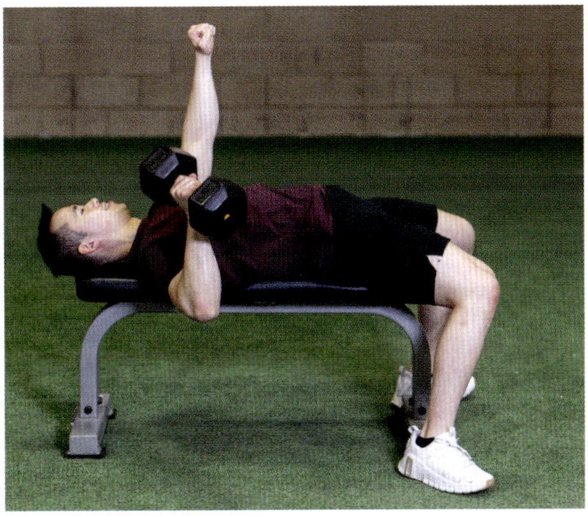

HALF-KNEELING SINGLE-ARM OVERHEAD PRESS

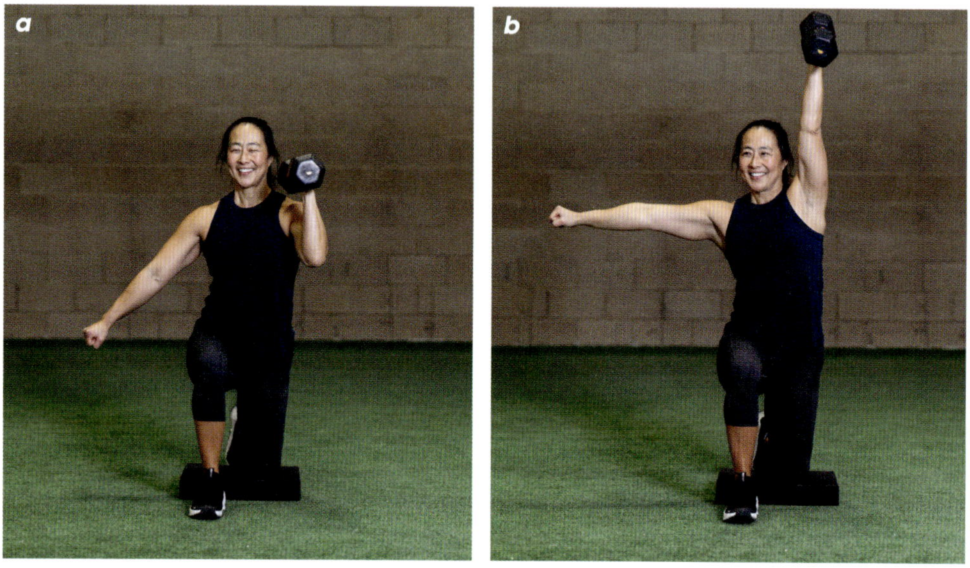

Benefits

The half-kneeling single-arm overhead press strengthens the shoulder and triceps while developing trunk stability and postural control. The half-kneeling stance limits lower body compensation, making it an effective way to develop pressing strength for beginners.

Instructions for the Client

1. Begin in a half-kneeling position, with the rear ankle dorsiflexed and toes tucked into the ground. Hold a dumbbell or kettlebell in front of your shoulder on the same side as the knee on the floor.
2. Maintain a stable torso position while pressing the arm vertically overhead. Lock the arm out fully at the top so that your biceps is lined up next to your ear.
3. Slowly lower the weight back to the starting position.
4. Complete the prescribed number of repetitions and repeat on the opposite side.

Variations

Regression: Half-Kneeling Angled Barbell Press

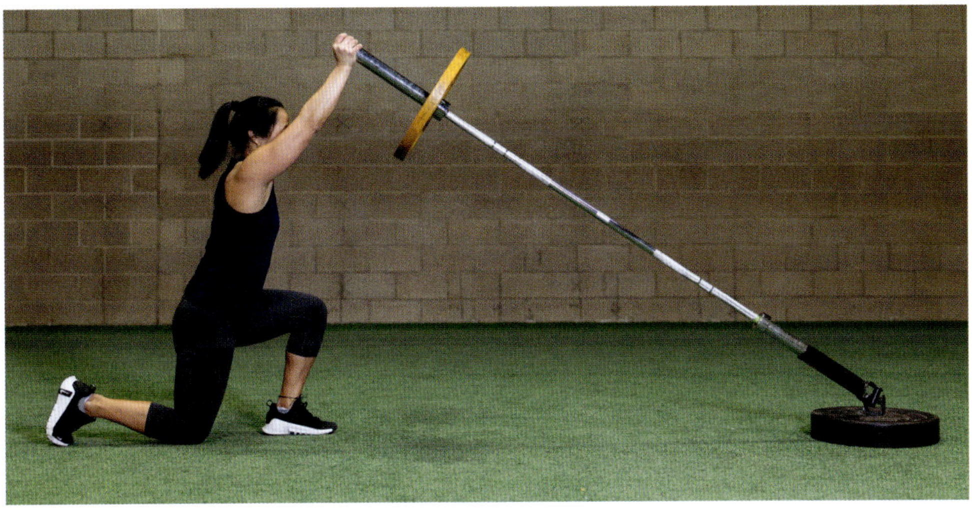

The half-kneeling angled barbell press is a regression from the overhead press, allowing the client to press at a forward angle that reduces shoulder mobility demands, making it a better option for those with limited shoulder range of motion.

Progression: Standing Single-Arm Overhead Press

The standing single-arm overhead press progresses the half-kneeling variation by increasing trunk stability demands. This exercise develops shoulder and triceps strength while also challenging core control in a fully upright position.

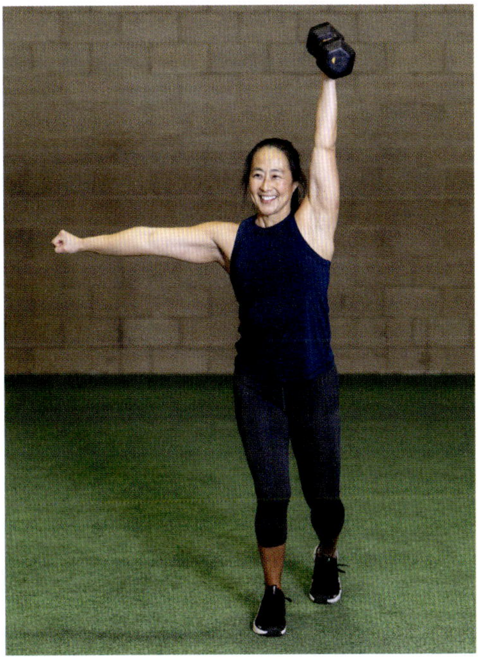

SINGLE-ARM DUMBBELL ROW

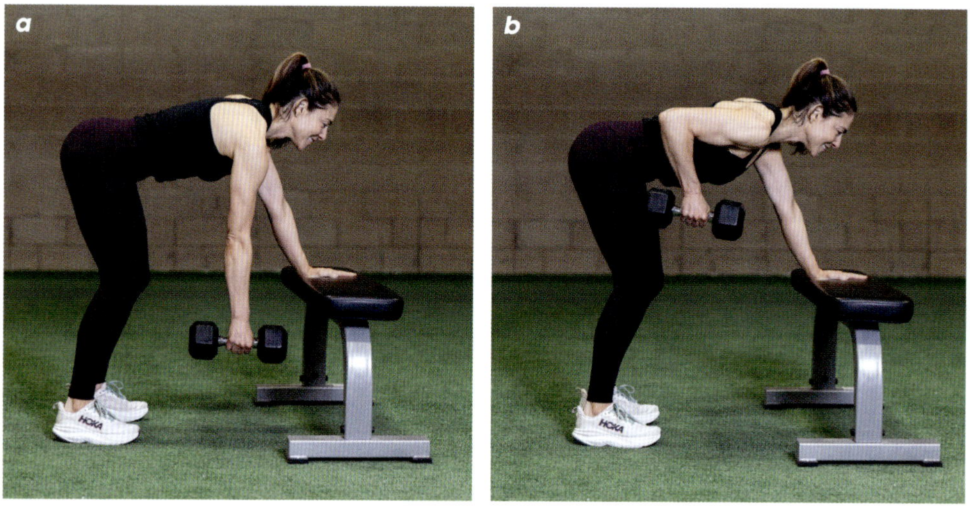

Benefits

The single-arm dumbbell row strengthens the upper back, lats, and biceps while also promoting scapular stability. The movement improves pulling strength while also supporting long-term shoulder health.

Instructions for the Client

1. Start by standing approximately 2 to 3 feet (0.6-0.9 m) from an exercise bench with your feet slightly wider than shoulder-width apart. Hinge at the hips with a flat back, and place one hand firmly on the bench.
2. Holding a dumbbell in the other hand, flex the elbow and pull the dumbbell upward until it reaches the pelvis.
3. Slowly lower the dumbbell back to the starting position while maintaining a neutral spine.
4. Complete the prescribed number of repetitions and repeat on the opposite side.

Variations

Regression: Half-Kneeling Cable Row

The half-kneeling cable row simplifies the development of pulling strength by decreasing the demand for mobility and postural control. This variation allows beginners to develop proper control before progressing to the single-arm dumbbell row.

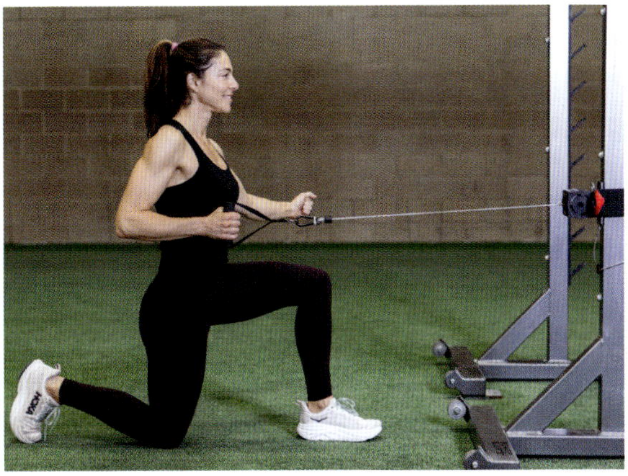

Progression: Dumbbell Row With Isometric Pause

The dumbbell row with an isometric pause progresses the standard row by requiring the client to hold the top position for 5 seconds. This increased time under tension reinforces scapular control and upper back strength.

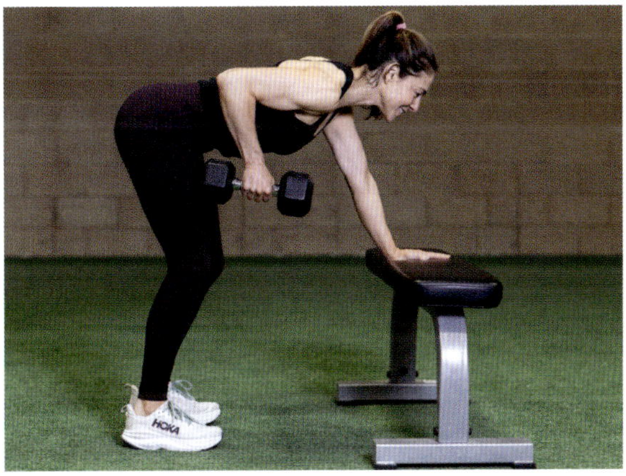

INVERTED ROW ON SUSPENSION TRAINER

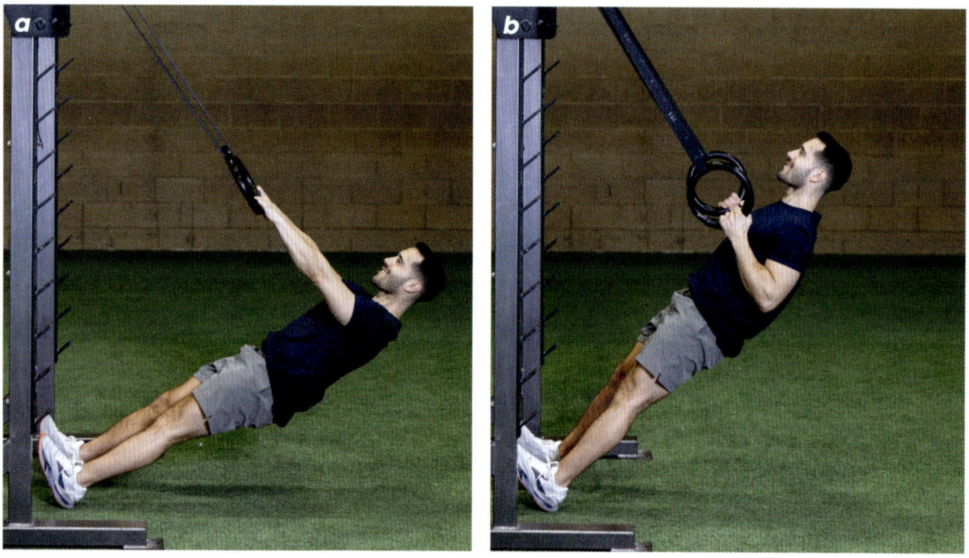

Benefits

The inverted row on suspension trainer strengthens the upper back, lats, and biceps while reinforcing scapular mechanics and trunk strength. The bodyweight pulling exercise supports shoulder health, can be learned easily by beginners, and is simple to progress by adjusting body angle and foot positioning.

Instructions for the Client

1. Set up a suspension trainer or rings in a rack so that the handles hang at waist height.
2. Grasp the handles and position your body at a roughly 45-degree angle underneath.
3. Extend your legs and dig your heels into the floor, and while keeping your body in a straight line from head to heels, brace your abdominals and glutes.
4. Pull your body upward by driving the elbows back and squeezing your shoulder blades together, rotating the arms into external rotation.
5. Pause briefly at the top and then lower yourself slowly to the starting position.
6. To increase difficulty, walk your feet forward to lower your body angle and create greater resistance. To decrease difficulty, walk the feet backward to incline your body angle and reduce resistance.

Variation

Progression: Feet-Elevated Inverted Row on Suspension Trainer

The feet-elevated inverted row on the suspension trainer increases difficulty by elevating the feet on a bench or box, which requires the client to lift a greater percentage of their body weight.

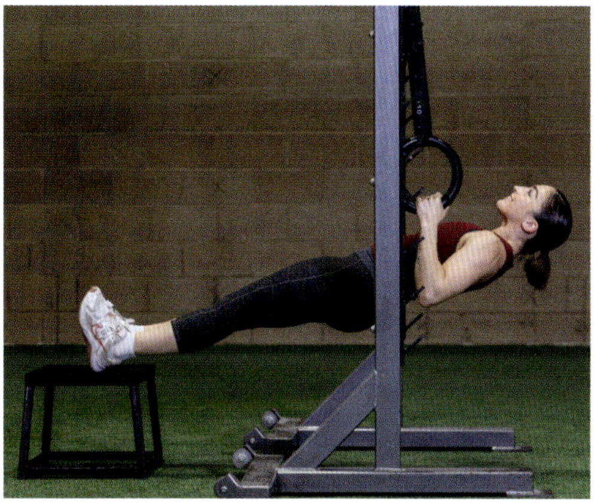

CHIN-UP

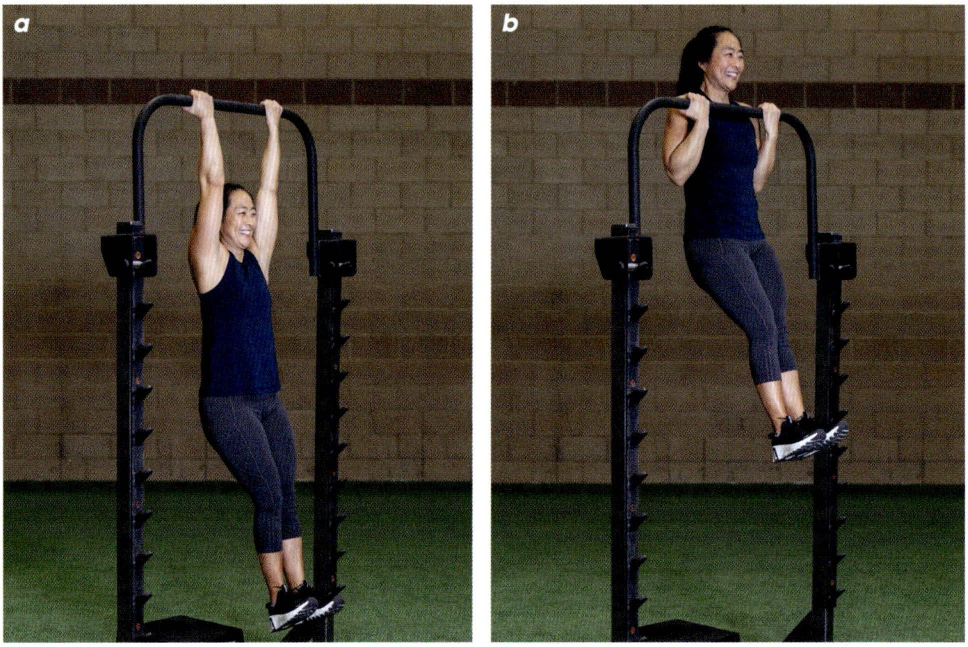

Benefits

The chin-up builds upper body strength in the lats, biceps, and upper back while also challenging core stability. The combination of developing upper body strength, shoulder mobility, and grip strength makes it one of the most effective upper body exercises for performance and longevity.

Instructions for the Client

1. Start in a full hanging position from a chin-up bar with your arms supine and palms facing toward you.
2. Forcefully pull yourself up to the bar by engaging your lats and upper back muscles while maintaining a plank-like position and minimizing any swing of your body. Pull all the way up until you get your collarbone to the bar.
3. Slowly lower yourself back down to the bottom under control until your arms are straight.
4. Repeat the exercise for the prescribed repetitions.

Variations

Regression: Half-Kneeling Single-Arm Cable Pulldown

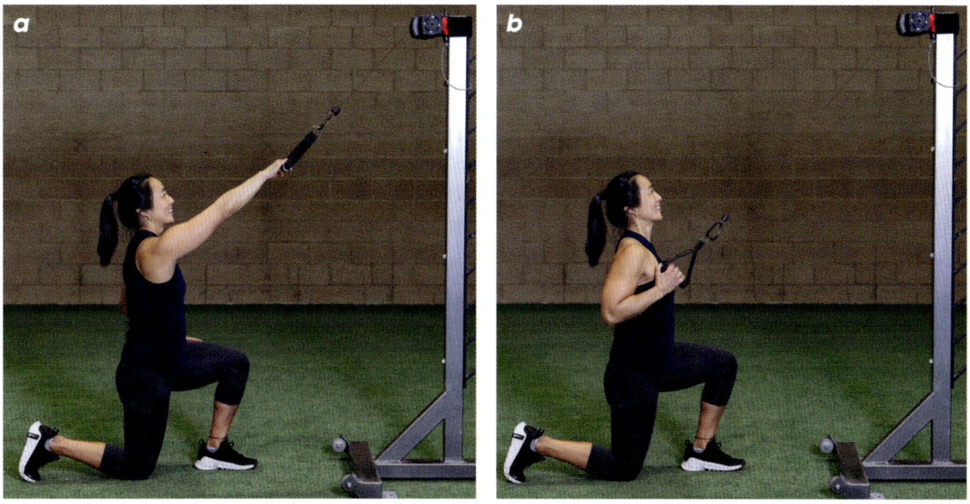

The half-kneeling single-arm cable pulldown serves as a regression from the chin-up because it allows the client to pull at a forward angle while reducing overall load, making it a better option for beginners or those with limited shoulder mobility.

Progression: Pull-Up

The pull-up progresses the chin-up by using a pronated grip, which places greater emphasis on the lats while demanding more shoulder mobility and reducing assistance from the biceps.

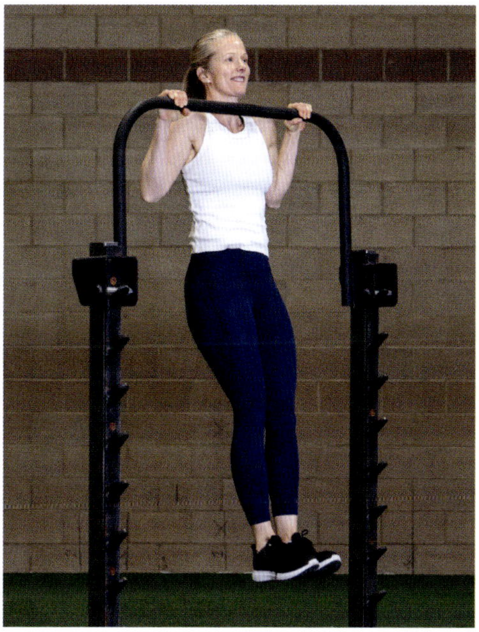

FRONT PLANK

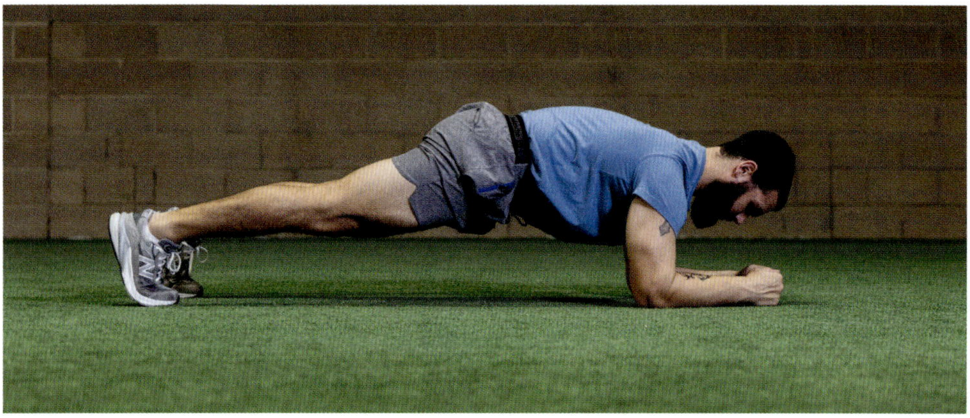

Benefits

The front plank is a sagittal plane core exercise that strengthens the abdominals, obliques, and deep core stabilizers. This should be used as a foundational exercise to develop trunk strength and lumbopelvic stability to support spinal health for activities of daily living.

Instructions for the Client

1. Begin by lying in a prone position with your elbows on the ground directly under your shoulders and forearms resting on the ground. Tuck your toes into the ground, squeeze your legs together, and contract your glutes tightly.
2. Lift your legs and hips off the ground so that you are supported entirely by your forearms and feet. Maintain active tension in your anterior abdominals so that you maintain a straight spinal alignment between your head, thoracic spine, and sacrum.
3. Actively focus on breathing throughout the exercise to engage your abdominal muscles, and hold the position for the prescribed amount of time.

Variations

Regression: Bear Plank

The bear plank serves as a regression from the front plank by reducing the demand on the anterior abdominal muscles. With the hips flexed to 90 degrees and arms positioned under the shoulders, this variation makes it easier for beginners to develop core stability before progressing to the front plank.

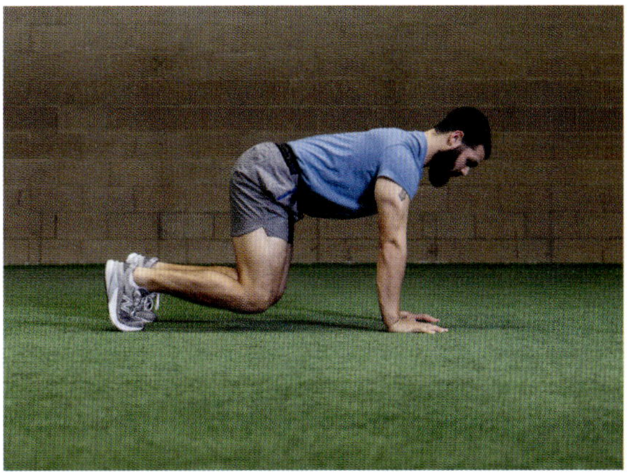

Progression: Kneeling Ball Rollout

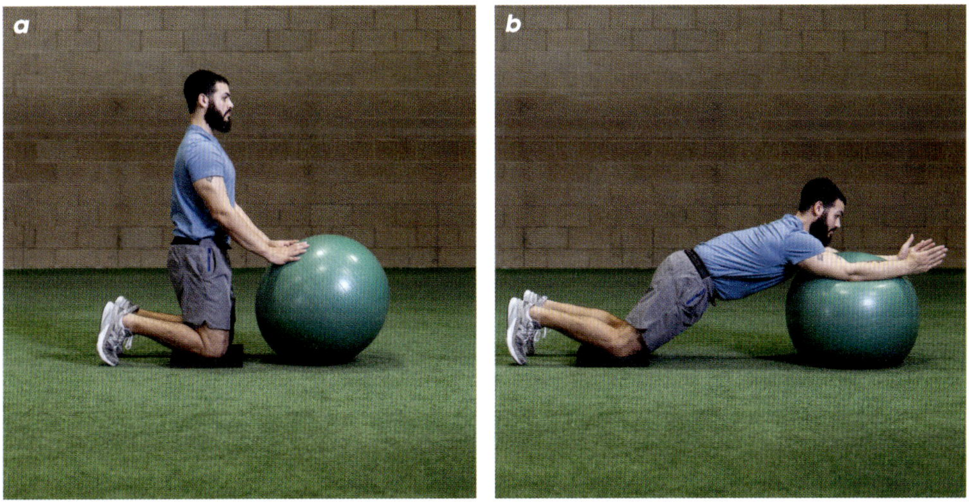

The kneeling ball rollout progresses the front plank by increasing the lever length and challenge to the anterior trunk musculature. The variation increases the dynamic eccentric demand, building greater abdominal strength and reinforcing spinal control under load.

HIGH PLANK SHOULDER TAPS

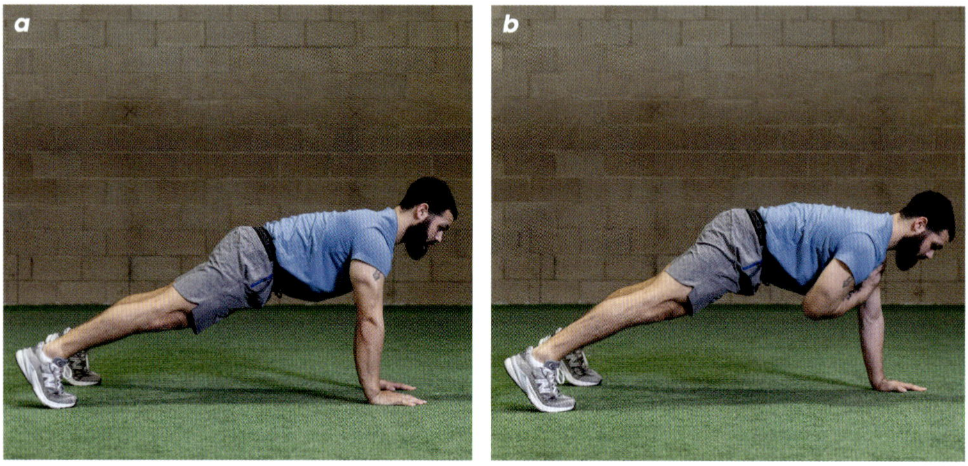

Benefits

High plank shoulder taps develop core strength by challenging the trunk to resist rotation and extension while the arms alternate support. This plank variation builds dynamic stability through the shoulders, hips, and trunk muscles.

Instructions for the Client

1. Begin in a high plank position with hands under shoulders, feet hip-width apart, and the body forming a straight line from head to heels.
2. Brace the core and squeeze the glutes to maintain stability.
3. Without letting the hips shift or rotate, lift one hand off the ground and tap the opposite shoulder.
4. Return the hand to the floor and repeat on the other side, alternating taps under control.
5. Continue for the prescribed number of repetitions.

Variations

Regression: High Plank Foot Lifts

High plank foot lifts reduce rotational demands on the trunk and shoulder musculature by keeping the hands fixed on the floor while lifting one foot at a time. This variation challenges trunk and shoulder stability with less rotational stress, making it a useful step before progressing to shoulder taps.

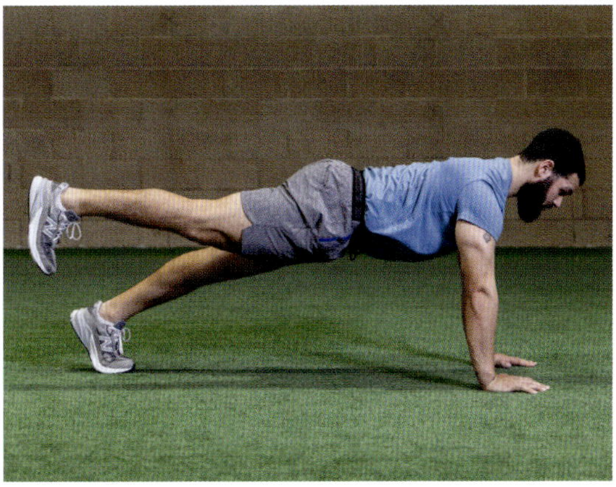

Progression: Plank Rows

Plank rows progress the high plank shoulder taps by adding external load and a pulling action at the shoulder. Using dumbbells, the client maintains a stable high plank position while rowing one weight up at a time. This increases the anti-rotational demand of the exercise by increasing the challenge in the shoulders, obliques, and anterior abdominals.

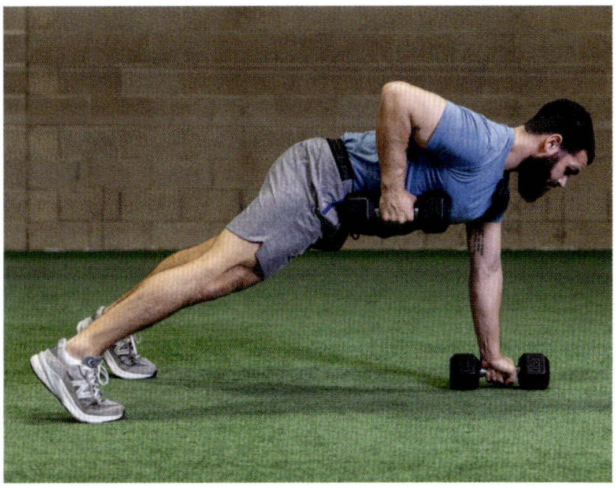

CORE

STRAIGHT-LEG SIT-UPS

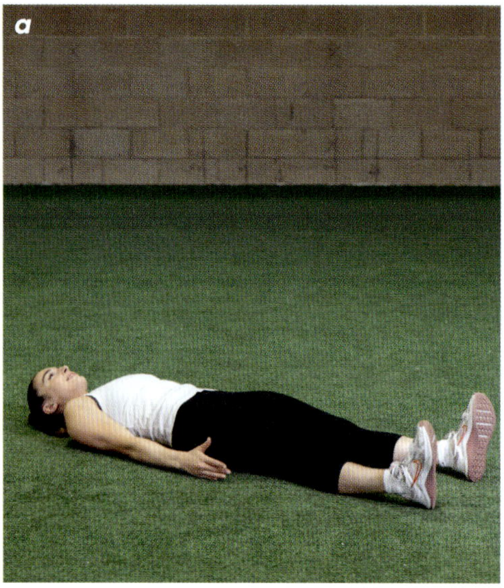

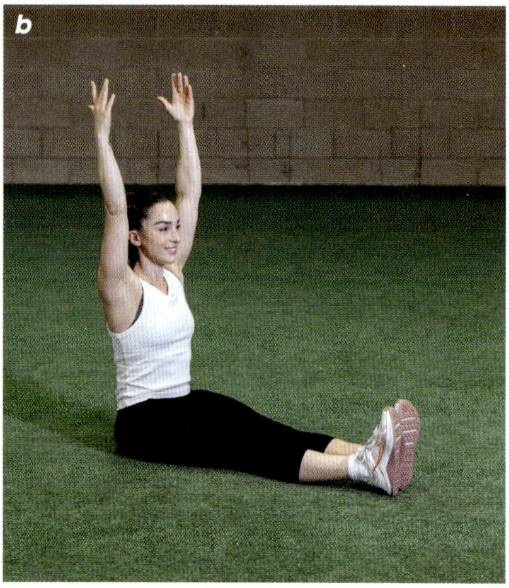

Benefits

Straight-leg sit-ups strengthen the abdominal and hip flexor muscles. Keeping the legs straight places a greater emphasis on the lower abdominal and hip flexor muscles.

Instructions for the Client

1. Lie on your back with both legs extended flat on the floor and your arms by your side.
2. Exhale as your slowly lift your trunk off the floor, reaching your arms upwards toward the ceiling while keeping your legs straight and feet in contact with the floor.
3. Continue rising up until you are sitting upright with your arms reaching overhead.
4. Slowly control the descent back to the floor, and return to the starting position.
5. Repeat for the prescribed number of repetitions.

Variation

Progression: One-Leg Bent Sit-Up

The one-leg bent sit-up increases the difficulty by flexing the hip on one side, creating an asymmetrical base of support and further challenging the abdominal muscles to lift the torso.

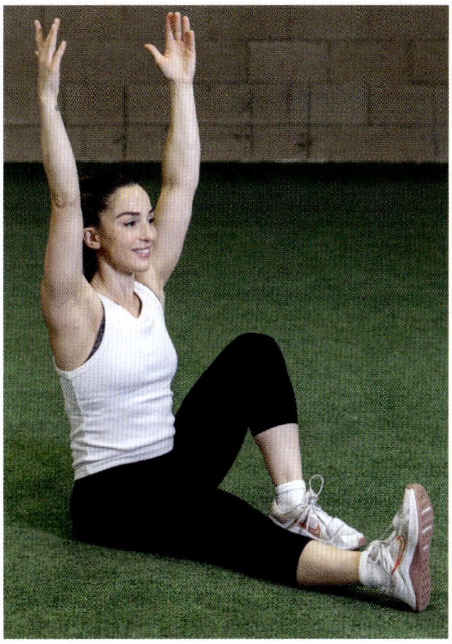

STANDING ANTIROTATION PRESS

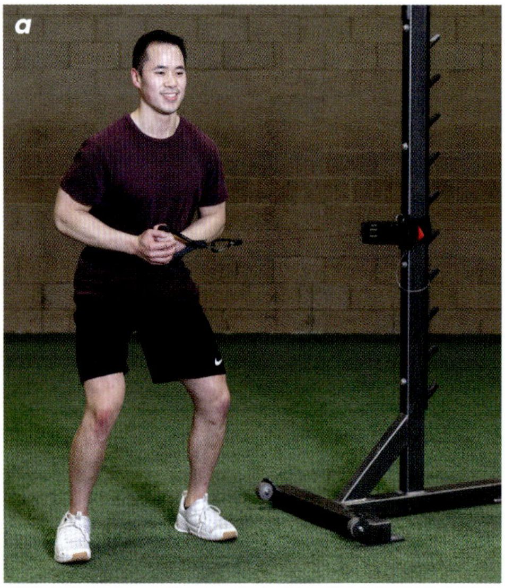

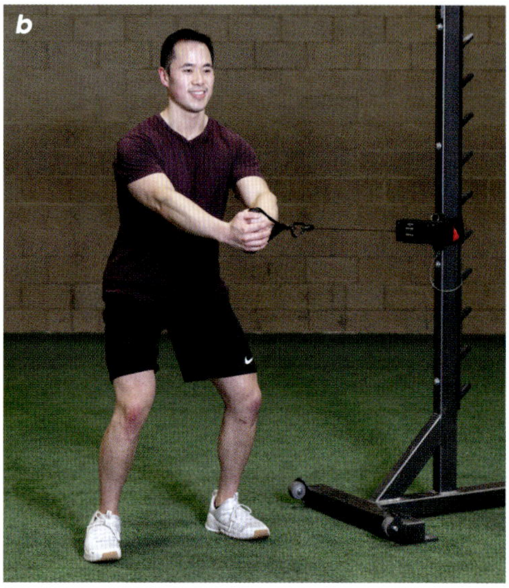

Benefits

The standing antirotation press strengthens the abdominals and obliques by resisting force in the transverse plane, improving trunk strength and stability for activities of daily living.

Instructions for the Client

1. Begin by standing tall with your feet shoulder-width apart and knees slightly bent with a cable machine at your side. Position the cable at chest height and grab the cable with both hands.
2. Exhale forcefully as you press the handle directly out in front of you, fully extending both arms. Resist the cable pulling you laterally, keeping your hands directly in front of you.
3. After a brief hold, bring the cable back in toward your chest and repeat for the prescribed repetitions.

Variations

Regression: Half-Kneeling Antirotation Press-Out

The half-kneeling antirotation press-out regresses the standing version by reducing the load and adding support from the ground. This position helps to develop lateral hip strength and trunk control, preparing the client to progress to the standing variation.

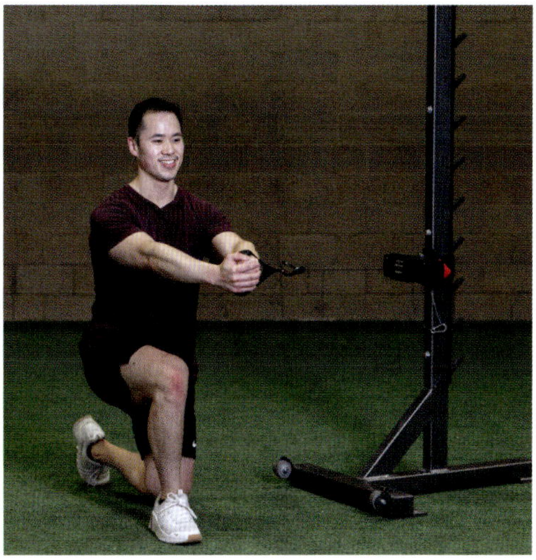

Progression: Staggered-Stance Antirotation Press-Out

The staggered-stance antirotation press-out progresses the bilateral standing variation by reducing ground support and increasing hip and trunk stability demand.

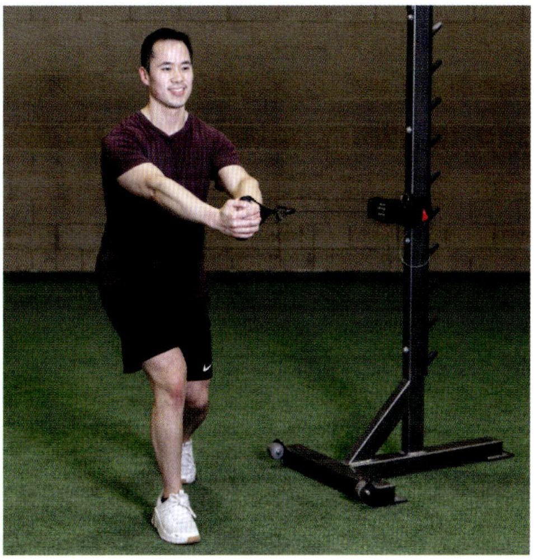

HALF-KNEELING CABLE CHOP

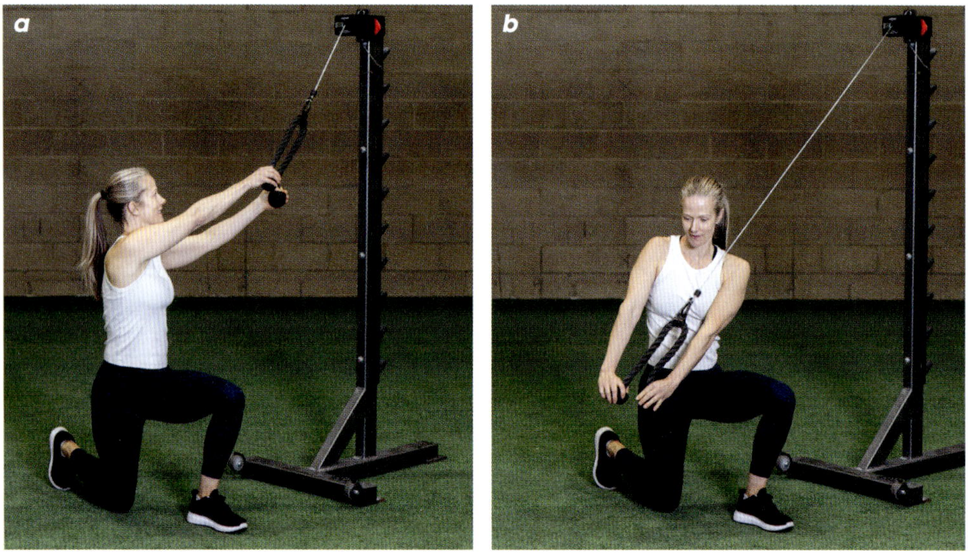

Benefits

The half-kneeling cable chop strengthens the abdominals and obliques while also improving hip stability. The half-kneeling stance reduces lower body compensation, helping clients build core strength, hip stability, and coordination for both athletic performance and daily movement.

Instructions for the Client

1. Begin in a half-kneeling position with a cable machine or band positioned above and next to the top side leg. On the downside leg, your knee should be positioned directly under your hip with your ankle dorsiflexed and toes tucked into the ground.
2. Grasp the rope handle of the cable with both hands and pull it downward diagonally to your chest. Press the handle downward and away from your body, fully extending your arms.
3. Focus on maintaining a tall and static position of your torso during the movement, resisting the pull of the cable.
4. Bring the cable back up, briefly pausing at your chest again before returning to the starting position.
5. Complete the prescribed number of repetitions and repeat on the opposite side.

Variations

Regression: Tall-Kneeling Cable Chop

The tall-kneeling cable chop regresses the half-kneeling variation by providing greater stability through both knees on the ground. This reduces balance and hip stability demands and allows clients to focus on maintaining trunk position and control before progressing to the half-kneeling variation.

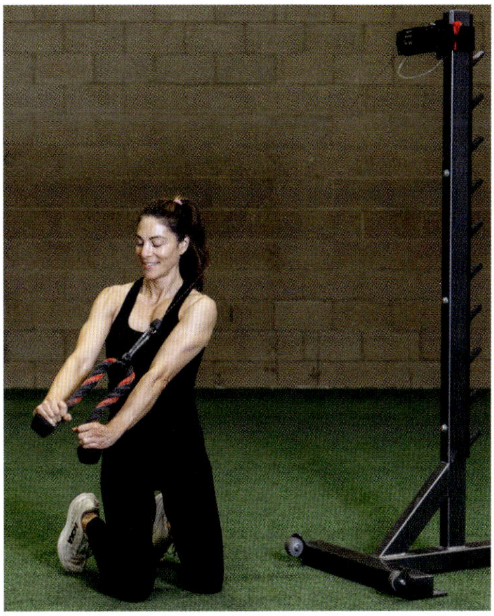

Progression: Standing Cable Chop

The standing cable chop progresses the half-kneeling variation by allowing greater external load and increased trunk and pelvic rotation, making it more transferable to both sport and daily activities.

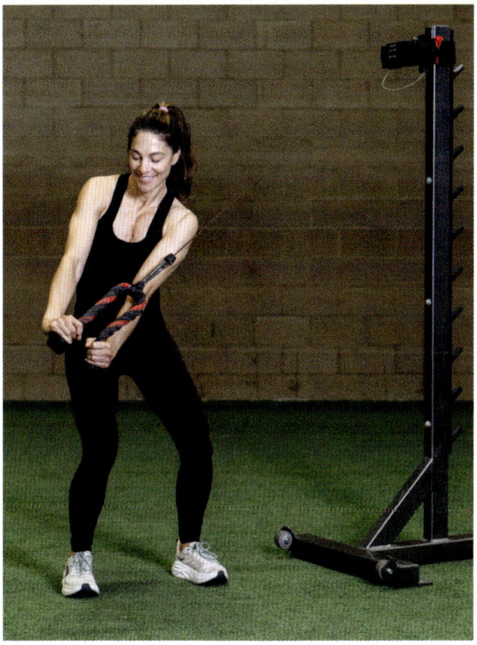

CORE

HALF-KNEELING CABLE LIFT

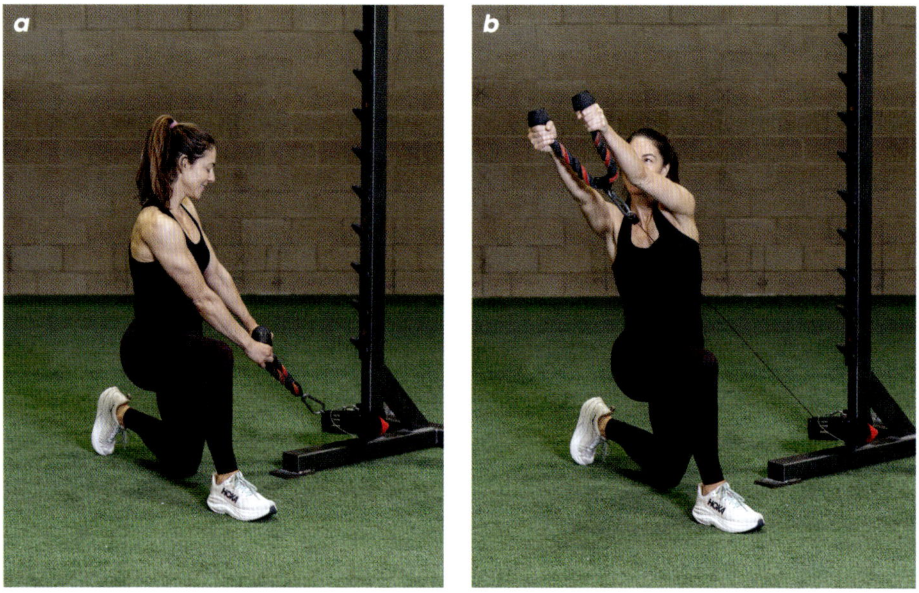

Benefits

The half-kneeling cable lift strengthens the abdominals, obliques, and hips while training the lower body to resist lateral flexion and rotation. The half-kneeling stance reduces lower body compensation, helping the client to build trunk and hip stability.

Instructions for the Client

1. Begin in a half-kneeling position with a cable machine or band positioned below and next to the downside leg. On the downside leg, your knee should be positioned directly under your hip with your ankle dorsiflexed and toes tucked into the ground.
2. Grasp the handle of the cable with both hands and pull it up diagonally to your chest. Press the handle up and away from your body, fully extending your arms.
3. Focus on maintaining a tall and static position of your torso during the movement, resisting the pull of the cable.
4. Bring the cable back down, briefly pausing at your chest again before returning to the starting position.
5. Complete for the prescribed number of repetitions and then repeat on the opposite side.

Variations

Regression: Tall-Kneeling Cable Lift

The tall-kneeling cable lift regresses the movement by providing more stability with both knees on the ground. This reduces the balance and hip stability demand and allows the client to work on developing strength and trunk stability before progressing to the half-kneeling version.

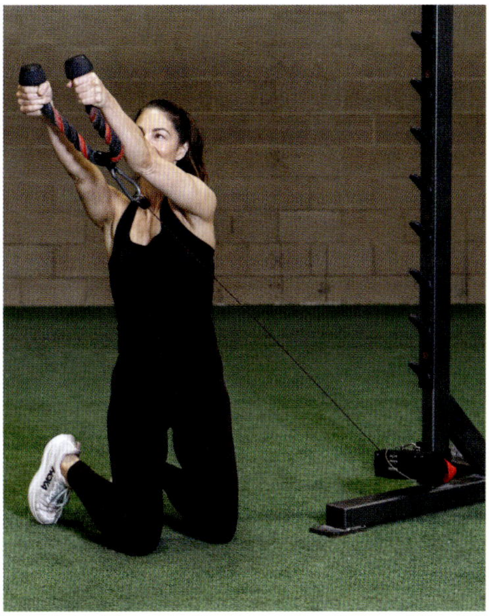

Progression: Standing Cable Lift

The standing cable lift progresses the exercise into a full body movement that integrates the lower body and increased trunk and pelvic rotation. This allows for greater external loading and transferability to daily life activities.

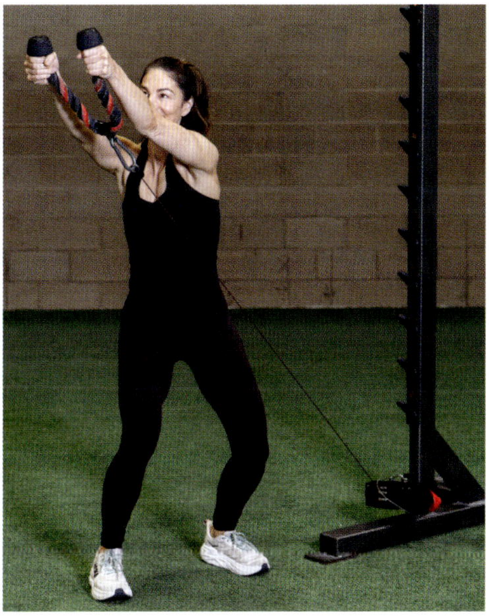

SIDE PLANK

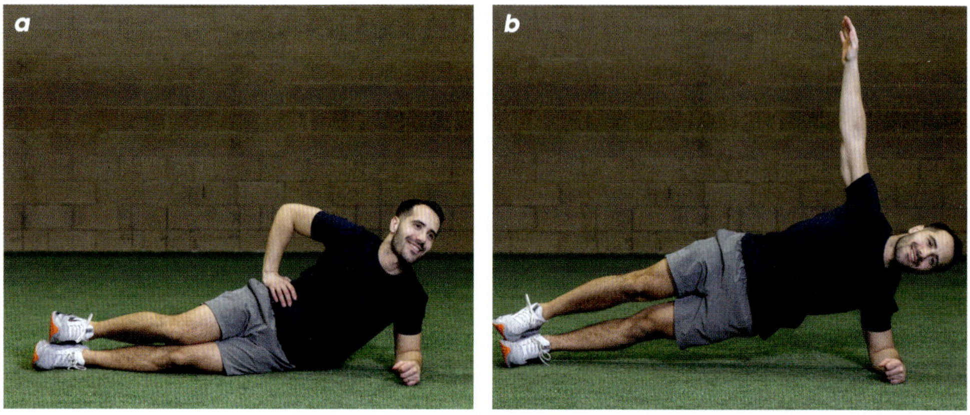

Benefits

The side plank strengthens the obliques and lateral hip muscles that develop trunk strength in the frontal plane to support spinal health and improve daily function.

Instructions for the Client

1. Begin in a side-lying position propped up on your forearm with your elbow lined up underneath your shoulder. Stack your legs on top of one another with your feet together.
2. Lift your hips up off the ground so that you are fully supported by your forearm and feet. Brace your abs tightly and maintain a straight line between your head, thoracic spine, and sacrum.
3. Focus on breathing in through your nose and out through your mouth throughout the exercise to encourage abdominal engagement.
4. Hold for the prescribed time and then repeat on the opposite side.

Variations

Regression: Short-Lever Side Plank

The short-lever side plank regresses the exercise by bending the knees to shorten the lever length. The decreased load on the core and hip muscles makes it a more accessible option for beginners to develop trunk strength before progressing to the side plank.

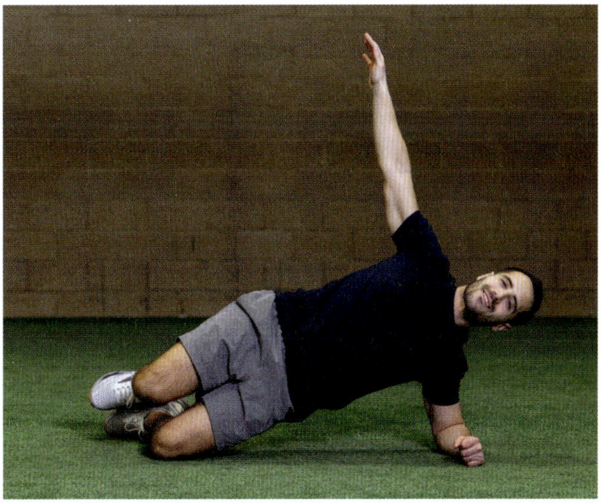

Progression: Feet-Elevated Side Plank

The feet-elevated side plank progresses the exercise by raising the legs on a bench or box, increasing the lever length and load. This variation further challenges the muscles of the shoulder, hips, and trunk to build greater core strength and stability.

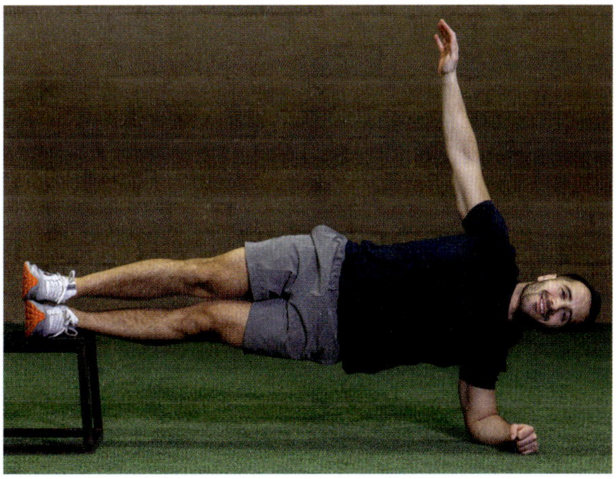

SUITCASE CARRY

Benefits

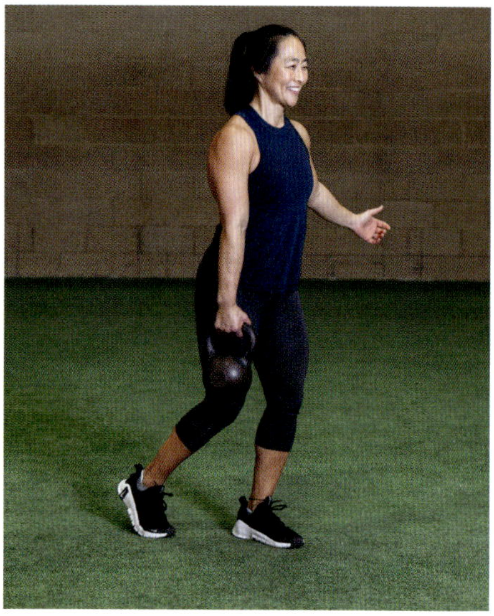

The suitcase carry strengthens the obliques, hips, and grip by resisting lateral flexion while walking with a weight on one side of the body. This anti-lateral flexion exercise improves core strength that transfers to daily physical activities.

Instructions for the Client

1. Begin by standing tall and holding a kettlebell or dumbbell in one hand at your side.
2. Walk slowly for the programmed distance while maintaining a tall posture, being sure to avoid bending laterally.
3. After walking the programmed distance, switch hands and repeat on the opposite side.

Variation

Progression: Single Kettlebell Rack Carry

The single kettlebell rack carry progresses the suitcase carry by moving the load in to the front rack position, increasing the demand for trunk strength and postural control.

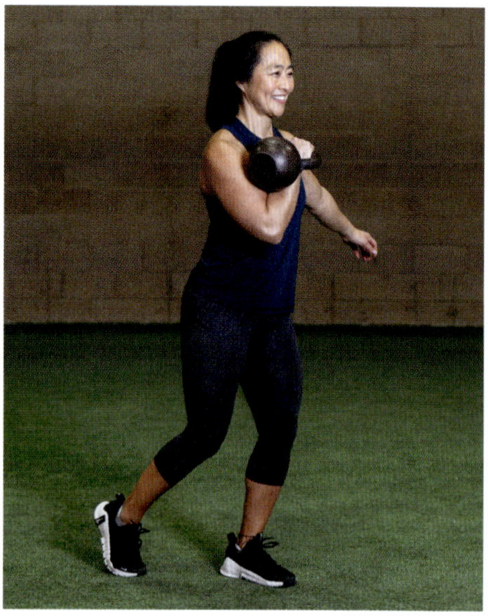

FARMER CARRY

Benefits

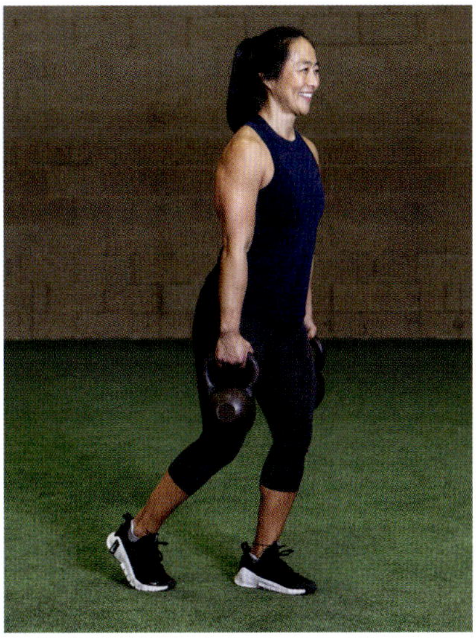

The farmer carry builds grip, trunk, and upper-back strength by walking while holding weights in both hands. This simple but highly effective exercise helps to improve full body strength and work capacity, making it transferrable to everyday physical activities.

Instructions for the Client

1. Begin by standing tall with equal-size kettlebells or dumbbells in each hand.
2. Walk the prescribed distance while maintaining a tall posture without flexing, extending, or laterally tilting your spine. Maintain active tension in your lats, rectus abdominis, and obliques.
3. Once you have walked the prescribed distance, turn around and walk back to the starting position.

Variation

Progression: Double Kettlebell Rack Carry

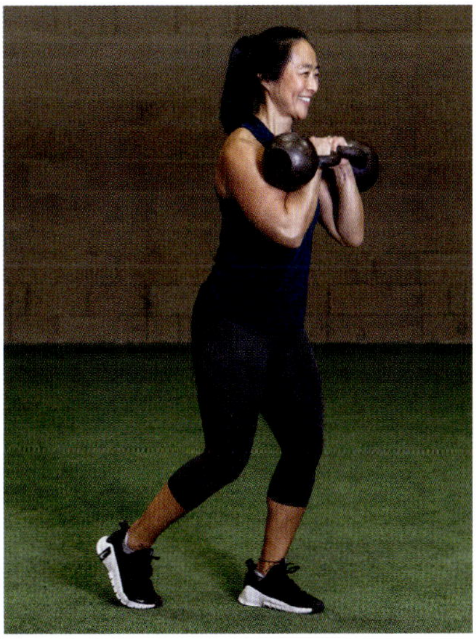

The double kettlebell rack carry progresses the farmer carry by moving the weights into the front rack position. This variation increases the demand on the trunk muscles, further developing core strength and stability.

Case Study: Laura's Strength Training Plan

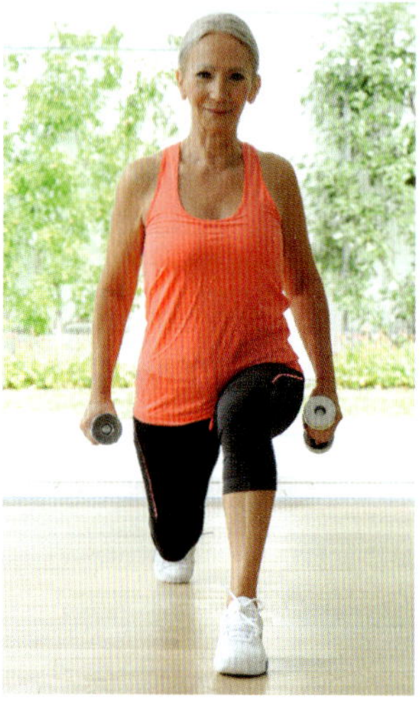

G&J Fey/Connect Images/Getty Images

Laura is a 57-year-old woman who is recreationally active but has not been following a structured strength training program. She joined the gym after being diagnosed with osteopenia and has noticed increasing difficulty with daily household tasks, such as carrying laundry and shoveling snow, due to a lack of strength.

During her intake assessment, we evaluated Laura's upper and lower body strength using a push-up test and a single-leg squat test. She was unable to complete a push-up, and performed three single-leg squats on her right leg and one on her left.

To increase muscular strength, improve bone density, and enhance her ability to perform daily activities, we recommend that Laura follow a full-body strength training program two or three days per week.

To develop upper body strength, Laura will perform exercises such as a dumbbell bench press, half-kneeling dumbbell overhead press, and incline push-ups. We will progressively lower the incline on her push-ups each week until she successfully can perform push-ups from the floor.

To improve lower body strength, Laura will start with knee and hip-dominant movements, including goblet squats, split squats, and single-leg deadlifts. After two months of foundational strength training, we will introduce single-leg squats to further develop her lower body strength and stability.

Strength training builds the foundation for a resilient body by improving force production, joint integrity, and tolerance to daily physical demands. However, strength alone is not enough to support long-term health and independence. To move through life with energy, recover between efforts, and support cardiovascular and metabolic health, a complete training program also must include conditioning. The next chapter focuses on cardiovascular training, outlining how aerobic and higher-intensity work complement strength training and help sustain movement, function, and independence across the life span.

Chapter 8

Cardiovascular Training

Cardiovascular disease (CVD) is often seen as a looming threat—and for good reason. It remains the leading cause of death worldwide for both men and women, making it a critical health concern for everybody reading this book (Martin et al., 2024). Each year, cardiovascular disease claims approximately 18 million lives, accounting for nearly 32 percent of all global deaths. In the United States alone, someone dies from heart disease every 33 seconds (World Health Organization, 2025).

While these statistics are alarming, there is good news: The most powerful tool for improving heart health and increasing life span is already within our reach: cardiovascular exercise.

Strength training is undeniably valuable for overall health, but if the goal is to maximize longevity, lifting weights alone is not enough—cardiovascular training is necessary too. However, because it can be uncomfortable and challenging, it is also the type of exercise most people neglect or avoid altogether.

THE CONSEQUENCES OF CARDIOVASCULAR INACTIVITY

Neglecting cardiovascular exercise has significant consequences on health. As aerobic fitness declines, so does overall metabolic health. Sedentary lifestyles and lack of cardiovascular exercise hinder the body's ability to regulate blood sugar, manage inflammation, and maintain healthy blood pressure and lipid levels. Over time, this deterioration in metabolic health contributes to the increasing epidemic of chronic diseases around the world.

Metabolic Dysfunction and Chronic Disease

Americans are facing a metabolic crisis largely driven by lifestyle behaviors. The decline of cardiovascular health is directly tied to metabolic dysfunction and the interplay of obesity, hypertension, atherosclerosis, insulin resistance, and chronic inflammation. Poor nutritional habits, combined with lack of proper exercise, create an internal environment in bodies that begins to dysregulate the ability to properly metabolize food, leading to plaque buildup, stiffening of the arteries, and excess strain on the heart.

Nearly half of all adults in the United States currently have hypertension, defined as a consistent blood pressure measured above 130/80 mm Hg (Fryar et al., 2021). And while just under 12 percent of Americans have been diagnosed with diabetes, nearly 40 percent of Americans have prediabetes, defined as fasting glucose ranging from 100 to 125 mg/dL or A1C values of 5.7 to 6.4 percent (Center for Disease Control, 2023). Together, high blood pressure and impaired glucose metabolism create a dangerous combination, leading to vascular damage, endothelial dysfunction, and an accelerated progression of heart disease.

Cardiovascular exercise is the most powerful tool for reducing the occurrence and severity of CVD due to its effect on interrelated risk factors such as obesity, hypertension, hyperlipidemia, and insulin resistance. In fact, low cardiorespiratory fitness has a statistically larger impact on longevity than traditional risk factors such as smoking, diabetes, coronary artery disease, and hypertension, primarily because exercise can reduce the occurrence of all those conditions other than cigarette smoking (Mandsager et al., 2018). The Cleveland Clinic (2021) estimates that 90 percent of heart disease could be eliminated simply by eating a healthy diet, consistently exercising, and not smoking.

Aerobic Decline With Aging

Like all physical attributes, aerobic fitness declines with age if not actively maintained, affecting health, performance, and longevity. In sedentary individuals, $\dot{V}O_2$max decreases by approximately 4 to 5 mL/kg/min per decade, significantly increasing the risk of cardiovascular disease, metabolic dysfunction, and loss of functional independence (Shephard, 2009).

However, maintaining aerobic health with age can have profound health benefits. Research suggests that for every 1 metabolic equivalent of task (MET) (3.5 mL/kg/min) increase in $\dot{V}O_2$max, the risk of CVD decreases by approximately 15 percent (Kodama, 2024). This highlights the importance of consistent aerobic training, not only for athletic performance but also for long-term health and disease prevention.

Even for those late to the game with aerobic exercise, it is never too late to begin improving cardiovascular fitness. Research shows that even those who start later in life can significantly improve both the structure and function of their heart through consistent cardiovascular training.

In a landmark two-year study out of the Institute for Exercise and Environmental Medicine, researchers found that sedentary 50-year-olds were able to reverse age-related changes in heart structure by following a structured program combining steady-state and interval training. Participants reduced stiffness in the left ventricle and myocardium while improving their $\dot{V}O_2$max by an average of 18 percent over the course of two years (Howden et al., 2018).

AEROBIC TRAINING AND COGNITIVE HEALTH

For many years, researchers viewed the brain and the rest of the body as separate entities. However, recent research has made it clear that cardiovascular exercise affects more than just muscles, lungs, and heart—it plays a crucial role in cognitive health and function as well.

Harvard professor of neurology Rudolph Tanzi sums it up well in his book *Decoding Darkness: The Search for the Genetic Causes of Alzheimer's Disease*, stating: "The bottom line is pretty irrefutable: what is good for the heart is good for the brain" (Tanzi and Parson, 2017, p. 201).

The emerging research on the impact of aerobic training can have on brains is truly astounding. Brains, like all the body's tissues, begin a progressive decline as people age, due partly to the natural aging process but largely due to lifestyle choices. Daily exercise and nutritional choices play a major role in the maintenance and regeneration of the brain and nervous system.

It has been well established that regular participation in aerobic exercise is vital to maintaining cognitive function as we age. Regular participation in all versions of cardiovascular exercise ranging from walking to moderate-intensity continuous training to high-intensity interval training (HIIT) has been shown to have a significant impact on the structure and function of brains (Erickson et al., 2011).

For many years, it was accepted that the brain would reduce in volume with age, and along with it would go much of the individual's cognitive function. However, researchers know now that people can do much to maintain their brain size and function by simply participating in aerobic exercise. In a study of 60- to 80-year-old sedentary participants engaging in three one-hour aerobic exercise sessions per week over a six-month period, researchers discovered that participants were able to increase their brain volume in the prefrontal and temporal cortices—the same regions that often are reported to show substantial age-related deterioration (Colcombe et al., 2006).

In response to cardiovascular strain, the body increases the blood flow to the brain and releases myokines such as brain-derived neurotrophic growth factor (BDNF). This powerful protein facilitates muscle-to-brain signaling, helping to guard the brain against neurodegeneration, enhance cognition, and improve neurological signaling. During cardiovascular exercise, BDNF is released from both the muscles and the brain, promoting the growth of the hippocampus, one of the regions of the brain most significantly affected by Alzheimer's disease (Seifert et al., 2010; Pajonk et al., 2010).

Simply put, the more people exercise, the more they nourish their brains. Aerobic exercise is one of the most powerful modifiable factors influencing cognitive function. Research shows that individuals with low cardiorespiratory fitness in midlife face nearly twice the risk of developing dementia later in life. The link between cardiovascular fitness measured by $\dot{V}O_2$max and a reduced risk of cognitive disease is clear. In fact, for every 1 MET (3.5 mL/kg/min) increase in $\dot{V}O_2$max, the risk of cognitive impairment decreases by 8 percent (Müller et al., 2017).

How Much Cardiovascular Exercise to Do

The U.S. Department of Health and Human Services recommends a baseline level of weekly cardiovascular exercise for overall health:

- 150 to 300 minutes of moderate-intensity aerobic exercise
- 75 to 150 minutes of vigorous-intensity aerobic exercise
- Or a combination of both

Moderate-intensity exercise is performed at 50 to 70 percent of maximum heart rate or a 5 to 6 out of 10 on the rate of perceived exertion (RPE) scale. Vigorous-intensity exercise exceeds 70 percent of maximum heart rate or rates 7 or higher on the RPE scale (U.S. Department of Health and Human Services, 2018). The flexibility of this recommendation allows individuals to tailor their exercise routine to their preferences, abilities, and schedule, making consistency easier to maintain.

Cardiovascular exercise is the most potent intervention people have to reduce the incidence of CVD, but the large majority of Americans are not getting enough. As it stands now, less than 50 percent of Americans are reaching the minimum recommended guideline. If strength training is the primary tool that helps people *live better*, cardiovascular training is the primary tool to help people *live longer*, and the research backs it up. Simply meeting these minimum guidelines can reduce all-cause mortality by 25 percent, with even greater benefits from additional activity beyond the minimum recommendation (Lee et al., 2022).

$\dot{V}O_2$MAX

$\dot{V}O_2$max is the maximum amount of oxygen, expressed in mL/kg/min, that an individual can take in and use during a bout of intense aerobic exercise. $\dot{V}O_2$max is widely considered the best measure of cardiorespiratory fitness. $\dot{V}O_2$max is most often measured in an exercise laboratory test using a graded treadmill or cycling test, during which participants progressively increase exercise intensity until volitional fatigue while a technician analyzes the oxygen and carbon dioxide in the participant's expired air to determine maximal oxygen consumption.

Research clearly demonstrates that $\dot{V}O_2$max is strongly correlated with both cardiorespiratory and all-cause mortality. Simply put, the higher a person's $\dot{V}O_2$max, the lower their risk of dying from heart disease or any cause. In a study of over 120,000 participants who underwent treadmill testing, researchers found that individuals with an "elite" $\dot{V}O_2$max for their age and sex were five times less likely to die over an 8.5-year follow-up compared to those in the "low" $\dot{V}O_2$max category. Even participants in the second-highest fitness category had a 29 percent higher risk of mortality compared to those in the elite group (Mandsager et al., 2018). Table 8.1 categorizes $\dot{V}O_2$max score by age and sex based on the data from Mandsager and colleagues (2018).

Although it is clear that $\dot{V}O_2$max is a powerful indicator of cardiovascular health and longevity, the problem with $\dot{V}O_2$max testing comes down to access and practicality. Proper $\dot{V}O_2$max testing requires a laboratory setting with an exercise physiologist and can be costly and impractical to execute for the average gymgoer. Furthermore, the data—although helpful to stratify risk—does not give a useful baseline measure from which trainers can prescribe future exercise sessions. Later in this chapter, I will outline how to use a max aerobic speed (MAS) test as a more practical measure for cardiorespiratory fitness that trainers can use as a baseline measure to program effective and appropriate cardiorespiratory training.

Table 8.1 Categorization of $\dot{V}O_2$max Score by Age and Sex

	Low	Below average	Above average	High	Elite
Men 18-19	37.8	45.2	48.6	56.7	57.0
Men 20-29	36.1	41.6	47.6	54.6	55.0
Men 30-39	35.0	38.8	45.2	52.2	52.5
Men 40-49	34.3	38.2	43.4	51.1	51.4
Men 50-59	28.7	34.6	39.6	48.6	49.0
Men 60-69	24.5	29.4	34.6	45.2	45.5
Men 70-79	21.0	24.2	29.4	39.9	40.2
Men ≥ 80	17.8	21.7	25.2	34.6	35.0
Women 18-19	35.0	38.5	45.2	52.2	52.5
Women 20-29	28.0	34.6	39.9	49.7	50.1
Women 30-39	27.0	32.6	37.8	47.6	47.9
Women 40-49	25.9	31.2	36.1	46.2	46.6
Women 50-59	24.5	28.0	34.6	45.2	45.5
Women 60-69	21.0	24.2	29.4	38.5	38.8
Women 70-79	17.5	20.7	24.2	34.6	35.0
Women ≥ 80	15.4	18.9	21.7	29.1	29.4

Adapted from K. Mandsager, S. Harb, P. Cremer, et al., "Association of Cardiorespiratory Fitness With Long-Term Mortality Among Adults Undergoing Exercise Treadmill Testing," *JAMA Network Open* 1, no. 6 (2018): e183605. Distributed under the terms of the Creative Commons Attribution 4.0 International License (http://creativecommons.org/licenses/by/4.0/).

CLIENT ASSESSMENT: RESTING HEART RATE

Resting heart rate is a key indicator of both aerobic fitness and cardiovascular health. Research shows that individuals with higher resting heart rates face an increased risk of CVD and all-cause mortality (Jensen et al., 2013). Additionally, an inverse relationship exists between resting heart rate and cardiorespiratory fitness—meaning that as fitness levels improve, resting heart rate tends to decrease (Gonzales et al., 2023).

Engaging in regular aerobic exercise can lower resting heart rate significantly by enhancing cardiac efficiency and increasing vagal tone. Tracking resting heart rate over time helps establish a baseline for aerobic fitness, guiding training decisions and monitoring stress levels in clients.

How to Test

1. Lie down on a flat surface, preferably wearing a chest strap heart rate monitor or, if necessary, a wrist monitor such as a smart watch.
2. Relax and lie still for at least 1 minute, then check your resting heart rate.
3. For the most accurate results, perform the test in a quiet area with minimal distractions, and avoid consuming stimulants or caffeine before the test.

Determining Results

Many sources describe a "normal" resting heart rate as 60 to 90 beats per minute, but in practice, clients should aim for a much lower resting heart rate for optimal cardiovascular health. If a client consistently presents with a resting heart rate greater than 60 beats per minute, it is often indictive of poor aerobic fitness or poor stress management. For these clients, prescribing low-intensity steady-state (LISS) cardiovascular training can improve cardiac output and efficiency (see the Low-Intensity Steady-State Cardiovascular Training section later in this chapter).

CLIENT ASSESSMENT: MAX AEROBIC SPEED TEST (MAS)

The two-mile MAS test on the air bike is a time trial test that is used to determine a baseline measure of aerobic power. By definition, MAS is the lowest exercise intensity at which an individual can reach $\dot{V}O_2max$ or the maximum sustained intensity at which that individual can exercise aerobically. The goal is to complete a 4- to 6-minute time trial as fast as possible at a sustained intensity. The two-mile air bike test is especially useful because it gives a baseline measure to test against to measure progress of aerobic fitness. It is recommended to use a test like this instead of $\dot{V}O_2max$ testing to measure aerobic fitness because it is more accessible and can be easily performed and consistently tested and measured in a normal gym setting. As shown in figure 8.1, the MAS test is best administered by a coach who can track data and provide continual encouragement.

How to Test

1. Have the client pedal lightly on the air bike for 3 minutes to warm up and determine the optimal seat height and distance that is most comfortable. Be sure that the client is wearing a heart rate monitor so that you can track heart rate during and after the test.
2. Once the bike is set up comfortably, let the client rest for a short period of time while you provide instructions.
3. Instruct the client to complete the two-mile distance at the fastest sustainable intensity. It is important that the client maintains a relatively consistent pacc and avoids sprinting and dropping throughout the test.

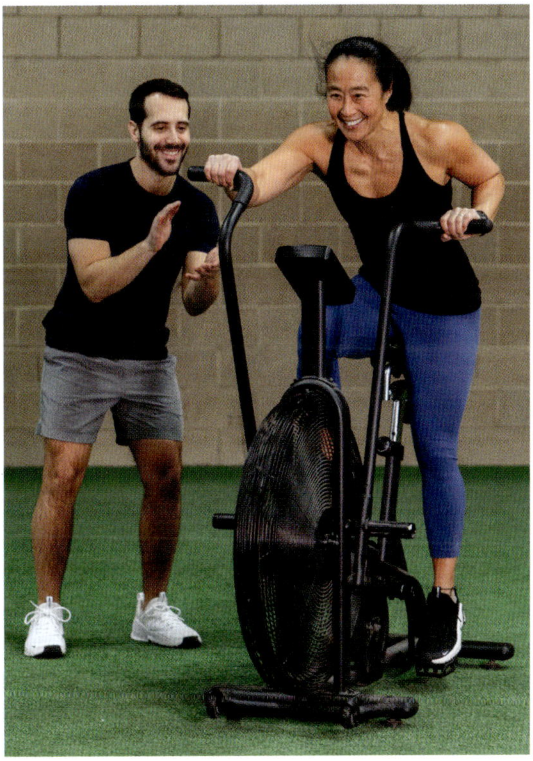

Figure 8.1 Max aerobic speed test with the coach administering the test to the athlete.

CLIENT ASSESSMENT: MAX AEROBIC SPEED TEST (MAS) *(continued)*

4. Consistently monitor and encourage the client throughout the time trial.
5. At completion of the test, record the client's time to completion as well as the average power output during the test measured in either revolutions per minute (RPM) or watts.

Determining Results

- *Time to completion:* Record the client's time and use it as a measure to assess progress when retesting in six to eight weeks. Table 8.2 provides age- and sex-specific performance benchmarks for the two-mile MAS test.
- *Max aerobic speed:* The client's average power measure recorded in either RPMs or watts over the course of the test is the MAS. This measure will be used to prescribe specific intensities for interval training.

Table 8.2 Age- and Sex-Specific Performance Bench Marks for the Two-Mile Max Aerobic Speed (MAS) Test

Male	15-25	26-35	36-45	46-55	56-65	66+
Elite	4:20	4:25	4:30	4:45	4:55	5:00
Excellent	4:35	4:45	4:40	4:50	5:00	5:20
Good	4:50	4:50	4:55	5:05	5:15	5:30
Fair	5:05	5:15	5:20	5:25	5:30	5:40
Needs improvement	5:40	5:50	6:00	6:10	6:20	6:30
Female	**15-25**	**26-35**	**36-45**	**46-55**	**56-65**	**66+**
Elite	5:00	5:00	5:10	5:20	5:30	5:45
Excellent	5:05	5:15	5:25	5:35	5:45	6:00
Good	5:15	5:25	5:35	5:45	5:55	6:05
Fair	5:25	5:35	5:45	5:55	6:05	6:15
Needs improvement	5:45	5:55	6:05	6:15	6:25	6:35

CLIENT ASSESSMENT: ONE-MINUTE HEART RATE RECOVERY

The speed at which heart rate drops in the minute following intense exercise is a strong indicator of both aerobic fitness and parasympathetic nervous system function. Clients who can rapidly lower their heart rate following a graded exercise test demonstrate a greater ability to shift from fight or flight (sympathetic activity) to rest and digest (parasympathetic activity), suggesting higher cardiovascular fitness and better nervous system balance.

Research also has shown a direct link between one-minute heart rate recovery and mortality. In a study of over 2,400 patients, researchers found that individuals with abnormal heart rate recovery—defined as a decrease of fewer than 12 beats per minute after a graded exercise test—not only had reduced exercise capacity but also faced up to four times the risk of death compared to those with normal heart rate recovery (Cole et al., 1999).

How to Test

1. Following the completion of the MAS test, record the peak heart rate achieved at the termination of the test.
2. Instruct the client to stay on the bike without moving and record how quickly the heart rate drops in the one minute following the cessation of exercise.

Determining Results

Although Cole et al. (1999) reported that a reduction of 13 beats per minute or more qualifies as "normal" heart rate recovery, we should aim for a much greater reduction in pursuit of cardiovascular fitness and longevity. In practice, a drop of 30 beats per minute is a much more appropriate target for determining a baseline of aerobic fitness and parasympathetic reactivation. If a client consistently displays a heart rate recovery of less than 30 beats per minute, it is recommended to prescribe LISS cardiovascular training to improve cardiac output and efficiency. Improvements in heart rate recovery gained as a result of low-intensity exercise will help the client recover better between high-intensity bouts of exercise during interval training.

LOW-INTENSITY STEADY-STATE CARDIOVASCULAR TRAINING

Low-intensity steady-state (LISS) cardiovascular training, often referred to as *zone 2 training*, is a low- to moderate-intensity, aerobic-focused form of conditioning typically performed at approximately 60 to 70 percent of an individual's maximum heart rate. A defining characteristic of LISS training is that the relatively low intensity allows participants to accumulate meaningful training volume while minimizing excessive fatigue and recovery cost.

Physiologically, LISS training supports improvements in aerobic metabolism, fat oxidation, and central cardiovascular function, including stroke volume and cardiac output. Like other forms of aerobic exercise, LISS contributes to mitochondrial adaptations; however, current evidence suggests that these adaptations are not unique to LISS and can also be achieved, often more robustly, through higher-intensity exercise when appropriately tolerated (Storoschuk et al., 2025).

By maintaining a steady, sustainable workload, LISS training prioritizes aerobic energy production and encourages the use of fat as a primary fuel source. This can support improvements in metabolic efficiency and insulin sensitivity, particularly in untrained or metabolically compromised individuals. While LISS does not appear to possess a unique advantage for stimulating mitochondrial biogenesis compared to higher-intensity training, it remains a valuable tool for building foundational aerobic capacity and improving overall work tolerance.

In addition to its metabolic effects, LISS exercise can induce favorable central cardiovascular adaptations. Sustained training at a moderate heart rate allows for prolonged ventricular filling with each cardiac cycle, creating an eccentric loading stimulus on the heart. Over time, this can contribute to improvements in stroke volume, cardiac efficiency, and reductions in resting heart rate.

Practical Application for Beginners and Deconditioned Clients

From a practical standpoint, LISS training is especially valuable for beginners and deconditioned individuals who may struggle to recover from repeated bouts of higher-intensity work. Clients with elevated resting heart rates, poor 60-second heart-rate recovery, or limited aerobic capacity often lack the foundational cardiovascular efficiency required to tolerate frequent interval training without excessive fatigue.

In these cases, accumulating low-intensity work can serve as an effective entry point. Regular exposure to LISS training helps improve cardiac output, autonomic balance, and recovery capacity, allowing clients to gradually lower resting heart rate and improve heart-rate recovery between efforts. As general aerobic fitness improves, these individuals are better equipped to tolerate and benefit from higher-intensity intervals without undue stress or setbacks.

For many beginners, building general aerobic capacity through LISS training first can enhance long-term adherence and create a physiological base that supports progression toward more demanding conditioning methods.

Programming Considerations

When using a heart-rate monitor, LISS training should be maintained at a steady, low to moderate intensity—generally around 60 to 70 percent of maximum heart rate for most clients. In the absence of heart rate data, intensity can be effectively regulated using the talk test, where the client can speak in short phrases comfortably but would struggle to carry on a prolonged conversation (Foster et al., 2008).

LISS training is typically performed in a continuous format using activities such as walking, incline walking, cycling, rowing, or elliptical training for durations ranging from 30 to 90 minutes, depending on the individual's training status and goals.

Due to the time commitment involved, extended LISS sessions are often best programmed separately from strength training sessions. Performing long bouts of low-intensity conditioning on the same day as strength training can increase overall fatigue and lengthen sessions unnecessarily. Scheduling LISS training on nonlifting days or lighter training days allows clients to accumulate aerobic volume while preserving recovery and performance in resistance training.

LISS TRAINING METHODS

It is essential to select training methods that align with a client's goals, preferences, and physical limitations in order to make LISS training both sustainable and effective. In this section are several practical and accessible ways to train at a low-intensity steady state, each offering unique benefits based on individual needs and circumstances.

Distance Running

The most commonly prescribed method for LISS training is continuous-distance running. Endurance athletes frequently use this approach to accumulate low-intensity volume and build a strong aerobic foundation for performance. While highly beneficial for competitive runners, it may not always be the most practical or effective option for the average fitness enthusiast seeking to improve general aerobic fitness.

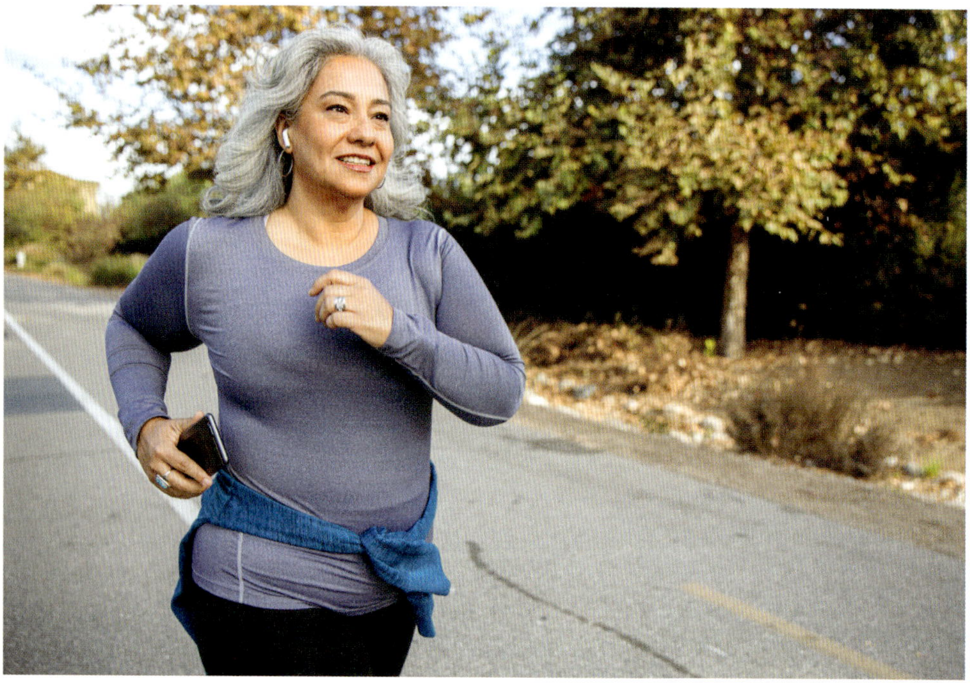

adamkaz/E+/Getty Images

One major drawback of long-distance running is the high potential for repetitive stress injuries due to the cumulative impact on the tendons and joints. Conditions such as patellofemoral pain, Achilles tendonitis, and plantar fasciitis are prevalent among runners, often stemming from poor mechanics, improper footwear, sudden increases in training volume, or inadequate recovery. Research indicates that nearly 50 percent of recreational runners in the United States sustain an injury each year, with a reinjury rate of up to 70 percent in the following year (Mechelen, 1992).

Given these risks, those in the general population looking to improve aerobic fitness should consider working with a running coach to refine their technique and training plan. Alternatively, exploring lower-impact methods of steady-state training such as uphill walking, rucking, or cycling can help reduce injury risk while still providing the same cardiovascular benefits.

Hiking or Uphill Walking

Hiking or uphill walking is an excellent alternative to distance running for developing low-intensity aerobic fitness. Walking uphill, whether outdoors on natural terrain or on an incline treadmill, adds a level of intensity that enhances cardiovascular endurance while minimizing the high-impact stress associated with running. This makes it a joint-friendly and accessible option for individuals of all fitness levels.

For those without access to hills or a treadmill, an effective alternative is walking with added resistance, such as a weighted backpack or weight vest. This practice is known as *rucking*. It increases the cardiovascular demand and muscular engagement of walking, making it a viable method to achieve an aerobic training effect.

Air Bike

The air bike is an excellent tool for low-intensity steady state due to its low impact on the joints, full body engagement, and ease of pace control. Most clients, regardless of physical limitations or injury history, can use the air bike comfortably. Additionally, the ability to monitor pacing in RPM, miles per hour, or watts helps users regulate their effort more effectively throughout the workout, ensuring they stay within the desired training zone.

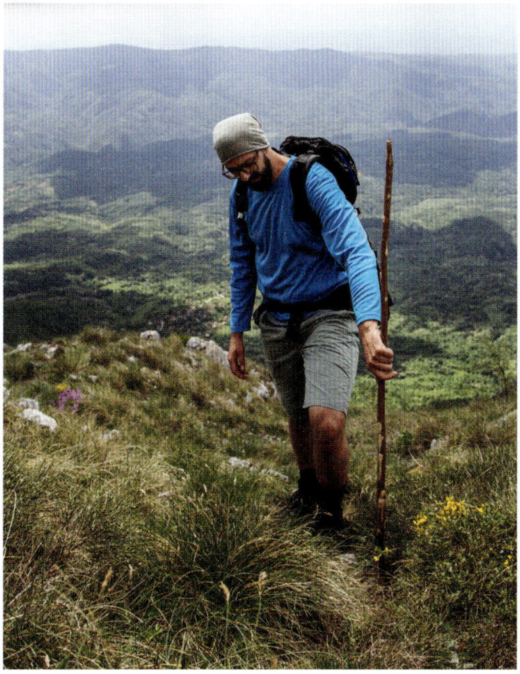

mmpile/E+/Getty Images

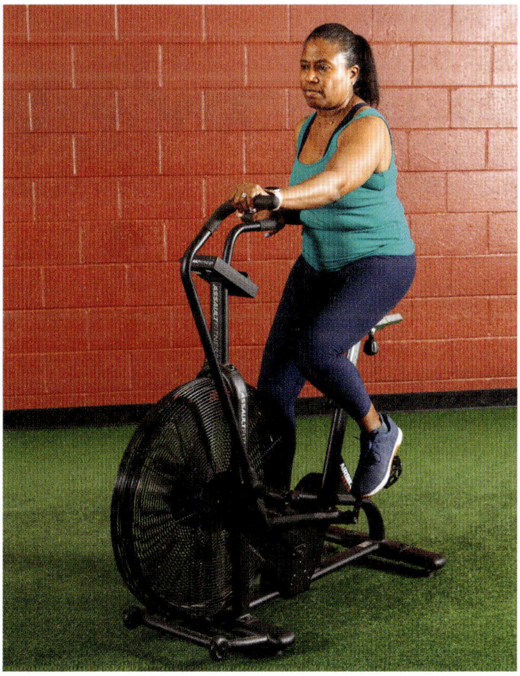

Elliptical

The elliptical is another effective method for developing low-intensity aerobic fitness. Like the air bike, it offers low-impact, full-body engagement while allowing users to control their pacing. While the elliptical is generally less muscularly demanding than the air bike, it provides the benefit of exercising in a standing position. This can be preferable for some clients and offers valuable variety of the exercise mode within a training program.

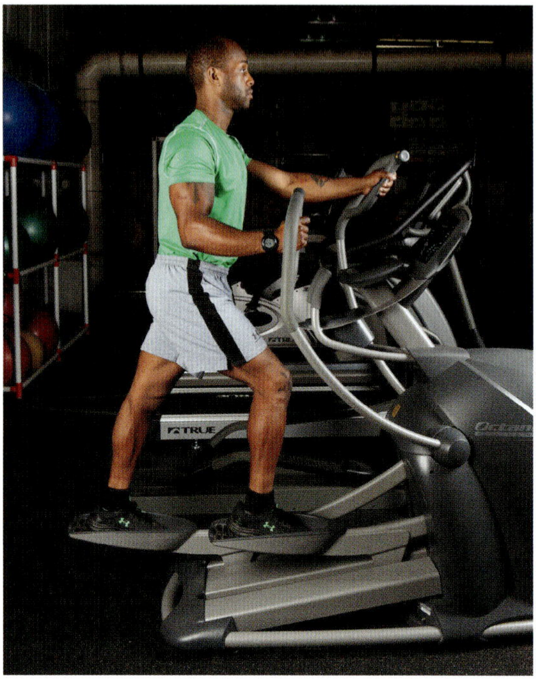

INTERVAL TRAINING

Interval training is an extremely popular and effective method that can be used to improve aerobic and anaerobic power. Interval training is especially valuable due to its time efficiency, maximizing the training effect with a minimal amount of time commitment. Given that lack of time is the most commonly cited reason for the average person not participating in an exercise routine, interval training presents a practical and efficient approach to improving cardiovascular health and fitness (Felicia et al., 2022).

Interval training, defined most simply, is "repeated bouts of relatively hard work interspersed with recovery periods of easier work or rest (Coates et al., 2023, p. 1). In the context of this text, we will discuss using HIIT, which consists of short bursts of activity ranging anywhere from 10 seconds to a few minutes in length performed at 75 to 90 percent of max heart rate.

HIIT is an extremely effective strategy for improving aerobic fitness, particularly for the average gymgoer, due to its time efficiency. Numerous studies have demonstrated that HIIT can provide similar, if not superior, benefits compared to moderate-intensity continuous exercise in a fraction of the time. One study compared 12 weeks of three weekly sessions of three 20-second all-out sprints with three weekly sessions of 45 minutes of continuous training at 70 percent max heart rate. Despite requiring five times less total exercise time, the HIIT protocol produced comparable improvements in $\dot{V}O_2$max, insulin sensitivity, and mitochondrial content (Gillen et al., 2016).

Given these findings, it is recommended that individuals who are struggling to meet minimum aerobic exercise guidelines use HIIT as a means to reach the weekly standard of 75 minutes of vigorous exercise recommended by the U.S. Department of Health and Human Services. HIIT is a practical and efficient option for those with limited time who are looking to improve their cardiovascular health.

The Air Bike for Interval Training

The primary recommended exercise mode for interval training in this book is the air bike. The air bike is highly effective due to its full body integration and low-impact design. Its low-impact nature makes it accessible for nearly all clients, regardless of their injury history or training status, allowing them to develop cardiovascular fitness without the risk of overuse injuries. Furthermore, the air bike engages both the upper and lower body, creating a greater metabolic demand compared to traditional cycling. Finally, tracking performance through metrics such as RPMs, miles per hour, or watts enables users to manage their effort more precisely, helping them maintain the intended training zone throughout the workout.

The 8-Minute Interval Workout

When time efficiency is a primary concern, a recommend starting point is the 8-minute interval workout as a means to start engaging in interval training for the beginner. The effectiveness and low time commitment required for this protocol make it a useful approach to add following a strength training workout or as a short stand-alone interval workout when time is limited.

After completing the MAS test on the air bike referenced previously, the trainer will have determined the MAS in RPMs. This is a crucial parameter in conditioning program design, because training at or above MAS serves as the key intensity factor for improving aerobic power (Baker, 2011).

For a beginner, start by selecting an intensity for the work periods that is equal to 110 percent of MAS. This will ensure that the client is working at an intensity that is high enough to ensure an aerobic power training effect but will be sustainable for all of the prescribed work bouts. For a more advanced trainee an intensity of 120 percent of MAS may be appropriate.

Here is an example.

MAS = 70 RPMs

Prescribed intensity: 70 RPMs × 1.10 = 77 RPMs

Once the intensity has been determined, the client begins the workout with 10-second-on and 20-second-off intervals by pedaling on the air bike at the assigned intensity for 10 seconds and resting for 20 seconds. Repeat this for eight rounds. Rest for two minutes, pedaling lightly, and then repeat the same protocol again for eight more rounds.

Follow the following progression shown one or two times per week, progressively adjusting the work-to-rest ratio to challenge the client's aerobic fitness. After eight weeks, repeat the same progression at 120 percent of MAS.

- *Week 1:* 10 seconds on and 20 seconds off × 8 repetitions (Complete one round only)
- *Week 2:* 10 seconds on and 20 seconds off × 8 repetitions
  - » Rest 2 minutes
  - » 10 seconds on and 20 seconds off × 8 repetitions
- *Week 3:* 10 seconds on and 20 seconds off × 8 repetitions
  - » Rest 2 minutes
  - » 10 seconds on and 20 seconds off × 8 repetitions
- *Week 4:* 15 seconds on and 15 seconds off × 8 repetitions
  - » Rest 2 minutes
  - » 10 seconds on and 20 seconds off × 8 repetitions
- *Week 5:* 15 seconds on and 15 seconds off × 8 repetitions
  - » Rest 2 minutes
  - » 15 seconds on and 15 seconds off × 8 repetitions
- *Week 6:* 15 seconds on and 15 seconds off × 8 repetitions
  - » Rest 2 minutes
  - » 15 seconds on and 15 seconds off × 8 repetitions
- *Week 7:* 20 seconds on and 10 seconds off × 8 repetitions
  - » Rest 2 minutes
  - » 15 seconds on and 15 seconds off × 8 repetitions
- *Week 8:* 20 seconds on and 10 seconds off × 8 repetitions
  - » Rest 2 minutes
  - » 20 seconds on and 15 seconds off × 8 repetitions

Longer Duration Intervals

As clients improve their cardiovascular fitness and increase tolerance to high volumes of interval-based training, it is recommended that they begin participating in extensive, longer duration intervals as a means to further increase aerobic power output. Generally speaking, the more time that clients accumulate training at or above their MAS, the more effectively they can increase it and as a result improve health and fitness.

Aim to increase the duration of intervals from the short 10-second and 20-second work bouts discussed earlier to longer intervals lasting anywhere from one to four minutes in duration. Implementing a few of the following methods can be a useful way to progressively develop cardiovascular fitness via longer interval methods.

Decreasing Duration Interval Training Accumulating more time training at or above MAS or $\dot{V}O_2$max is believed to be one of the most effective ways to increase aerobic capacity (Vaccari et al., 2023). For novice trainees, training at such a high intensity for extended periods of time can be exhausting and unsustainable; however, decreasing duration interval training has been proven to be an effective strategy and practical for trainees to begin accumulating more time near their $\dot{V}O_2$max without excessive perceived exertion.

In this method, both work and rest intervals are progressively shortened with each successive repetition. This approach helps maintain a higher intensity throughout the workout, keeping effort levels near $\dot{V}O_2$ peak and potentially eliciting greater metabolic adaptations. Research has shown that this strategy enables trainees to sustain a greater relative intensity compared to traditional interval structures, such as long intervals lasting three minutes or short intervals of 30 seconds (Vaccari, 2020).

The interval protocols that follow can be used to program high-intensity decreasing duration interval training.

Beginner Decreasing Duration Interval Protocol Start with the protocol shown here for beginners. All repetitions should performed at or above their MAs intensity determined in RPMs or watts during their MAS test on the air bike.

- *Work bout #1:* 90 seconds
- *Rest period #1:* 60 seconds
- *Work bout #2:* 60 seconds
- *Rest period #2:* 40 seconds
- *Work bout #3:* 40 seconds
- *Rest period #3:* 30 seconds
- *Work bout #4:* 30 seconds
- *Rest period #4:* 20 seconds
- *Work bout #5:* 20 seconds
- *Rest period #5:* 10 seconds
- *Work bout #6:* 10 seconds

Advanced Decreasing Duration Interval Protocol Once clients have shown that they can comfortably and repeatedly perform the previous protocol, begin introducing the longer duration protocol that follows. All repetitions should be performed at or above a client's MAS intensity determined in RPMs or watts during the MAS test on the air bike.

- *Work bout #1:* 180 seconds
- *Rest period #1:* 120 seconds
- *Work bout #2:* 120 seconds
- *Rest period #2:* 80 seconds
- *Work bout #3:* 60 seconds

- *Rest period #3:* 40 seconds
- *Work bout #4:* 40 seconds
- *Rest period #4:* 25 seconds
- *Work bout #5:* 30 seconds
- *Rest period #5:* 20 seconds
- *Work bout #6:* 30 seconds

One-Minute-On and One-Minute-Off Max Aerobic Speed Intervals

Another effective HIIT protocol for the air bike involves intervals of one minute of work and one minute of rest to build glycolytic capacity. This method will help clients to accumulate more total training time at their MAS intensity while developing peripheral adaptations to improve their ability to manage local muscle fatigue.

Clients should perform these intervals at their MAS intensity, measured in RPMs or watts, as determined by their MAS test. In the first week, start with five one-minute intervals, each followed by one minute of rest. Each week, add one additional interval until the client successfully completes 10 intervals at the prescribed intensity. At that point, retest MAS and adjust the training intensity based on the new results.

Tempo Running

Tempo runs are a form of moderate-intensity, interval-based running designed to develop work capacity and enhance overall aerobic fitness. They are particularly effective for general-population clients because they offer a structured approach to running without the excessive volume of long-distance training or the high velocities of sprinting. This makes tempo runs more accessible while also reducing the risk of injury, making them a practical and sustainable option for improving basic aerobic fitness.

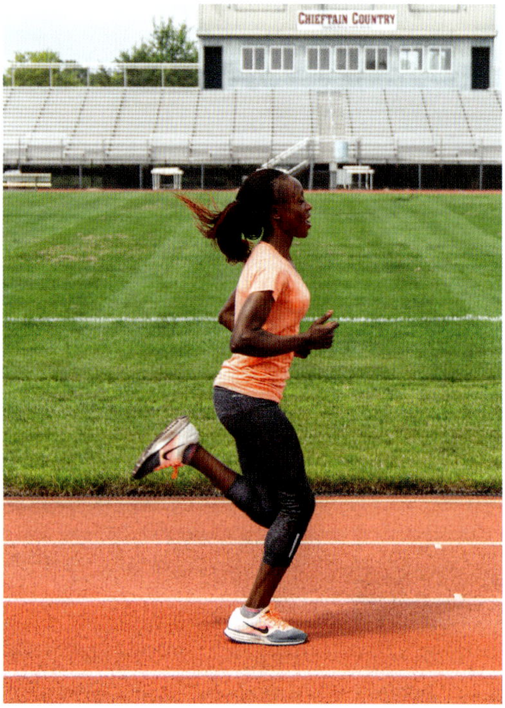

Tempo runs can be performed either on a track, in an open field, or on a treadmill.

TEMPO RUN ON A TRACK OR FIELD

1. Run at roughly 75 percent effort so you are neither jogging nor sprinting at full speed for a distance of 75 yards (69 m).
2. Walk back to the starting line, allowing yourself to rest for at least one minute or until your heart rate drops back below 70 percent max heart rate.
3. Repeat this process, progressively building your volume and following the progression listed here:
   - *Week 1:* 6 reps
   - *Week 2:* 8 reps
   - *Week 3:* 10 reps
   - *Week 4:* 12 reps
   - *Week 5:* 14 reps
   - *Week 6:* 16 reps

TEMPO RUN ON A TREADMILL

1. Set the speed on the treadmill to about 75 percent of your maximal running speed.
2. Run continuously at that designated pace for 15 to 20 seconds.
3. Step off the treadmill and rest for at least one minute or until your heart rate drops back below 70 percent max heart rate.
4. Repeat this process, progressively building your volume and following the progression listed here:
   - *Week 1:* 6 reps
   - *Week 2:* 8 reps
   - *Week 3:* 10 reps
   - *Week 4:* 12 reps
   - *Week 5:* 14 reps
   - *Week 6:* 16 reps

BALANCING CARDIOVASCULAR TRAINING ACROSS THE WEEK

For many coaches and trainees alike, it can be confusing to determine how and when to apply the wide range of cardiovascular conditioning options discussed in this chapter, particularly when considering the competing physical demands of strength training. Adding to this confusion are the many conflicting viewpoints surrounding conditioning, with some coaches strongly advocating for low-intensity aerobic work and others favoring high-intensity interval training as the primary solution.

For general-population clients, the reality is much simpler: All cardiovascular exercise is beneficial. Any form of cardiovascular training, when performed consistently, will have a positive impact on cardiovascular health, metabolic function, and longevity.

Rather than debating which single method is best, it is far more productive to consider how different conditioning methods can complement one another over the course of a training week.

From a practical standpoint, short bouts of high-intensity interval training are easiest to place at the end of strength training sessions. These protocols provide a strong cardiovascular stimulus while remaining time efficient, allowing them to be incorporated without requiring a separate training session. In contrast, longer-duration, lower-intensity aerobic work is often best performed on days when strength training is not scheduled. This approach allows clients to accumulate meaningful aerobic volume without compromising recovery or extending already long training sessions.

The most important factor in developing cardiovascular fitness is accumulating time spent moving at a variety of intensities. Exposure to multiple intensity levels helps build well-rounded aerobic adaptations and improves resilience to a broad range of cardiovascular stressors.

When deciding how to structure cardiovascular conditioning for a client, the most important questions to ask are not physiological, but practical:

- *What can this person do?* This includes injury history, orthopedic or skill limitations, and current fitness level.
- *What will this person actually do?* This includes time availability, access to equipment, personal preferences, and lifestyle.

With these constraints in mind, cardiovascular training can be organized into three simple intensity categories. Each serves a distinct purpose, and together they create a balanced, effective, and sustainable conditioning program.

The Three Intensity Zones

Easy (Low Intensity)

- Low-intensity steady-state aerobic exercise

Moderate (Moderate Intensity)

- Extensive interval training
- Tempo running

Hard (High Intensity)

- High-intensity interval training

Figure 8.2 illustrates this three-zone model and shows how the cardiovascular training methods discussed in this chapter fit within each intensity category.

The exact balance between these zones does not need to be rigid. It should fluctuate from week to week based on energy levels, life stress, recovery capacity, and individual goals. Over time, the objective is to increase gradually both total aerobic volume and tolerance to higher intensities without sacrificing consistency or enjoyment.

When cardiovascular training is viewed through this broader lens, it becomes less about choosing the right method and more about building a complete engine that supports health, performance, and resiliency over the long term.

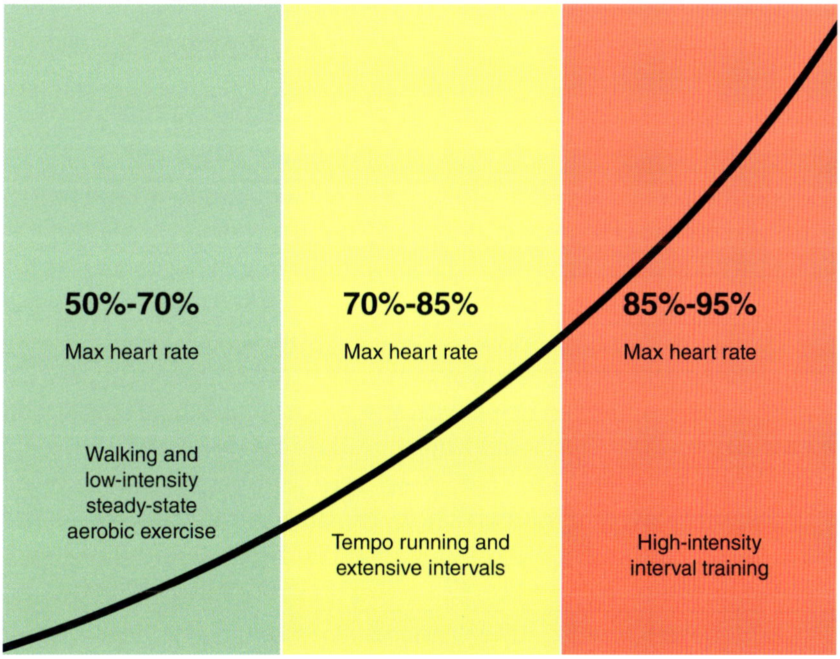

Figure 8.2 Zone intensity model for categorizing cardiovascular exercise.

Case Study: Victor's Cardiovascular Training Plan

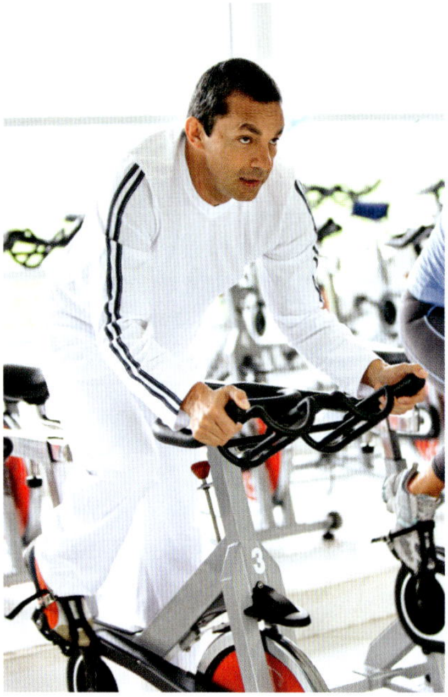

Andres Rodriguez/fotolia.com

My client, Victor, is a 61-year-old sedentary man who joined the gym to improve his body composition and cardiovascular health. He had a resting heart rate of 80 beats per minute, indicating low cardiac output and aerobic fitness. Victor previously attempted HIIT but found that he became exhausted after just a few repetitions, making it unsustainable for him.

To better assess his cardiovascular fitness, we conducted a two-mile MMAS test on the air bike to determine his MAS and one-minute heart rate recovery. This assessment helped us establish the optimal intensity for his intervals, ensuring they were both effective and manageable while also evaluating his recovery capacity between efforts.

Victor completed the two-mile test in six minutes, maintaining a MAS of 52 RPMs. His one-minute heart rate recovery posttest was 20 beats in 60 seconds.

To improve his aerobic fitness, we recommended that Victor engage in 60 to 120 minutes per week of zone 2 training outside of his structured gym sessions. For each session, he can choose his preferred mode of exercise such as brisk walking, biking, or using an elliptical. Regular zone 2 training helps him increase cardiac output, lower his resting heart rate, and improve heart rate recovery.

Additionally, we introduced short-duration intervals (10 seconds on and 20 seconds off). Victor began these intervals at 110 percent of his MAS, which equates to 57 to 58 RPM. This intensity was both effective and sustainable, allowing him to complete the training safely while building cardiovascular fitness.

PART IV

THE LONGEVITY PRESCRIPTION

Chapter 9

Laying the Groundwork

So far, this book has provided insights into how to help clients exercise effectively to enhance their health and longevity. Unfortunately, if our goal as trainers is to improve the health or the health habits of those we coach, knowing how to exercise is only part of the challenge. The real difficulty lies in actually doing it. There is no big secret regarding exercise and physical activity. The great paradox is that while nearly everyone understands that exercise is beneficial, most people still struggle to maintain a regular routine.

In a nationwide poll examining fitness awareness as a predictor of initiating and adhering to an exercise program, 63 percent of respondents were classified as "Uninitiated Believers." These individuals recognize that exercise holds value and know they should be exercising, yet they lack consistent dedication to a program (Tharrett, 2017, p. 49). This statistic implies that roughly 167 million Americans over the age of 18 are aware of the need to exercise regularly but find it challenging to commit to a consistent routine. Additionally, research shows that 50 percent of people who begin exercising often quit within six months (Linke et al., 2011).

Given this data, it is clear that the primary barrier for many individuals who are not physically active is not their belief in the importance of exercise but rather how to get started and stick with it.

Why is it so difficult to start and stick with an exercise program? Beginning a fitness journey can be intimidating, confusing, and, above all, challenging. Meaningful progress requires a sustained effort over time, and the payoff is rarely immediate. Early improvements are often subtle, while soreness, fatigue, and changes to daily routine are felt right away. The gap between effort and visible results is where many people lose momentum, not because exercise does not work but because it works much slower than people expect.

Additionally, the mainstream fitness industry often promotes extreme approaches and promises of rapid transformations. This leads to unrealistic expectations, which can result in frustration, burnout, injury, and ultimately, giving up altogether. In a culture that values quick fixes, it is no surprise that many struggle to maintain a long-term commitment to fitness. Building strength, improving health, and transforming your body demands patience, resilience, and a willingness to embrace the process for what it truly is: a lifelong journey, not a short sprint.

When it comes to many aspects of life, particularly exercise, people tend to overestimate the results they expect in the short term while underestimating what can be achieved over time. This pattern aligns with Amara's law, attributed to futurist Roy Amara, which suggests that we often overestimate short-term change and underestimate long-term impact (Ratcliffe, 2016).

In the context of exercise, this short-term mindset—combined with high expectations—often leaves gymgoers feeling discouraged when rapid results fail to appear, prompting them to abandon their routines before meaningful adaptations occur. With continued consistency, however, the long-term rewards of exercise typically far exceed initial expectations. Figure 9.1 illustrates Amara's law as applied to adaptation to an exercise routine.

My good friend and mentor, Michael Boyle, put it brilliantly: "Training is like farming." That is, you cannot speed up the process. No matter how hard someone works, results will not come in days but in weeks and months. Another great analogy is to think of exercising like long-term investing. At first, one's efforts may feel small and unrewarding—just like contributing $100 a week to a retirement account. After a month or even a year, the returns seem modest. But stay consistent and those small investments can grow into something significant over time as a result of compounding interest. The same goes for fitness: Steady, regular workouts may not yield dramatic results immediately, but over months and years, they compound into lasting health and resilience.

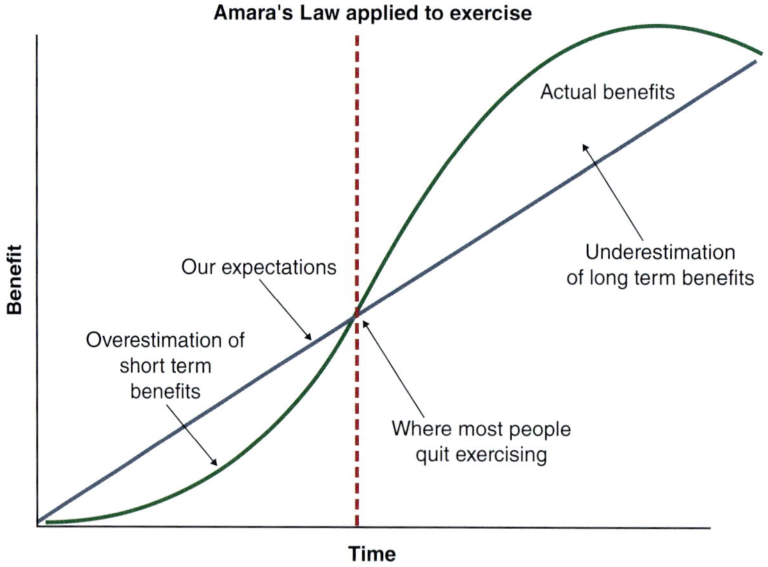

Figure 9.1 Amara's law applied to exercise.

CREATING THE CLIENT-COACH RELATIONSHIP

Fortunately, fitness professionals are uniquely positioned to influence the health and fitness habits of the people they work with. Personalized coaching, whether one-on-one or in a group setting, can significantly affect personal attitudes and adherence to fitness programs, helping clients build long-term sustainable exercise habits (McClaran, 2003).

Establishing a strong client–coach relationship is the cornerstone to creating an environment for client behavior change. The old saying "People don't care how much you know until they know how much you care" rings true when it comes to building a foundation on which a coach can help clients improve their health. The first priority of any coach should be to learn as much as possible about their clients and their personal motivations for joining an exercise program. In this process, the coach can establish trust and buy-in around the exercise program.

Introductory Interview

At the outset of any training program, the coach should conduct an intake interview to allow clients to share their motivations for exercising. The coach should ask open-ended questions that cannot be answered with a simple yes or no. This approach encourages clients to share more information about themselves. Following are some suggested intake questions:

- What motivated you to come to the gym and start an exercise program?
- What are some of your past experiences with exercise?
- What does your current weekly exercise routine consist of?
- How would you define success after training with me for six months?
- What is a realistic weekly commitment to exercise for you?
- What, if any, barriers do you feel might prevent you from committing to a consistent exercise program?

Asking questions in this manner provides valuable information to the coach about the client's motivations, past experiences and perceptions of exercise, long-term goals, and a realistic understanding of what the client can commit to.

Identifying a Client's "Why"

Once a client's goals have been established, it is essential for the coach to demonstrate clearly how the training program is aligned with those goals. This connection builds trust and helps the client see purpose in their effort.

As coaches, we often have a deep passion for exercise and find joy in the process of training. But most clients do not share that same love for the work itself. For them, exercise is a tool, not a passion. They show up not because they relish the exercises but because they value the results: feeling better, moving more easily, and enjoying the social experience of being around their coach and peers.

This distinction is critical. What motivates a coach is often very different from what drives a client. Research supports this: Most people begin exercising due to **extrinsic motivators**—to look better, perform better, or improve objective markers like body weight, blood pressure, and cholesterol (Ryan et al., 1997). Yet these external goals often are not enough to sustain long-term commitment. Even clients who see early results may lose motivation if the deeper "why" behind their training remains unrecognized or unaddressed.

Long-term adherence to exercise is more often fueled by intrinsic motivators—things such as feeling physically better, a sense of community, positive emotional associations, or the simple joy of reclaiming control over one's health (Ryan et al., 1997). When clients hire a trainer, they are seeking a result that holds personal meaning. That goal might be as specific as playing tennis into their 80s or as simple as getting out of bed without pain. Whether they articulate it clearly, there is always a deeper reason behind their decision to train. The coach's role is to uncover that reason and keep it central to the training program.

Research in positive psychology provides valuable insights into how we can influence our clients' mindset regarding exercise, helping them stay motivated and committed to their fitness routines. In his book *Before Happiness*, positive psychologist Shawn Achor discusses "meaning markers," which he describes as the emotional road signs behind our goals that are essential for sustained motivation, resilience, and happiness. He states that we experience up to three times higher levels of motivation, engagement, and productivity when our work aligns with our positive meaning markers (Achor, 2013). With this in mind, we can apply the same approach to help clients discover more meaning in their exercise routines, fostering greater motivation, consistency, and commitment.

Road Maps and Recaps for Training Success

After identifying a clients' big-picture goals, we should work with them to create a **road map** to success. In this process, we actively talk through the training plan—starting from where they are right now—and outline how their training will evolve over time to move them toward their long-term goals. We should explain how the program will adapt at different stages, providing a clear sense of progression and growth.

A key part of this conversation is connecting the exercises, milestones, and phases of training back to what is personally meaningful to them. By tying the structure of the program to their own motivations—their meaning markers—the journey becomes more than just checking boxes on a workout sheet. It becomes a personal investment. This approach helps clients feel like active participants in their own health journey rather than passive passengers. It provides them with a sense of ownership, a long-term vision, and the reassurance that the program is thoughtfully designed to help them achieve what matters most to them.

Once training is underway, we should actively look for opportunities to identify and highlight **meaning markers** throughout the process by using recaps at the end of each training session or training phase. These moments help redirect our clients' attention toward the progress they are making, even when it might feel slow or difficult. Intentionally emphasizing the positive aspects of the journey is crucial because the human brain is naturally wired with a negativity bias—a tendency to give more weight to negative emotions and experiences than to positive ones. While this bias was once an important survival mechanism, it can become a major roadblock for anyone trying to build and sustain a new habit today.

By regularly using recaps to spotlight improvements, milestones, and small wins, we help counteract this bias, reinforce positive momentum, and keep clients motivated over the long term.

GETTING STARTED IN THE GYM

The first 30 days of starting an exercise routine with a new client are crucial. During this critical period, clients constantly evaluate—whether consciously or subconsciously—whether they made the right decision in choosing to exercise.

They may think the following:

- Is this trainer any good?
- Did I take on too much?
- Am I going to get hurt?
- Do I even like this gym?

It is essential for the coach to navigate this period of transition effectively, turning the client from someone who is temporarily interested in exercise into a long-term committed exerciser. The most important thing to remember for successfully onboarding a new client into an exercise routine goes against the conventional approach to fitness: Make it easy.

During the first 30 days, our goal should be to provide clients with as many successful experiences as possible, demonstrating that they are capable and comfortable with the training process. Instead of pursuing intensity and complexity from day one, focus on stacking early wins. Start small to build confidence, and gradually increase the challenge. Every positive experience clients have in the gym reinforces the new identity they are trying to create. Each time they show up for a workout, they affirm the person they aspire to become. The reason most people never become consistent exercisers is because they quit too early—long before that new identity has had a chance to take root.

If we build an initial program that is too hard, it will often leave clients feeling overwhelmed by soreness, fatigue, and frustration and put them at risk for injury early in the process. Instead, intentionally design a program with basic exercise progressions with relatively low volume and intensity that they will be able to successfully complete. It is important to remember that the program always can be made harder if it is too easy, but starting out with too much challenge quickly can get the trainer into trouble.

Introductory Training Session

After having an initial conversation with a client about their injury history, training background, and long-term goals, the next step is to guide the client through an introductory workout. This session is crucial for both the coach and the client, because it lays the groundwork for a successful training relationship.

For the client, this introductory workout provides an opportunity to understand what it is like to train with this particular trainer, become familiar with the components of the exercise program, and start building confidence in the gym.

For the coach, the first training session serves as a fact-finding mission. It allows us to complement the subjective information gathered during the conversation with practical insights about the client's movement and feelings throughout the workout. This experience helps us identify which exercises may be suitable or unsuitable for the client moving forward.

During this introductory workout we should look to introduce foundational movement patterns to identify basic competency and identify where there may be pain or potential mobility or stability limitations. The chart in figure 9.2 demonstrates examples of basic movement patterns that can be used during an introductory workout to introduce the client to the training program while assessing movement quality.

Exercise category	Exercise	Movement quality
Movement prep	Shoulder floor slide	Overhead shoulder flexion and external rotation
Movement prep	Band-assisted leg lower	Hip separation
Movement prep	Wall ankle mobility	Ankle dorsiflexion
Movement prep	Bilateral hip lift	Hip extension
Movement prep	Standing toe touch	Spinal flexion and posterior hip shifting
Strength	Squat press-out	Hip mobility and squat motor control
Strength	Split squat	Unilateral strength and hip stability
Strength	Push-up or incline push-up	Upper body pushing strength and antiextension trunk strength
Strength	Reaching single-leg deadlift	Single-leg hip stability
Strength	Half-kneeling cable row	Upper body pulling strength
Strength	Standing hip hinge	Hip hinge motor control
Strength	Bear plank	Antiextension trunk strength

Figure 9.2 Movements that can be used in an introductory workout to assess movement quality and strength.

The purpose of an introductory workout should not be to exhaust or overly challenge the client. Instead, it should serve as an opportunity for the coach to gather information and observe how the client moves and feels, physically and psychologically, throughout the training program. After the introductory workout, the coach can evaluate which elements of the program should be progressed and which aspects should be maintained or regressed based on the client's performance and feedback.

Do No Harm

Referring to the original Hippocratic Oath, the foremost principle for health practitioners is to "do no harm." Unfortunately, coaches often make poor choices regarding exercise selection, intensity, and volume, which can result in client injuries and pain. If a client is injured while under our supervision, it is ultimately our responsibility. Injuring a client will not only derail the training process and increase the likelihood of dropout but could even result in legal consequences for the coach. With this in mind, it is essential to prioritize caution when selecting exercises and designing programs.

Clients can achieve significant progress with basic exercise progressions and small, incremental improvements each week. Keep in mind that clients will have diverse medical and injury histories that need to be considered when deciding on exercise selection. The key principle for fitness professionals is that clients should never be exercising in pain. Coaches can ask clients a straightforward question to assess whether an exercise is suitable for them: "Does it hurt?"

The answer should be a clear yes or no.

If the response is yes, we must choose an alternative exercise that helps develop the client's fitness without causing pain. Using the system of progressions and regressions outlined in the earlier chapters in this book, another exercise option always should be available that can enhance fitness without discomfort.

Referring Out

As fitness professionals, we must maintain clear boundaries regarding our scope of practice, particularly when it comes to injury and pain management. If clients experience pain, injury, or any medical issues during training, coaches should always refer them to licensed medical professionals instead of attempting to treat the issue themselves. A helpful guiding phrase to remember is, "When in doubt, refer out." Personal trainers should also strive to build professional relationships with physical therapists, doctors, psychologists, and dietitians. This collaboration will create a comprehensive health network for their clients to ensure they receive proper professional care.

It is inevitable that the clients that we are coaching will experience pain at some point during the training process. However, this does not mean we should cease all exercise. Instead, we should be prepared to modify the training program to accommodate their limitations. Simple adjustments can be made to exercises, such as reducing load, speed, and range of motion or incorporating external stability, to create conditions for pain-free workouts.

If clients feel pain in a segment of the body, we can alter the movement pattern to allow them to continue loading the general area while changing the load distribution across the joints to ensure the movement is pain free. Additionally, if a client is injured and cannot use a limb due to immobilization or medical guidelines, we should still train the contralateral limb. This approach can help prevent atrophy and leverage the cross-education effect, which minimizes strength losses during immobilization (Altheyab et al., 2024). The chart in figure 9.3 provides examples of how to modify exercise selections to work around pain.

Reduce load		
Goblet squat	Switch to	Bodyweight squat press-out
Reduce speed		
Split squat	Switch to	Split squat isometric hold
Reduce impact		
Continuous hurdle jump	Switch to	Box jump
Add stability		
Bodyweight squat press-out	Switch to	Suspension trainer assisted squat
Pain during knee dominant exercise		
Goblet squat	Switch to	Kettlebell deadlift
Pain during horizontal pushing exercise		
Dumbbell bench press	Switch to	Dumbbell row
Unable to use one leg due to injury		
Split squat	Switch to	Single-leg squat
Unable to use one arm due to injury		
Push-up	Switch to	One-arm dumbbell press

Figure 9.3 Guidelines for basic exercise modification.

Case Study: Suki

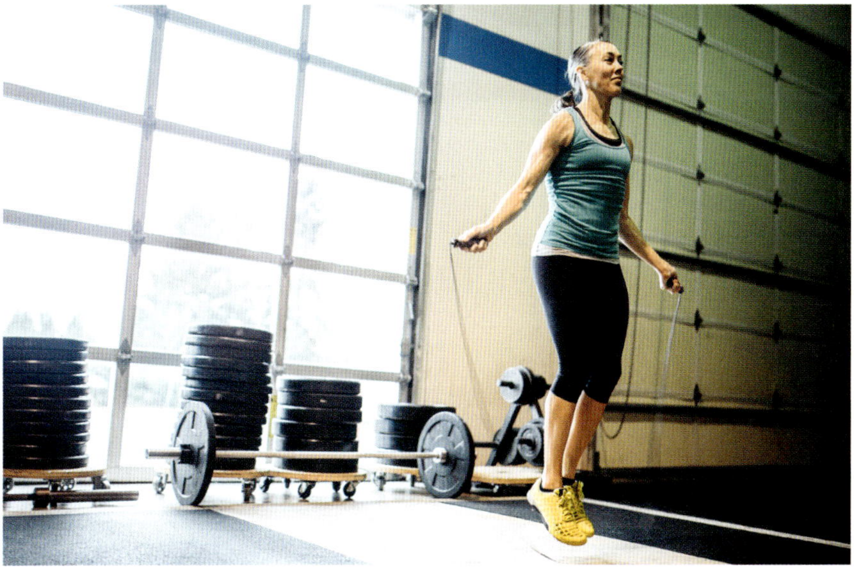

RyanJLane/Getty Images

Suki is a 48-year-old woman with a full-time desk job and significant family responsibilities. Although she understood the benefits of exercise, she had a long history of starting programs only to abandon them within a few weeks. She described herself as inconsistent and was apprehensive about getting hurt or struggling with the program.

During her intake interview, Suki explained that her primary motivation was improving her energy, reducing daily aches, and maintaining independence as she aged. She wanted to keep up with her family and avoid the physical decline she had observed in her parents. Identifying this deeper "why" helped establish trust and provided a clear anchor for her training program.

Given her background, the initial goal was adherence, not intensity. We designed a simple, twice-per-week introductory program focused on basic movement patterns, conservative loading, and short, manageable sessions. The priority during the first month was to make training feel achievable, comfortable, and repeatable.

Early sessions included a brief dynamic warm-up, fundamental strength exercises such as goblet squats, supported split squats, incline push-ups, and rows, along with low-intensity cardiovascular work. Exercises were selected to build confidence, assess movement

(continued)

Case Study: Suki *(continued)*

quality, and avoid unnecessary soreness or pain. Any movement that caused discomfort was immediately modified, reinforcing the principle of "do no harm."

Throughout the onboarding phase, the coach emphasized small wins and used brief recaps at the end of each session to highlight progress, counteracting Suki's tendency to focus on perceived shortcomings. As consistency improved, a clear road map was introduced, outlining how volume, load, and complexity would gradually progress over time.

After several months, Suki had improved her strength, mobility, and cardiovascular capacity, but more importantly, she had built a consistent exercise habit. By prioritizing simplicity, early success, and meaningful coaching interactions, this approach laid the foundation for sustainable training and long-term health.

Chapter 10

Designing a Program for Health and Longevity

The preceding chapters have covered the essential building blocks of a fitness program for health and longevity: mobility, warm-up, power, strength, conditioning, and general physical activity. Each of these components is valuable on its own, but their true power comes from how they are combined into a complete system.

For most coaches, the challenge is not understanding the individual parts. The real challenge is figuring out how to assemble them into a program that is practical, commercially viable, and repeatable—something that can be delivered in the familiar 60-minute training session while still driving meaningful long-term results.

This is where coaching truly becomes an art. Our role as coaches is to translate broad scientific principles and public health recommendations into programs that real people can follow. We need programs that fit into busy schedules, respect recovery needs, and still deliver enough stimulus to move the needle on health and longevity.

The good news is that building effective programs does not have to be complicated. By anchoring our design to the established minimum guidelines for physical activity and layering in the essential qualities of functional training, we can create a framework that is simple, sustainable, and scalable.

START WITH THE GUIDELINES

Let's revisit the minimum recommended levels of physical activity outlined in the Physical Activity Guidelines for Americans (Piercy et al., 2018):

- 150–300 minutes per week of moderate-intensity aerobic activity, or
- 75–150 minutes per week of vigorous-intensity aerobic activity, or
- an equivalent combination of the two, plus muscle-strengthening activities for all major muscle groups at least two days per week

These public recommendations provide a broad framework, but it is our job as coaches to translate them into programs that clients realistically can follow. Importantly, the guidelines say nothing about mobility or power training, two elements that are rarely emphasized in public health messaging but are critical for preserving independence and quality of life. Including them ensures clients are not just checking the box on exercise but building true resilience.

It is also worth noting that beginners do not need to hit the full guidelines right away. For someone just starting out, the priority should be establishing consistency, not chasing numbers. Our role is to scale the prescription so clients feel successful, not overwhelmed, and then help them progressively build toward these targets over time. In practice, most beginners do best starting with a simple two-day-per-week program that blends mobility, power, strength, and conditioning into a 60-minute session. This provides an efficient foundation while establishing a sustainable exercise habit that can expand to greater volumes and intensities as they adapt.

WEEKLY STRUCTURE

For the majority of clients, the most effective and realistic approach is a full body functional training program performed two to three times per week. This frequency allows them to meet the strength guidelines, train all major movement patterns, and make meaningful progress, all while leaving room for adequate recovery.

On the days between strength and high-intensity interval sessions, encourage clients to be active at a lower intensity. This could mean lower-intensity steady state cardio such as cycling, jogging, or swimming or recreational activities such as hiking, tennis, or pickleball. These sessions not only support recovery but also help clients accumulate the aerobic volume needed to meet the guidelines without feeling like they are living in the gym.

By centering programs around two to three full body sessions and layering in lower-intensity activity on off days, coaches can give clients a structure that is both effective and sustainable—a foundation strong enough to support health and longevity over the long term. Figure 10.1 provides a framework for a balanced weekly training structure that is both sustainable and meets the minimum recommended physical activity guidelines.

Sample weekly program (Meeting minimum exercise guidelines)		
Sunday	60-minute brisk walk, hike, or recreational activity	
Monday	Full body training + HIIT intervals	
Tuesday	30-minute steady-state cardio	
Wednesday	Full body training + HIIT intervals	
Thursday	60-minute brisk walk, hike, or recreational activity	
Friday	Full body training + HIIT intervals	
Saturday	Rest	zzZ

Figure 10.1 A sample of a well-rounded weekly program that includes both full body strength training and cardiovascular exercise.

TRAINING IS A RECIPE, NOT A MENU

Michael Boyle famously said, "Training is a recipe, not a menu." A functional training program works because of the interaction of all its parts. Clients do not get to pick their favorites and skip the rest; each ingredient plays a role in creating the final product. Mobility, power, strength, and conditioning each contribute something unique to the bigger picture of health and resilience.

As coaches, our responsibility is to deliver this recipe in a way that is practical: a balanced program that fits into the constraints of a 60-minute session, whether in a group or one-on-one setting.

When designing programs for the general population, the goal is not to maximize one quality in isolation but to build a resilient, well-rounded foundation. Unlike bodybuilding or competitive weightlifting, the focus is not aesthetics or competition but health, independence, and quality of life.

Programs should be progressive, sustainable, and adaptable. The framework remains the same—mobility, movement prep, power, strength, conditioning—but the details can shift based on a client's needs, goals, and experience level. This balance of structure and flexibility is what allows trainers to reliably prescribe exercise as medicine in a way clients can sustain for the long haul.

THE FRAMEWORK OF A SESSION

The order of a training session matters. A well-structured workout should gradually build in intensity, starting with low-load preparation and progressing toward the most demanding work. This sequencing allows the body to gradually increase activity in the nervous system and raise body temperature. The result is better performance, reduced injury risk, and higher-quality movement throughout the session.

Every session should ramp up systematically in the following order:

1. *Mobility:* Encourage joint range of motion, improve tissue quality, and prepare the body
2. *Warm-up and movement prep:* Increase body temperature, stimulate the central nervous system, rehearse movement patterns, and reinforce motor control and movement skills
3. *Power:* Preserve and develop muscular power and deceleration skills
4. *Strength:* Develop strength and muscle mass in all major movement patterns
5. *Conditioning:* Develop aerobic power and capacity for metabolic health and performance

This sequence ensures clients move from low-intensity preparation to higher-intensity demands in a safe and progressive way.

Along with understanding the individual components of the program, coaches also need to understand how to fit all of this into the typical 60-minute training session. By allocating time intentionally, we can ensure each component is addressed without overwhelming the client or running over time. Providing this training prescription in a reliable, predictable, and commercially viable format allows for consistency and sustainability. A typical breakdown might look like table 10.1.

Table 10.1 Time Allocation for Each Section of Program Session

Component	Time
Foam roll, stretch	Approximately 10 minutes
Motor control and active warm-up	Approximately 5 minutes
Power	Approximately 5 minutes
Strength training	Approximately 30 minutes
Conditioning	Approximately 10 minutes

This structure gives each component enough time to have an impact while keeping the session efficient. It also leaves room for flexibility; a coach can expand or contract sections based on a client's needs, training age, or group dynamics while still keeping the recipe intact.

BEGINNER INTRODUCTORY PROGRAM

When novice, untrained clients first begin training, coaches often overestimate how much exercise they can tolerate and underestimate how little it takes to make them sore or fatigued. For clients with little to no training history, it is best to start with an introductory program that emphasizes familiarity and success over intensity.

This phase serves two purposes: First, it allows the client to get comfortable in the gym environment, learn basic movements, and build initial confidence. Second, it provides the coach with a rolling assessment. By watching how clients move and respond to training in real time, coaches can gather more meaningful information than a single snapshot assessment.

Before even implementing the more formal assessments outlined earlier in this book, it is recommended to begin with a four-week introductory phase for the untrained client. It establishes a safe and manageable starting point while giving coaches the information they need to individualize the next stage of training.

In this introductory phase, training volume is low and intensity is moderate, gradually building work capacity over the four weeks. The focus should remain on low-complexity exercises and less intense conditioning, allowing clients to find success early and progressively adapt to participating in structured exercise. Throughout this process, it is imperative for the coach to check in consistently, asking how clients felt during and after sessions, monitoring for soreness or pain, and seeking feedback on perceived difficulty. This information is invaluable for adjusting the program and planning the next stage of training.

The program in table 10.2 starting on page 259 is an example of a two-day-per-week functional training plan designed for novice clients. On days outside the gym, coaches should encourage additional low-intensity activity, such as steady-state cardiovascular exercise, recreational sports, or focused mobility work to support recovery, build aerobic capacity, and reinforce healthy movement habits.

INTERMEDIATE THREE-PHASE PROGRAM

Clients who have completed the introductory phase or those with prior training experience can progress to a three-phase intermediate program. This model gradually increases exercise variation, load, and volume within the warm-up, strength, power, and conditioning components. It is important to emphasize that this program is intended as a general template, not a rigid prescription, for balanced training. Coaches should always adapt programs to the individual by applying the progression and regression principles outlined in the previous chapters.

The intermediate program found in tables 10.3 through 10.5 starting on page 262 represents the core framework of training for health and longevity, the structure most clients will follow for the majority of their time in the gym.

Ultimately, the goal of any well-designed program is not perfection, novelty, or complexity; it is consistency and effectiveness. What matters most is not how sophisticated a program looks on paper but whether it can be executed week after week and sustained over time.

Coaching and programming exist at the intersection of art and science. The science provides the principles; the art lies in applying them to real people with real constraints.

The role of the coach, therefore, is not simply to write programs but to design and continually refine them based on an individual's history, goals, and day-to-day readiness. Programs must be flexible enough to accommodate setbacks, changing schedules, and fluctuations in motivation while still providing a meaningful training stimulus.

The framework presented in this book is intended to give trainers a practical starting point for building programs that both improve performance and meaningfully influence both the length and quality of their clients' lives. Using the strategies outlined throughout this text, the goal is not to create rigid templates but to empower trainers to make informed adjustments and sound decisions that meet the specific needs of each client.

Exercise should be viewed not as a short-term intervention but as a long-term, meaningful investment in health. A program only works if it can be repeated, adapted as life inevitably changes, and sustained long enough to close the gap between life span and health span.

When movement is prescribed with intention, balancing strength, power, cardiovascular fitness, mobility, and everyday physical activity, it becomes more than a collection of exercises; it becomes a practical delivery system for movement as medicine.

The responsibility of coaches and practitioners, then, is not to chase novelty but to build systems that foster adherence, resilience, and durability. Applied consistently over time, thoughtful exercise programming becomes a foundation for health, function, and longevity. In the end, the best program is the one that helps people keep moving today, next year, and for the rest of their lives.

Table 10.2 Beginner Two-Day Introductory Program

Day 1				
Movement preparation				
Foam rolling	Glutes (p. 41)	Calves (p. 48)	Posterior shoulder (p. 46)	
	Thoracic spine (p. 45)	Adductors (p. 43)	Lumbar (p. 44)	
	Quads (p. 42)	Lats (p. 46)		
Mobility	90/90 hip stretch (p. 52)			1 min each
	Spiderman stretch (p. 53)			1 min each
	Adductor rocking stretch (p. 54)			10 reps each
	Wide split thoracic rotation (p. 56)			10 reps each
	Shoulder articular rotations (p. 57)			10 reps each
	Active lumbar flexion and extension (p. 62)			10 reps
	Wall ankle mobility (p. 59)			10 reps each
Motor control	Bilateral hip lift (p. 70)			10 reps
	Band-assisted leg lower (p. 76)			10 reps each
	Shoulder floor slide (p. 72)			10 reps
Patterning	Squat press-out (p. 78)			5 reps
	Split squat (p. 80)			5 reps each
	Lateral squat (p. 82)			5 reps each
	Chest-loaded bilateral hip hinge (p. 84)			5 reps
Multiplanar active warm-up	**Perform all drills 10 yards (meters) down and back.*			
	Forward A-skip (p. 91)			
	High knee run (p. 93)			
	Heel to butt (p. 94)			
	Lateral shuffle (p. 95)			
	Carioca (p. 96)			
	Backpedal (p. 97)			
Power	Box jump (p. 120): 2 sets × 5 reps			
	Tall-kneeling medicine ball chest pass (p. 138): 2 × 8 reps			

(continued)

Table 10.2 Beginner Two-Day Introductory Program *(continued)*

Day 1 *(continued)*				
Movement preparation				
Day 1, block 1	**Week 1**	**Week 2**	**Week 3**	**Week 4**
A1: Chest-loaded hip hinge (p. 187) or kettlebell deadlift (p. 186)	2×8 reps	3×8 reps	3×8 reps	3×10 reps
A2: Bear plank (p. 203)	2×15 sec	3×15 sec	3×20 sec	3×20 sec
A3: Spiderman stretch (p. 53)	2×30 sec each	2×30 sec each	2×30 sec each	2×30 sec each
Day 1, block 2				
B1: Incline push-up (p. 191)	2×6 reps	3×6 reps	3×8 reps	3×8 reps
B2: Half-kneeling cable row (p. 197)	2×6 reps each	3×6 reps each	3×8 reps each	3×8 reps each
Day 1, block 3				
C1: Bodyweight split squat (p. 175)	2×5 reps each	3×5 reps each	3×6 reps each	3×8 reps each
C2: Tall-kneeling cable chop (p. 211)	2×8 reps each	2×10 reps each	2×10 reps each	2×12 reps each
Day 1 conditioning				
Steady-state air bike (p. 231)	6 min	8 min	10 min	10 min

Day 2				
Movement preparation				
Foam rolling	Glutes (p. 41)	Calves (p. 48)	Posterior shoulder (p. 46)	
	Thoracic spine (p. 45)	Adductors (p. 43)	Lumbar (p. 44)	
	Quads (p. 42)	Lats (p. 46)		
Mobility	90/90 hip stretch (p. 52)			1 min each
	Spiderman stretch (p. 53)			1 min each
	Adductor rocking stretch (p. 54)			10 reps each
	Wide split thoracic rotation (p. 56)			10 reps each
	Shoulder articular rotations (p. 57)			10 reps each
	Active lumbar flexion and extension (p. 62)			10 reps
	Wall ankle mobility (p. 59)			10 reps each

Day 2		
Movement preparation		
Motor control	Bilateral hip lift (p. 70)	10 reps
	Band-assisted leg lower (p. 76)	10 reps each
	Shoulder floor slide (p. 72)	10 reps
Patterning	Squat press-out (p. 78)	5 reps
	Split squat (p. 80)	5 reps each
	Lateral squat (p. 82)	5 reps each
	Chest-loaded bilateral hip hinge (p. 84)	5 reps
Ladder drills	**Perform all drills forward and backward on ladder.*	
	1-2 stick (p. 99)	
	In-in-out-out forward/backward (p. 102)	
	In-in-out-out sideways (p. 104)	
	Cross in front (p. 100)	
	Cross behind (p. 101)	
Power	Lateral bound and stick (p. 124): 2 sets × 5 reps each	
	Standing medicine ball slam (p. 143): 2 sets × 8 reps	

Day 2, block 1	**Week 1**	**Week 2**	**Week 3**	**Week 4**
A1: Squat with medicine ball press-out (p. 173) or goblet squat (p. 172)	2 × 8 reps	3 × 8 reps	3 × 8 reps	3 × 10 reps
A2: Short-lever side plank (p. 215)	2 × 15 sec each	3 × 15 sec each	3 × 20 sec each	3 × 20 sec each
A3: Wide split thoracic rotation (p. 56)	2 × 8 reps each	2 × 8 reps each	2 × 8 reps each	2 × 8 reps each
Day 2, block 2				
B1: Two-arm standing cable press (p. 193)	2 × 6 reps	3 × 6 reps	3 × 8 reps	3 × 8 reps
B2: Half-kneeling single-arm cable pulldown (p. 201)	2 × 6 reps each	3 × 6 reps each	3 × 8 reps each	3 × 8 reps each
Day 2, block 3				
C1: Bodyweight reaching single-leg deadlift (p. 181)	2 × 8 reps each	3 × 8 reps each	3 × 8 reps each	3 × 10 reps each
C2: Half-kneeling antirotation press-out (p. 209)	2 × 8 reps each	2 × 10 reps each	2 × 10 reps each	2 × 12 reps each
Day 2 conditioning				
Incline treadmill walk (p. 230)	6 min	8 min	10 min	10 min

Table 10.3 Three-Day Program: Phase 1

Day 1				
Movement preparation				
Foam rolling	Glutes (p. 41)	Calves (p. 48)	Posterior shoulder (p. 46)	
	Thoracic spine (p. 45)	Adductors (p. 43)	Lumbar (p. 44)	
	Quads (p. 42)	Lats (p. 46)		
Mobility	90/90 hip stretch (p. 52)			1 min each
	Spiderman stretch (p. 53)			1 min each
	Adductor rocking stretch (p. 54)			10 reps each
	Wide split thoracic rotation (p. 56)			10 reps each
	Shoulder articular rotations (p. 57)			10 reps each
	Active lumbar flexion and extension (p. 62)			10 reps
	Wall ankle mobility (p. 59)			10 reps each
Motor control	Bilateral hip lift (p. 70)			10 reps
	Band-assisted leg lower (p. 76)			10 reps each
	Shoulder floor slide (p. 72)			10 reps
Patterning	Squat press-out (p. 78)			10 reps
	Split squat (p. 80)			5 reps each
	Lateral squat (p. 82)			5 reps each
	Chest-loaded bilateral hip hinge (p. 84)			10 reps
Multiplanar active warm-up	**Perform all drills 10 yards (meters) down and back.*			
	Forward A-skip (p. 91)			
	Lateral A-skip (p. 92)			
	High knee run (p. 93)			
	Heel to butt (p. 94)			
	Lateral shuffle (p. 95)			
	Carioca (p. 96)			
	Backpedal (p. 97)			
Power	Box jump (p. 120): 3 sets × 5 reps			
	Tall-kneeling medicine ball chest pass (p. 138): 3 × 10			

Day 1, block 1	Week 1	Week 2	Week 3	Week 4
A1: Kettlebell deadlift (p. 146)	3 × 8 reps	3 × 8 reps	3 × 10 reps	3 × 10 reps
A2: Bear plank (p. 203)	3 × 25 sec	3 × 25 sec	3 × 30 sec	3 × 30 sec
A3: Wall quad stretch (p. 55)	2 × 30 sec each	2 × 30 sec each	2 × 30 sec each	2 × 30 sec each
Day 1, block 2				
B1: Dumbbell bench press (p. 192)	3 × 8 reps	3 × 8 reps	3 × 10 reps	3 × 10 reps
B2: Half-kneeling cable row (p. 197)	3 × 8 reps each	3 × 8 reps each	3 × 10 reps each	3 × 10 reps each
Day 1, block 3				
C1: Goblet split squat (p. 174)	3 × 6 reps each	3 × 8 reps each	3 × 10 reps each	3 × 10 reps each
C2: Tall-kneeling cable chop (p. 211)	3 × 6 reps each	3 × 8 reps each	3 × 10 reps each	3 × 12 reps each
C3: Farmer carry (p. 217)	3 × 40 yd (37 m)	3 × 40 yd (37 m)	3 × 40 yd (37 m)	3 × 40 yd (37 m)
Day 1 conditioning				
10 sec and 20 sec bike intervals at 110%-120% of max aerobic speed (p. 233)	8 reps	10 reps	12 reps	14 reps

Day 2				
Movement preparation				
Foam rolling	Glutes (p. 41)	Calves (p. 48)	Posterior shoulder (p. 46)	
	Thoracic spine (p. 45)	Adductors (p. 43)	Lumbar (p. 44)	
	Quads (p. 42)	Lats (p. 46)		
Mobility	90/90 hip stretch (p. 52)			1 min each
	Spiderman stretch (p. 53)			1 min each
	Adductor rocking stretch (p. 54)			10 reps each
	Wide split thoracic rotation (p. 56)			10 reps each
	Shoulder articular rotations (p. 57)			10 reps each
	Active lumbar flexion and extension (p. 62)			10 reps
	Wall ankle mobility (p. 59)			10 reps each

(continued)

Table 10.3 Three-Day Program: Phase 1 *(continued)*

Day 2 *(continued)*		
Movement preparation		
Motor control	Bilateral hip lift (p. 70)	10 reps
	Band-assisted leg lower (p. 76)	10 reps each
	Shoulder floor slide (p. 72)	10 reps
Patterning	Squat press-out (p. 78)	10 reps
	Split squat (p. 80)	5 reps each
	Lateral squat (p. 82)	5 reps each
	Chest-loaded bilateral hip hinge (p. 84)	10 reps
Ladder drills	**Perform all drills forward and backward on ladder.*	
	1-2 stick (p. 99)	
	In-in-out-out forward/backward (p. 102)	
	In-in-out-out sideways (p. 104)	
	Cross in front (p. 100)	
	Cross behind (p. 101)	
Power	Lateral bound and stick (p. 124): 3 sets × 5 reps each	
	Half-kneeling medicine ball side toss (p. 140): 3 sets × 5 reps each	

Day 2, block 1	**Week 1**	**Week 2**	**Week 3**	**Week 4**
A1: Bodyweight jump squat (p. 148)	3 × 5 reps	3 × 5 reps	3 × 5 reps	3 × 5 reps
A2: Short-lever side plank (p. 215)	3 × 25 sec each	3 × 25 sec each	3 × 30 sec each	3 × 30 sec each
A3: Wide split thoracic rotation (p. 56)	3 × 5 reps each	3 × 5 reps each	3 × 5 reps each	3 × 5 reps each
Day 2, block 2				
B1: Half-kneeling angled barbell press (p. 195)	3 × 6 reps each	3 × 8 reps each	3 × 10 reps each	3 × 10 reps each
B2: Half-kneeling single-arm cable pulldown (p. 201)	3 × 6 reps each	3 × 8 reps each	3 × 10 reps each	3 × 12 reps each
Day 2, block 3				
C1: Goblet lateral squat (p. 178)	3 × 6 reps each	3 × 8 reps each	3 × 10 reps each	3 × 10 reps each
C2: Half-kneeling antirotation press-out (p. 209)	3 × 6 reps each	3 × 8 reps each	3 × 10 reps each	3 × 12 reps each
C3: Single-leg hip lift (p. 71)	3 × 8 reps each	3 × 8 reps each	3 × 10 reps each	3 × 10 reps each
Day 2 conditioning				
Tempo run (p. 236)	6 reps	8 reps	10 reps	12 reps
Rest until heart rate drops to 60% of max heart rate.				

Day 3				
Movement preparation				
Foam rolling	Glutes (p. 41)	Calves (p. 48)	Posterior shoulder (p. 46)	
	Thoracic spine (p. 45)	Adductors (p. 43)	Lumbar (p. 44)	
	Quads (p. 42)	Lats (p. 46)		
Mobility	90/90 hip stretch (p. 52)			1 min each
	Spiderman stretch (p. 53)			1 min each
	Adductor rocking stretch (p. 54)			10 reps each side
	Wide split thoracic rotation (p. 56)			10 reps each
	Shoulder articular rotations (p. 57)			10 reps each
	Active lumbar flexion and extension (p. 62)			10 reps
	Wall ankle mobility (p. 59)			10 reps each
Motor control	Bilateral hip lift (p. 70)			10 reps
	Band-assisted leg lower (p. 76)			10 reps each
	Shoulder floor slide (p. 72)			10 reps
Patterning	Squat press-out (p. 78)			10 reps
	Split squat (p. 80)			5 reps each
	Lateral squat (p. 82)			5 reps each
	Chest-loaded bilateral hip hinge (p. 84)			10 reps each
Dynamic (5 min)	**Perform all drills 10 yards (meters) down and back.*			
	Forward A-skip (p. 91)			
	Lateral A-skip (p. 92)			
	High knee run (p. 93)			
	Heel to butt (p. 94)			
	Lateral shuffle (p. 95)			
	Carioca (p. 96)			
	Backpedal (p. 97)			
Power	Single-leg box hop (p. 128): 3 sets × 5 reps each			
	Kneeling medicine ball overhead throw (p. 142): 3 sets × 10 reps			

(continued)

Table 10.3 Three-Day Program: Phase 1 *(continued)*

Day 3 *(continued)*				
Movement preparation				
Day 3, block 1	**Week 1**	**Week 2**	**Week 3**	**Week 4**
A1: Goblet squat (p. 172)	3 × 8 reps	3 × 8 reps	3 × 10 reps	3 × 10 reps
A2: Bear plank (p. 203)	3 × 25 sec	3 × 25 sec	3 × 30 sec	3 × 30 sec
A3: Spiderman stretch (p. 53)	2 × 30 sec each	2 × 30 sec each	2 × 30 sec each	2 × 30 sec each
Day 3, block 2				
B1: Reaching single-leg deadlift (p. 85)	3 × 6 reps each	3 × 8 reps each	3 × 10 reps each	3 × 10 reps each
B2: Inverted row on suspension trainer (p. 198)	3 × 8 reps each	3 × 8 reps each	3 × 10 reps each	3 × 10 reps each
Day 3, block 3				
C1: Push-up (p. 86)	3 × 6 reps	3 × 8 reps	3 × 10 reps	3 × 10 reps
C2: Tall-kneeling cable lift (p. 213)	3 × 6 reps each	3 × 8 reps each	3 × 10 reps each	3 × 12 reps each
C3: Straight-leg sit-ups (p. 206)	3 × 6 reps	3 × 8 reps	3 × 10 reps	3 × 12 reps
Day 3 conditioning				
10 sec on and 20 sec off bike intervals at 110%-120% of max aerobic speed (p. 233)	8 reps	10 reps	12 reps	14 reps

Table 10.4 Three-Day Program: Phase 2

Day 1				
Movement preparation				
Foam rolling	Glutes (p. 41)	Calves (p. 48)	Posterior shoulder (p. 46)	
	Thoracic spine (p. 45)	Adductors (p. 43)	Lumbar (p. 44)	
	Quads (p. 42)	Lats (p. 46)		
Mobility	90/90 hip stretch (p. 52)			1 min each
	Spiderman stretch (p. 53)			1 min each
	Adductor rocking stretch (p. 54)			10 reps each
	Wide split thoracic rotation (p. 56)			10 reps each
	Shoulder articular rotations (p. 57)			10 reps each
	Active lumbar flexion and extension (p. 62)			10 reps
	Wall ankle mobility (p. 59)			10 reps each

Day 1		
Movement preparation		
Motor control	Single-leg hip lift (p. 71)	10 reps each
	Unassisted leg lower (p. 77)	10 reps each
	Shoulder wall slide (p. 73)	10 reps
Patterning	Light Zercher squat (p. 79)	10 reps
	Reverse lunge (p. 81)	5 reps each
	Lateral lunge (p. 83)	5 reps each
	Reaching single-leg deadlift (p. 85)	10 reps each
Multiplanar active warm-up	**Perform all drills 10 yards (meters) down and back.*	
	Forward A-skip (p. 91)	
	Lateral A-skip (p. 92)	
	High knee run (p. 93)	
	Heel to butt (p. 94)	
	Lateral shuffle (p. 95)	
	Carioca (p. 96)	
	Backpedal (p. 97)	
Power	Hurdle jump and stick (p. 119): 3 sets × 5 reps	
	Standing medicine ball chest pass (p. 137): 3 sets × 10 reps	

Day 1, block 1	Week 1	Week 2	Week 3	Week 4
A1: Kettlebell swing (p. 145)	3 × 8 reps	3 × 8 reps	3 × 10 reps	3 × 10 reps
A2: Front plank (p. 202)	3 × 20 sec	3 × 25 sec	3 × 30 sec	3 × 30 sec
A3: Wall quad stretch (p. 55)	2 × 30 sec each	2 × 30 sec each	2 × 30 sec each	2 × 30 sec each
Day 1, block 2				
B1: Dumbbell bench press (p. 192)	3 × 8 reps	3 × 8 reps	4 × 6 reps	4 × 6 reps
B2: Single-arm dumbbell row (p. 196)	3 × 8 reps each	3 × 8 reps each	4 × 6 reps each	4 × 6 reps each
B3: Kettlebell deadlift (p. 146)	3 × 8 reps	3 × 8 reps	4 × 6 reps	4 × 6 reps
Day 1, block 3				
C1: Two-dumbbell rear-foot-elevated split squat (p. 175)	3 × 8 reps each	3 × 8 reps each	4 × 6 reps each	4 × 6 reps each
C2: Half-kneeling cable chop (p. 210)	3 × 6 reps each	3 × 8 reps each	3 × 10 reps each	3 × 12 reps each
C3: Farmer carry (p. 217)	3 × 40 yd (37 m)	3 × 40 yd (37 m)	3 × 40 yd (37 m)	3 × 40 yd (37 m)
Day 1 conditioning				
15 sec and 15 sec bike intervals at 110%-120% of max aerobic speed (p. 233)	12 reps	14 reps	16 reps	16 reps

(continued)

Table 10.4 Three-Day Program: Phase 2 *(continued)*

Day 2				
Movement preparation				
Foam rolling	Glutes (p. 41)	Calves (p. 48)	Posterior shoulder (p. 46)	
	Thoracic spine (p. 45)	Adductors (p. 43)	Lumbar (p. 44)	
	Quads (p. 42)	Lats (p. 46)		
Mobility	90/90 hip stretch (p. 52)			1 min each
	Spiderman stretch (p. 53)			1 min each
	Adductor rocking stretch (p. 54)			10 reps each
	Wide split thoracic rotation (p. 56)			10 reps each
	Shoulder articular rotations (p. 57)			10 reps each
	Active lumbar flexion and extension (p. 62)			10 reps
	Wall ankle mobility (p. 59)			10 reps each
Motor control	Single-leg hip lift (p. 71)			10 reps each
	Unassisted leg lower (p. 77)			10 reps each
	Shoulder wall slide (p. 73)			10 reps
Patterning	Light Zercher squat (p. 79)			10 reps
	Reverse lunge (p. 81)			5 reps each
	Lateral lunge (p. 83)			5 reps each
	Reaching single-leg deadlift (p. 85)			10 reps each
Ladder drills	**Perform all drills forward and backward on ladder.*			
	1-2 stick (p. 99)			
	In-in-out-out forward/backward (p. 102)			
	In-in-out-out sideways (p. 104)			
	Cross in front (p. 100)			
	Cross behind (p. 101)			
Power	45-degree bound and stick (p. 123): 3 sets × 5 reps each			
	Standing medicine ball side toss (p. 139): 3 sets × 5 reps each			

Day 2, block 1	Week 1	Week 2	Week 3	Week 4
A1: Dumbbell jump squat and stick (p. 147)	3 × 5 reps	3 × 5 reps	3 × 5 reps	3 × 5 reps
A2: Side plank (p. 214)	3 × 20 sec each	3 × 25 sec each	3 × 30 sec each	3 × 30 sec each
A3: Wide split thoracic rotation (p. 56)	3 × 5 reps each	3 × 5 reps each	3 × 5 reps each	3 × 5 reps each

Day 2, block 2				
B1: Half-kneeling single-arm overhead press (p. 194)	3 × 8 reps each	3 × 8 reps each	4 × 6 reps each	4 × 6 reps each
B2: Chin-up (p. 200)	3 × 5 reps	3 × 6 reps	3 × 7 reps	3 × 8 reps
B3: Skater squat (p. 182)	3 × 5 reps each	3 × 6 reps each	3 × 7 reps each	3 × 8 reps each
Day 2, block 3				
C1: Goblet lateral lunge (p. 179)	3 × 8 reps each	3 × 8 reps each	4 × 6 reps each	4 × 6 reps each
C2: Standing antirotation press (p. 208)	3 × 6 reps each	3 × 8 reps each	3 × 10 reps each	3 × 12 reps each
C3: Single-leg shoulder-elevated hip lift (p. 184)	3 × 8 reps each	3 × 8 reps each	3 × 10 reps each	3 × 10 reps each
Day 2 conditioning				
Tempo run (p. 236)	12 reps	12 reps	14 reps	14 reps
Rest until heart rate drops to 60% of max heart rate.				

Day 3				
Movement preparation				
Foam rolling	Glutes (p. 41)	Calves (p. 48)	Posterior shoulder (p. 46)	
	Thoracic spine (p. 45)	Adductors (p. 43)	Lumbar (p. 44)	
	Quads (p. 42)	Lats (p. 46)		
Mobility	90/90 hip stretch (p. 52)			1 min each
	Spiderman stretch (p. 53)			1 min each
	Adductor rocking stretch (p. 54)			10 reps each
	Wide split thoracic rotation (p. 56)			10 reps each
	Shoulder articular rotations (p. 57)			10 reps each
	Active lumbar flexion and extension (p. 62)			10 reps
	Wall ankle mobility (p. 59)			10 reps each
Motor control	Single-leg hip lift (p. 71)			10 reps each
	Unassisted leg lower (p. 77)			10 reps each
	Shoulder wall slide (p. 73)			10 reps
Patterning	Light Zercher squat (p. 79)			10 reps
	Reverse lunge (p. 81)			5 reps each
	Lateral lunge (p. 83)			5 reps each
	Reaching single-leg deadlift (p. 85)			10 reps each

(continued)

Table 10.4 Three-Day Program: Phase 2 *(continued)*

Day 3 *(continued)*				
Movement preparation				
Dynamic (5 min)	**Perform all drills 10 yards (meters) down and back.*			
	Forward A-skip (p. 91)			
	Lateral A-skip (p. 92)			
	High knee run (p. 93)			
	Heel to butt (p. 94)			
	Lateral shuffle (p. 95)			
	Carioca (p. 96)			
	Backpedal (p. 97)			
Power	Linear hurdle hop and stick (p. 127): 3 sets × 5 reps each			
	Standing medicine ball overhead throw (p. 141): 3 sets × 10 reps			
Day 3, block 1	**Week 1**	**Week 2**	**Week 3**	**Week 4**
A1: Offset kettlebell front squat (p. 173)	3 × 6 reps each	3 × 8 reps each	3 × 8 reps each	3 × 10 reps each
A2: High plank shoulder taps (p. 204)	3 × 6 reps each	3 × 8 reps each	3 × 10 reps each	3 × 12 reps each
A3: Spiderman stretch (p. 53)	2 × 30 sec each	2 × 30 sec each	2 × 30 sec each	2 × 30 sec each
Day 3, block 2				
B1: One-kettlebell single-leg deadlift (p. 180)	3 × 8 each	3 × 8 each	4 × 6 each	4 × 6 each
B2: Inverted row on suspension trainer (p. 198)	3 × 8 reps	3 × 8 reps	4 × 6 reps	4 × 6 reps
B3: Push-up (p. 86)	3 × 6 reps	3 × 8 reps	3 × 10 reps	3 × 12 reps
Day 3, block 3				
C1: Single-leg squat to box (p. 176)	3 × 5 reps each	3 × 6 reps each	3 × 7 reps each	3 × 8 reps each
C2: Half-kneeling cable lift (p. 212)	3 × 6 reps each	3 × 8 reps each	3 × 10 reps each	3 × 12 reps each
C3: One-leg bent sit-up (p. 207)	3 × 6 reps each	3 × 8 reps each	3 × 10 reps each	3 × 12 reps each
Day 3 conditioning				
15 sec and 15 sec bike intervals at 110%-120% of max aerobic speed (p. 233)	12 reps	14 reps	16 reps	16 reps

Table 10.5 Three-Day Program: Phase 3

Day 1				
Movement preparation				
Foam rolling	Glutes (p. 41)	Calves (p. 48)	Posterior shoulder (p. 46)	
	Thoracic spine (p. 45)	Adductors (p. 43)	Lumbar (p. 44)	
	Quads (p. 42)	Lats (p. 46)		
Mobility	90/90 hip stretch (p. 52)			1 min each
	Spiderman stretch (p. 53)			1 min each
	Adductor rocking stretch (p. 54)			10 reps each
	Wide split thoracic rotation (p. 56)			10 reps each
	Shoulder articular rotations (p. 57)			10 reps each
	Active lumbar flexion and extension (p. 62)			10 reps
	Wall ankle mobility (p. 59)			10 reps each
Motor control	Single-leg hip lift (p. 71)			10 reps each
	Prone hip flexion (p. 75)			10 reps each
	Shoulder wall slide (p. 73)			10 reps
Patterning	Sandbag offset-loaded squat (p. 79)			5 reps each
	Forward lunge (p. 81)			5 reps each
	Diagonal lunge (p. 83)			5 reps each
	Triplanar reaching single-leg deadlift (p. 85)			5 reps each
Multiplanar active warm-up	**Perform all drills 10 yards (meters) down and back.*			
	Forward A-skip (p. 91)			
	Lateral A-skip (p. 92)			
	High knee run (p. 93)			
	Heel to butt (p. 94)			
	Lateral shuffle (p. 95)			
	Carioca (p. 96)			
	Backpedal (p. 97)			
Power	Hurdle jump with mini bounce (p. 121): 3 sets × 5 reps			
	Two-point sprint start chest pass (p. 138): 3 sets × 5 reps each			

(continued)

Table 10.5 Three-Day Program: Phase 3 *(continued)*

Day 1, block 1	Week 1	Week 2	Week 3	Week 4
A1: Single-arm kettlebell swing (p. 146)	4 × 6 reps each	4 × 8 reps each	4 × 8 reps each	4 × 10 reps each
A2: Kneeling ball rollout (p. 203)	3 × 6 reps	3 × 8 reps	3 × 10 reps	3 × 12 reps
A3: Wall quad stretch (p. 55)	2 × 30 sec each	2 × 30 sec each	2 × 30 sec each	2 × 30 sec each
Day 1, block 2				
B1: Single-arm dumbbell bench press (p. 193)	4 × 6 reps each	4 × 8 reps each	4 × 8 reps each	4 × 10 reps each
B2: Dumbbell row with isometric pause (p. 197)	4 × 6 reps each	4 × 8 reps each	4 × 8 reps each	4 × 10 reps each
B3: Trap bar deadlift (p. 187)	4 × 6 reps	4 × 6 reps	4 × 8 reps	4 × 8 reps
Day 1, block 3				
C1: Goblet slide board reverse lunge (p. 177)	4 × 6 reps each	4 × 8 reps each	4 × 8 reps each	4 × 10 reps each
C2: Standing cable chop (p. 211)	3 × 6 reps each	3 × 8 reps each	3 × 10 reps each	3 × 12 reps each
C3: Double kettlebell rack carry (p. 217)	3 × 40 yd (37 m)	3 × 40 yd (37 m)	3 × 40 yd (37 m)	3 × 40 yd (37 m)
Day 1 conditioning				
20 sec and 10 sec bike intervals at 110%-120% of max aerobic speed (p. 233)	16 reps	16 reps	16 reps	16 reps

Day 2				
Movement preparation				
Foam rolling	Glutes (p. 41)	Calves (p. 48)	Posterior shoulder (p. 46)	
	Thoracic spine (p. 45)	Adductors (p. 43)	Lumbar (p. 44)	
	Quads (p. 42)	Lats (p. 46)		
Mobility	90/90 hip stretch (p. 52)			1 min each
	Spiderman stretch (p. 53)			1 min each
	Adductor rocking stretch (p. 54)			10 reps each
	Wide split thoracic rotation (p. 56)			10 reps each
	Shoulder articular rotations (p. 57)			10 reps each
	Active lumbar flexion and extension (p. 62)			10 reps
	Wall ankle mobility (p. 59)			10 reps each

Day 2		
Movement preparation		
Motor control	Single-leg hip lift (p. 71)	10 reps each
	Prone hip flexion (p. 75)	10 reps each
	Shoulder wall slide (p. 73)	10 reps
Patterning	Sandbag offset-loaded squat (p. 79)	5 reps each
	Forward lunge (p. 81)	5 reps each
	Diagonal lunge (p. 83)	5 reps each
	Triplanar reaching single-leg deadlift (p. 85)	5 reps each
Ladder drills	**Perform all drills forward and backward on ladder.*	
	1-2 stick (p. 99)	
	In-in-out-out forward/backward (p. 102)	
	In-in-out-out sideways (p. 104)	
	Cross in front (p. 100)	
	Cross behind (p. 101)	
Power	45-degree bound with a mini bounce (p. 125): 3 sets × 5 reps each	
	Medicine ball shuffle side toss (p. 140): 3 sets × 5 reps each	

Day 2, block 1	Week 1	Week 2	Week 3	Week 4
A1: Continuous dumbbell jump squats (p. 148)	3 × 5 reps	3 × 5 reps	3 × 5 reps	3 × 5 reps
A2: Feet-elevated side plank (p. 215)	3 × 20 sec each	3 × 25 sec each	3 × 30 sec each	3 × 30 sec each
A3: Wide split thoracic rotation (p. 56)	3 × 5 reps each	3 × 5 reps each	3 × 5 reps each	3 × 5 reps each
Day 2, block 2				
B1: Standing single-arm overhead press (p. 195)	4 × 6 reps each	4 × 8 reps each	4 × 8 reps each	4 × 10 reps each
B2: Pull-up (p. 201)	3 × 5 reps	3 × 6 reps	3 × 7 reps	3 × 8 reps
B3: Sandbag Zercher loaded skater squat (p. 183)	3 × 8 reps each	3 × 8 reps each	4 × 6 reps each	4 × 6 reps each

(continued)

Table 10.5 Three-Day Program: Phase 3 *(continued)*

Day 2 *(continued)*				
Movement preparation				
Day 2, block 3				
C1: Goblet lateral lunge (p. 179)	4 × 6 reps each	4 × 8 reps each	4 × 8 reps each	4 × 10 reps each
C2: Staggered-stance antirotation press-out (p. 209)	3 × 6 reps each	3 × 8 reps each	3 × 10 reps each	3 × 12 reps each
C3: Sliding leg curl (p. 188)	3 × 6 reps	3 × 6 reps	3 × 8 reps	3 × 10 reps
Day 2 conditioning				
Tempo run (p. 236)	12 reps	14 reps	14 reps	14 reps
Rest until heart rate drops to 60% of max heart rate.				

Day 3				
Movement preparation				
Foam rolling	Glutes (p. 41)	Calves (p. 48)	Posterior shoulder (p. 46)	
	Thoracic spine (p. 45)	Adductors (p. 43)	Lumbar (p. 44)	
	Quads (p. 42)	Lats (p. 46)		
Mobility	90/90 hip stretch (p. 52)			1 min each
	Spiderman stretch (p. 53)			1 min each
	Adductor rocking stretch (p. 54)			10 reps each
	Wide split thoracic rotation (p. 56)			10 reps each
	Shoulder articular rotations (p. 57)			10 reps each
	Active lumbar flexion and extension (p. 62)			10 reps
	Wall ankle mobility (p. 59)			10 reps each
Motor control	Single-leg hip lift (p. 71)			10 reps each
	Prone hip flexion (p. 75)			10 reps each
	Shoulder wall slide (p. 73)			10 reps
Patterning	Sandbag offset-loaded squat (p. 79)			5 reps each
	Forward lunge (p. 81)			5 reps each
	Diagonal lunge (p. 83)			5 reps each
	Triplanar reaching single-leg deadlift (p. 85)			5 reps each

Day 3				
Movement preparation				
Dynamic	**Perform all drills 10 yards (meters) down and back.*			
	Forward A-skip (p. 91)			
	Lateral A-skip (p. 92)			
	High knee run (p. 93)			
	Heel to butt (p. 94)			
	Lateral shuffle (p. 95)			
	Carioca (p. 96)			
	Backpedal (p. 97)			
Power	Hurdle hop with mini bounce (p. 129): 3 sets × 5 reps each			
	Medicine ball overhead throw with step (p. 142): 3 sets × 5 reps each			

Day 3, block 1	Week 1	Week 2	Week 3	Week 4
A1: Double kettlebell front squat (p. 173)	3 × 8 reps	3 × 8 reps	4 × 6 reps	4 × 6 reps
A2: Plank rows (p. 205)	3 × 6 reps each	3 × 8 reps each	3 × 10 reps each	3 × 12 reps each
A3: Spiderman stretch (p. 53)	2 × 30 sec each	2 × 30 sec each	2 × 30 sec each	2 × 30 sec each
Day 3, block 2				
B1: Two-kettlebell single-leg deadlift (p. 181)	4 × 6 reps each	4 × 8 reps each	4 × 8 reps each	4 × 10 reps each
B2: Inverted row on suspension trainer (p. 198)	4 × 6 reps	4 × 8 reps	4 × 8 reps	4 × 10 reps
B3: Weighted push-up (p. 191)	3 × 10 reps	3 × 10 reps	3 × 12 reps	3 × 12 reps
Day 3, block 3				
C1: Single-leg squat to box (p. 176)	3 × 8 reps each	3 × 8 reps each	4 × 6 reps each	4 × 6 reps each
C2: Standing cable lift (p. 213)	3 × 6 reps each	3 × 8 reps each	3 × 10 reps each	3 × 12 reps each
C3: One-leg bent sit-up (p. 207)	3 × 12 reps each	3 × 14 reps each	3 × 14 reps each	3 × 15 reps each
Day 3 conditioning				
1 min on and 1 min off bike intervals at 100% of max aerobic speed (p. 233)	5 reps	6 reps	7 reps	8 reps

ABOUT THE AUTHOR

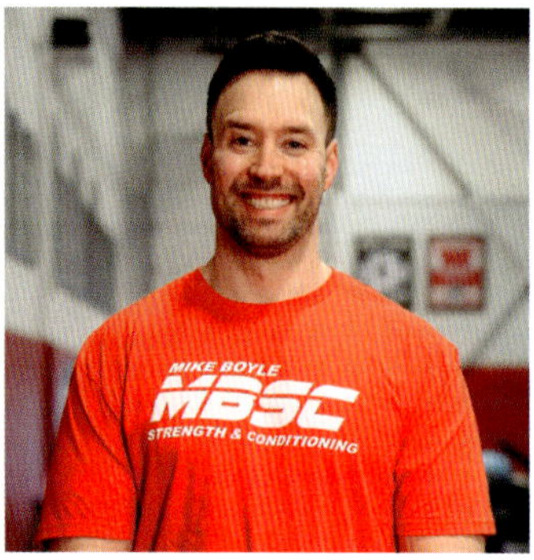

Kevin Carr is a strength and conditioning coach and manager at Mike Boyle Strength and Conditioning (MBSC) as well as a massage therapist and cofounder of Movement as Medicine, a massage and movement therapy clinic in Woburn, Massachusetts. He is the creator of the Certified Functional Strength Coach certification. He has a bachelor's degree in kinesiology from the University of Massachusetts at Amherst and a license in massage therapy from Cortiva Institute in Watertown, Massachusetts.

Carr amassed a wealth of experience in the field of sport performance and personal training while working at MBSC and has traveled all over the world to educate thousands of coaches and therapists about the MBSC coaching system. He has coached everyone from U.S. Olympians looking for a competitive edge to the average person looking to shed some pounds, move better, and improve their health.